Psychiatric Mental Health Nursing Research Digest

Joyce J. Fitzpatrick, PhD, RN, FAAN, is Professor of Nursing, Frances Payne Bolton School of Nursing at Case Western Reserve University in Cleveland, Ohio, where she was Dean from 1982 to 1997. Dr. Fitzpatrick is widely published in nursing literature, having received the American Journal of Nursing Book of the Year Award ten times. She is the Editor of the *Annual Review of Nursing Research* series, now in its eighteenth volume, and in 1997 she was appointed Editor of the National League for Nursing's journal *Nursing and Health Care Perspectives*. She also is Consulting Editor of the Springer journal *Nursing Leadership Forum*. Dr. Fitzpatrick was president of the American Academy of Nursing from 1997–99.

Patricia A. Wilke, MSN, RN, is an Advanced Practice Nurse in psychiatry at University Hospitals of Cleveland. She is the Family Education Coordinator on the inpatient older adult and adult psychiatric units and facilitates process oriented groups with patients and their families. She is a student in the Doctor of Nursing program at Case Western Reserve University.

Psychiatric Mental Health Nursing Research Digest

Joyce J. Fitzpatrick
PhD, RN, FAAN
Editor

Patricia A. Wilke
MSN, RN
Associate Editor

Springer Publishing Company

Springer Publishing Company, Inc.
536 Broadway
New York, NY 10012-3955

Acquisitions Editor: Sheri Sussman
Production Editor: Janice G. Stangel
Cover design by Susan Hauley

01 02 03 04 05 / 5 4 3 2 1

Library of Congress Cataloging-in-Publication Data

Psychiatric mental health nursing research digest / Joyce J. Fitzpatrick, Patricia A. Wilke, editors.
p. ; cm.
Includes bibliographical references and index.
ISBN 0-8261-1393-1
1. Psychiatric nursing—Research. I. Fitzpatrick, Joyce J., 1944– II. Wilke, Patricia A.
[DNLM: 1. Psychiatric Nursing. 2. Mental Disorders—nursing. 3. Nursing Research. WY 160 P972065 2001]
RC440.P7425 2001
610.73'68—dc21

2001017013
CIP

Printed in the United States of America by Sheridan

CONTENTS

Contributors *viii*

Preface *xiii*

1. HEALTH PROMOTION AND RISK REDUCTION

Introduction, Joyce J. Fitzpatrick 3
Biofeedback Training, Helen Kogan Budzynski 4
Child and Adolescents Mental Health Interventions, Diane Magyary 9
Child Failure to Thrive, Heidi vonKoss Krowchuk 14
Comfort, Katharine Kolcaba 17
Community Mental Health, Grayce M. Sills 20
Consultation-Liaison Nursing, Marianne Miles 22
Creative Arts as Nursing Intervention, Elissa Emerson 26
Cultural Aspects of Psychiatric Mental Health Nursing and Research, Kathryn Hopkins Kavanagh 29
Empathy, Joan L. Bottorff 33
Family Caregiving of the Mentally Ill, Alice R. Kempe 35
Forensic Psychiatric Care and Juvenile Justice, Deborah Shelton 39
Grandmother Caregivers, Carol M. Musil 43
Grief, Alice S. Demi 46
Individual Nursing Therapy, Rauda Gelazis 49
Interpersonal Communication, Carol W. Kennedy and Bonnie J. Garvin 52
Mental Disorders Prevention, Sandra Graham McClowry 56
Mental Health in Public Sector Primary Care, Emily J. Hauenstein 59
Mental Health Policy: Relevance for Psychiatric Nursing, Research Jeanne A. Clement 63
Mental Health Services Research, Jeanne C. Fox 66
Minority Issues in Mental Health, Diana Lynn Morris 67
Music Therapy, Marion Good 76
No-Suicide Contracts, Barbara L. Drew 78
Nurse-Patient Communication, Joan L. Bottoroff 81
Nurse-Patient Interaction, Joan L. Bottoroff 84
Nurse-Patient Relationship, Joan L. Bottoroff 86
Peplau's Theoretical Model, Nelma B. Shearer and Pamela G. Reed 88
Pregnancy: Anxiety and Conflict, Regina Lederman 91
Primary and Mental Health Services Integration, Diane Magyary 95

Psychodrama in Nursing, Linnea Carlson-Sabelli 99
Psychosocial Adjustment and the Family, Carol Noll Hoskins 102
Psychosocial Interventions, Graham J. McDougall 109
Quality of Life, Carol E. Smith and Carol Gaskamp 112
Relaxation Techniques, Mariah Snyder 113
Resourcefulness, Jaclene A. Zauszniewski 115
Self-efficacy, Graham J. McDougall 119
Smoking Cessation, Mary Ellen Wewers 122
Stress, Brenda L. Lyon 125
Stress Management, Brenda L. Lyon 127
Violence as a Nursing Area of Inquiry, Jacquelyn Campbell, Joan Kub, and Linda Lewandowski 128
Workplace Mistreatment, Lois Price Spratlen 133
Workplace Violence, Jane Lipscomb 134
Young Women and Depression, Emily J. Hauenstein 138

II. PATHOLOGIC CONDITIONS AND NURSING INTERVENTION

Introduction, Patricia A. Wilke 145
Acute Confusion/Delirium, Marquis D. Foreman and Patricia Vermersch 147
Alcoholism, Eleanor J. Sullivan 151
Bipolar Disorders, Graham J. McDougall 153
Child Abuse and Neglect, Jennifer Harrison Elder 157
Childhood Cancer Experience and Sibling Psychosocial Adaptation, Lt. Colonel John S. Murray 160
Childhood Psychopathology, Wanda K. Mohr 163
Chronic Mental Illness, Catherine F. Kane 167
Cognitive Impairment in Older Adults: Psychosocial Interventions, Graham J. McDougall 170
Coronary Artery Bypass Graft (CABG) Surgery: Psychological Sequelae, Susan McCrone and Elizabeth Lenz 175
Correctional Mental Health: A Research Agenda, David G. Allen, David Lovell, and Lorna A. Rhodes 180
Depression Among Older Adults, May L. Wykle and Jaclene A. Zauszniewski 184
Depression in Families, Terry A. Badger 188
Drug Abuse, Eleanor J. Sullivan 191
Eating Disorders, Karen Farchaus Stein and Monica White 193
Health Concerns of Women with Severe and Persistent Mental Illness, Debra E. Lyon, Catherine Kane, and Barbara J. Parker 197

HIV Symptom Management and Quality of Life, Kenn M. Kirksey, Angela L. Hudson, Eli Haugen Bunch, and William L. Holzemer 201
Homeless Health, Mary J. McNamee and Ada M. Lindsey 204
Homelessness and Related Mood Disorders, Alice R. Kempe 208
Mentally Ill Adults with Coexisting Substance Disorders: Dual Diagnosis, Bethany J. Phoenix 216
Schizophrenia Nursing Research, Sarah P. Farrell
Schizophrenia: Symptom Detection and Self-Management, Frederica O'Connor 218
Seclusion and Restraint, Ruby J. Martinez and Mary Adamson 221
Substance Abuse and Addiction Among Registered Professional Nurses, Madeline A. Naegle 224
Suicide, Alice S. Demi 227
Traumatic Events: Individual and Collective Responses, Shirley A. Murphy 230
Youth Suicide Prevention in the American Indian and Alaska Native Community, Carolyn J. Strickland 234
References 239

Index *293*

CONTRIBUTORS

Mary Adamson, MS, RN
Assistant Nurse Manager
Colorado Mental Health Institute at Fort Logan
Denver, CO

David G. Allen, PhD, RN, FAAN
Professor
Psychosocial & Community Health
School of Nursing
University of Washington
Seattle, WA

Terry A. Badger, PhD, RN, CS
Associate Professor
The University of Arizona
College of Nursing
Tucson, AZ

Joan L. Bottorff, PhD, RN
Associate Professor and NHRDP Health Researcher
University of British Columbia
School of Nursing
Vancouver, BC

Helen Kogan Budzynski, RN, PhD, FAAN
Professor
University of Washington School of Nursing
Psychosocial and Community Health
Seattle, WA

Eli Haugen Bunch, DNSc, RN
Associate Professor
Institute of Nursing Science
University of Oslo
Oslo, Norway

Jacquelyn C. Campbell, PhD, RN, FAAN
Professor
Johns Hopkins University
School of Nursing
Baltimore, MD

Linnea Carlson-Sabelli, PhD, RN, CCS TEP
Director, Psychodrama Program
Rush University College of Nursing
Chicago, ILL

Jeanne A. Clement, EdD, RN, CS, FAAN
Associate Professor, Nursing and Psychiatry
College of Nursing
The Ohio State University
Columbus, OH

Alice S. Demi, DNS, RN, FAAN
Professor
Georgia State University
School of Nursing
Atlanta, GA

Barbara L. Drew, PhD, RN
Senior Staff Scientist
MetroHealth Medical Center
Cleveland, OH

Jennifer Harrison Elder, PhD, RN
Associate Professor
University of Florida
College of Nursing
Gainesville, FLA

Elissa Emerson, PhD, RN, CS-P, FNP
Assistant Professor
Howard University
Washington, DC

Sarah P. Farrell, PhD, RN, CS
Assistant Professor
University of Virginia
Charlottesville, VA

Joyce J. Fitzpatrick, PhD, RN, FAAN
Elizabeth Brooks Ford Professor
Case Western Reserve University
Frances Payne Bolton School of Nursing
Cleveland, OH

Marquis D. Foreman, PhD, RN, FAAN
Associate Professor
University of Illinois at Chicago
College of Nursing
Chicago, ILL

Jeanne C. Fox, PhD, RN, FAAN
Director, SRMHRC
University of Virginia
SE Rural Research Center
Charlottesville, VA

Bonnie J. Garvin, PhD, RN
Professor
Ohio State University
College of Nursing
Columbus, OH

Carol Gaskamp, MA, RN
Associate Professor
Kansas Newman College
Division of Nursing
Wichita, KS

Rauda Gelazis, PhD,RN,CS,CTN
Associate Professor
Ursuline College
Pepperpike, OH

Deborah Gross, DNSc, RN, FAAN
Professor
Rush University
College of Nursing
Chicago, IL

Emily J. Hauenstein, PhD, RN, CS
Associate Professor
University of Virginia
School of Nursing
Charlottesville, VA

William L. Holzemer, PhD, RN, FAAN
Professor & Chair
Department of Community Health Systems
University of California, San Francisco
San Francisco, CA

Carol Noll Hoskins, PhD, RN, FAAN
Professor
New York University
New York, NY

Angela L. Hudson, PhD, RN
Postdoctoral Fellow
Department of Community Health Systems
University of California, San Francisco
San Francisco, CA

Catherine F. Kane, PhD, RN, FAAN
Associate Professor
University of Virginia School of Nursing
Charlottesville, VA

Kathryn Hopkins Kavanagh, PhD, RN
Associate Professor & Coordinator NAU Nursing (Navajo-Hopi)
Northern Arizona University, NAU/ Nursing, Sage Memorial Hospital
Ganado, AZ

Alice R. Kempe Ph.D., RN, C.S.
Associate Professor
Ursuline College
Pepperpike, OH

Carol W. Kennedy, PhD, RN, CS
Professor
Ohio State University
Columbus, OH

Kenn M. Kirksey, PhD, RN
Postdoctoral Fellow
University of California, San Francisco
San Francisco, CA

Katharine Y. Kolcaba, PhD, RN
Assistant Professor
University of Akron
College of Nursing
Akron, OH

Heidi vonKoss Krowchuck, PhD, RN
Associate Professor
The University of North Carolina at Greensboro
School of Nursing
Greensboro, NC

Joan Kub, PhD, RN
Assistant Professor
Johns Hopkins University
School of Nursing
Baltimore, MD

Regina Lederman, PhD, RN
Professor
School of Nursing and Dept. of Preventive Medicine & Community Health
Division of Sociomedical Sciences
University of Texas at Galveston
Galveston, TX

Elizabeth Lenz, PhD, RN, FAAN
Associate Dean for Research and
Anna C. Maxwell Professor of Nursing Research
Columbia University
School of Nursing
New York, NY

Linda Lewandowski, PhD, RN
Assistant Professor
Johns Hopkins University
School of Nursing
Baltimore, MD

Ada M. Lindsey, RN, PhD, FAAN
Dean and Professor
University of Nebraska Medical Center
College of Nursing
Omaha, NE

Jane Lipscomb, PhD, RN, FAAN
Associate Professor
University of Maryland
School of Nursing
Baltimore, MD

David Lovell, PhD, MSW
Research Assistant Professor, Nursing
Psychosocial and Community Health
University of Washington
Seattle, WA

Brenda L. Lyon, DNS, RN, FAAN
Associate Professor
Indiana University School of Nursing
Adult Health Nursing
Indianapolis, IN

Debra E. Lyon, PhD, RN, CS
Assistant Professor
University of Virginia School of Nursing
Charlottesville, VA

Diane Magyary, PhD, RN, ARNP
Professor
University of Washington
School of Nursing
Seattle, WA

Ruby J. Martinez, PhD, RN, CS
Assistant Professor
University of Colorado School of Nursing
Denver, CO

Sandra Graham McClowry, PhD, RN, FAAN
Associate Professor
New York University
New York, NY

Susan McCrone, PhD, RN, CS-P
Associate Professor and Chair
Department of Health Promotion/Risk Reduction
West Virginia University School of Nursing
Morgantown, WV

Graham J. McDougall, Jr., PhD, RN, CS
Associate Professor
The University of Texas at Austin
School of Nursing
Austin, TX

Mary J. McNamee, PhD, RN
Assistant Dean and Assistant Professor
University of Nebraska Medical Center
College of Nursing
Omaha, NE

Marianne Miles, PhD, RN, CS
Nurse Psychotherapist
University of Rochester Medical Center
Rochester, NY

Wanda K. Mohr, PhD, RN, FAAN
Associate Professor
Indiana University
Indianapolis, IN

Diana Lynn Morris, PhD, RN, FAAN
Associate Professor of Nursing
Senior Faculty Associate, University Center on Aging and Health
Case Western Reserve University
Cleveland, OH

Shirley A. Murphy, PhD, RN, FAAN
Professor
School of Nursing
University of Washington
Seattle, WA

Lt. Colonel John S. Murray, PhD, RNC, CPNP, CS
Military Consultant to the Surgeon General for Pediatric Nursing
The United States Sir Force
74MDG
Wright-Patterson AFB, OH

Carol M. Musil, PhD, RN
Associate Professor
Case Western Reserve University
Frances Payne Bolton School of Nursing
Cleveland, OH

Madeline A. Naegle, PhD, RN, CS, FAAN
Associate Professor
New York University
New York, NY

Frederica W. O'Connor, PhD, RN
Associate Professor
University of Washington
School of Nursing
Seattle, WA

Barbara J. Parker, PhD, RN, FAAN
Professor
University of Virginia School of Nursing
Charlottesville, VA

Bethany J. Phoenix, PhD, RN
Assistant Clinical Professor
University of California, San Francisco School of Nursing
Department of Community Health Systems
San Francisco, CA

Pamela G. Reed, PhD, RN, FAAN
Professor and Associate Dean for Academic Affairs
University of Arizona
College of Nursing
Tucson, AZ

Lorna A. Rhodes, PhD
Associate Professor, Anthropology
University of Washington
Seattle, WA

Nelma B. Shearer, MEd, MS
University of Arizona
College of Nursing
Tucson, AZ

Deborah Shelton, PhD, RN
Associate Professor
Howard University
Washington, DC

Grayce M. Sills, PhD, RN, FAAN
Professor Emerita
The Ohio State University
College of Nursing
Columbus, OH

Carol E. Smith, RN, PhD
Professor
University of Kansas
School of Nursing
Kansas City, KS

Mariah Snyder, PhD, RN, FAAN
Professor
University of Minnesota
School of Nursing
Minneapolis, MN

Lois Price Spratlen, PhD, RN, FAAN
Professor, School of Nursing
University Ombudsman
Ombudsman for Sexual Harassment
University of Washington
Seattle, WA

Karen F. Stein, PhD, RN
Associate Professor
The University of Michigan
School of Nursing
Ann Arbor, MI

C. June Strickland, Ph.D., R.N.
Assistant Professor
University of Washington School of Nursing
University of Washington
Seattle, WA

Eleanor J. Sullivan, PhD, RN, FAAN
Professor
University of Kansas
School of Nursing
St. Louis, MO

Patricia E. H. Vermeersch, PhD, RN
Adjunct Assistant Professor
Wright State University
School of Nursing and Health
Dayton, OH

Mary Ellen Wewers, PhD, RN, MPH, ANP
Professor
Ohio State University
College of Nursing
Columbus, OH

Monica White
Baccalaureate Student
University of Michigan
Ann Arbor, MI

Patricia A. Wilke, MSN, RN
ND Student
Case Western Reserve University
Frances Payne Bolton School of Nursing
Cleveland, OH

May L. Wykle, PhD, RN, FAAN
Professor and Associate Dean for Community Affairs
Case Western Reserve University
Frances Payne Bolton School of Nursing
Cleveland, OH

Jaclene A. Zauszniewski, PhD, RNC
Associate Professor
Case Western Reserve University
Frances Payne Bolton School of Nursing
Cleveland, OH

PREFACE

The *Psychiatric Mental Health Nursing Research Digest* represents an important resource for the care of persons with psychiatric illnesses. The publication is timely. In late 1999, the Surgeon General, Dr. David Satcher, issued a major report on mental health in which he called for attention to mental health and illness as key areas for scientific investigation (Satcher, 1999). As nurses expand evidence-based practice and look for proven ways to enhance care, we also must aim to achieve the highest level of science possible. This *Digest* represents an important contribution to the expansion of the science and the link between science and professional practice for psychiatric mental health nurses. The psychiatric mental health nurses who have authored the individual entries are in the forefront on this nursing specialty; they are content experts who are aware of the state of the science in the selected areas. In the introduction to each section, we have highlighted the entries and described the relevance of this set of research entries to psychiatric mental health nursing. Thus, it is our expectation that this Digest will be useful to both clinicians and researchers.

It is readily apparent how much our knowledge base has grown over the past several years. Through new research, we now know that far better care is possible and should be expected. We believe that this *Digest* provides information that forms the foundation for better care. In the future, as new knowledge is generated through nursing and health care research, we can expect even more significant breakthroughs. As our science base continues to evolve in both sophistication and breadth, avenues such as the *Psychiatric Mental Health Nursing Research Digest* will keep both clinicians and researchers apprised of our scientific and clinical progress. Each author was asked to identify and describe the most significant research in the selected area. All entries were kept to the succinct style originally used in the *Encyclopedia of Nursing Research* (Fitzpatrick, 1998), and references were limited to those that were deemed classic in the research area or representative of the most recent research in the topic area.

It is our goal to guide both future research in psychiatric mental health nursing and professional nursing care of those with mental health or psychiatric problems. Also, the *Digest* is designed to help beginning students in psychiatric mental health nursing, improve their understanding of the field, and to lead advanced students in psychiatric mental health nursing to research questions and future examples of evidence-based practice.

JOYCE J. FITZPATRICK, Editor

Part I

HEALTH PROMOTION AND RISK REDUCTION

INTRODUCTION

Health promotion is one of the most significant topics in the overall field of health care today. In the case of mental health, health promotion and risk reduction activities are extremely important. Nurses are often in the best positions to initiate interventions related to mental health and the prevention of mental illness, as they are front line providers and therefore in contact with individuals and their families in a large number and wide variety of settings.

This section of the *Digest* includes one of the largest areas of nursing research and practice in this specialty field. Nursing interventions that are highlighted here include those that are related generally to the field of mental health and illness, such as biofeedback training, child and adolescent mental health interventions, music therapy, comfort and empathy, relaxation, and stress management, for example. In addition to these general interventions that would be implemented by mental health professionals in many disciplines, there are specific interventions that are targeted to psychiatric mental health nurses. These include nurse-patient communication, interpersonal communication, nurse-patient interaction, the nurse-patient relationship, individual nursing therapy, consultation-liaison nursing, the use of creative arts in nursing, and psychodrama in nursing. The authors of these entries have addressed the specific ways in which these interventions are used in nursing research and professional practice.

The centerpiece of this section, and of the whole field of psychiatric mental health nursing, is the work of Peplau, who added much to nursing knowledge of the understanding and care of psychiatric patients. Peplau's primary contribution to the field is in the description of the nurse client relationship, an aspect of nursing that is further elaborated in this section.

A series of entries focused more generally on conditions and intervention strategies for both mental and physical health and illness also are included in this section. Examples of these entries are quality of life, stress, self-efficacy, resourcefulness, grief, psychosocial interventions, and smoking cessation.

Several interventions focused on the family are included. These entries describe research on family care-giving, grandmother caregivers, child failure to thrive, depression among young women, pregnancy as a time of anxiety and conflict, and psychosocial adjustment and the family.

Interventions targeted at the highest risk behaviors in psychiatric care, situations in which the patient might harm self or others, are included. These are the entries on violence, including workplace mistreatment and workplace violence, and no-suicide contracts in the therapeutic care of patients.

Several descriptions in this section are focused on the integration of primary and mental health services and the prevention of mental disorders. Sills describes the arena of community mental health, Morris delineates minority issues in mental health, and Kavanagh describes the more general area of cultural aspects of mental health nursing research. McClowry describes mental disorders prevention. Forensic psychiatric care, with particular attention to juvenile justice, is discussed by Shelton. Again, in the broad mental health research arena, Allen delineates mental health services research from a systems perspective, Clement details mental health policy and the relevance for psychiatric nursing, Hauenstein describes mental health and its relationship to primary care in the public sector, and Magyary describes the need for integration of primary health and mental health services.

In summary, health promotion and risk reduction within the field of psychiatric mental health nursing includes many dimensions. The area is rich with information regarding research and clinical evaluations conducted by nurses and other health professionals. It also represents one of the most fruitful areas for potential research.

JOYCE J. FITZPATRICK

BIOFEEDBACK TRAINING

Biofeedback is training in the use of information linked with training in sensitivity to the body state. Patients learn to achieve awareness of the contrast between the ill and the healthy mind/body state. Patients are taught mastery in self-regulation to maintain the healthy state. The kind of information that is cogent is that which can be used for patients to monitor themselves. The premier tool of patient training for self-management of health is offering patients the capacity to track body processes that indicate health and illness. Thus, feedback of physical/emotional signals (biofeedback) to patients is by far the most potent kind of information for self-management of health care.

Feedback of biological and psychological status is not new, but the complexity of indicators of health status now available to patients is vastly proliferated. A decade ago minimal knowledge was available about processes that led to illness and indicators by which to judge the maladaptation. Information is now available about how illness develops in the body. Now, any number of self-management skills can be instituted to interfere with the illness process. For example, a person may monitor bone density, thus tracing or preventing the osteoporosis process, or monitor electroencephalographic (EEG) patterns, thus preventing memory loss. Health professionals know more about the mechanisms of body processes—what produces, prevents, or reverses the disease process. The challenge is to program that knowledge and provide technical and counseling expertise so that patients acquire solid skills in self-management of mind and body.

Psychophysiology is the clinical science that provides the basis for understanding health and disease processes in biofeedback and other self-management skills. This topic initially highlights the central neurocognitive processes that join emotions and cognitive activity with physiological processes. Next, biofeedback will be reported in the context of a larger framework of self-management training, in which a programmatic approach is developed for self-regulation of specific symptom patterns depictive of neural disregulation. Were space available, the cogency of biofeedback for a cadre of chronic functional disorders could be outlined that would capture the pertinence and importance of biofeedback and self-management in future health care.

Psychophysiology—the Interface Between Mind and Body

Biofeedback/self-management interventions are relevant for any dysfunction in which cognitive-emotional and physiological processes produce neural arousal or activation. These neural processes, when dysfunctional, can be demonstrated in neuroendocrine excesses or deficits, immune suppression, cerebral hypoperfusion, EEG hypostimulation or hyperstimulation, and reactions in numerous peripheral organ responses, such as the skin, the cardiovascular system, and neural pathways. Neural dysfunction also can be diffusely manifested as general symptoms of fatigue, cognitive impairment, confusion, chronic pain, and insomnia. It is now understood that neural dyscontrol lies at the heart of most chronic manifestations for which no specific etiological origin has been delineated (Benarroch, 1993). These disease conditions are called diseases of disregulation, a state during which the brain's integrative functions, providing neural control of management of body processes, have gone awry. The enlarging field of psychophysiology provides understandings about how the brain-body interface becomes disregulated.

In a regulated state the brain and body maintain a homeostatic balance, adapting brain activity with biochemical action; hormonal flow; neural, respiratory, and circulatory activity; and peripheral organ performance. Continuous adaptations will prevent long-term disregulation. The brain is the major organ needed for adaptation. Consider the dynamic efforts taking place: cognitive-emotional information flow and the generation of the more subtle cellular and chemical adaptive activity. A stress response or its counterpart, adaptation, is determined by this brain processing.

The homeostatic model traces an adaptive state, whereas the disregulated model is known as a stress response. It is suggested that under stress, the homeostatic pattern achieved by prior adaptation is overridden, producing a tenuous and dysfunctional pattern of psychophysiological stress reaction. Over a prolonged time, chronic disease develops. Thus, in most chronic major illnesses there can be traced a configuration of symptoms that are neurally mediated, overlaying and interacting with a pathophysiological process of the original disease (Steptoe, 1991; Wolf, 1981).

More and more disease conditions are viewed with recognition of this dynamic, interactive dyscontrol. Hypertension, irritable bowel syndrome, chronic fatigue, and fibromyalgia, among other disorders, are examples of disregulation. Even diabetes, arthritis, and a large number of collagen diseases, such as lupus erythematosis, and neuromuscular diseases such as multiple sclerosis are discovered to be outcomes of the autoimmune process triggered by immunological disregulation and its neural control. Certainly, psychiatric disorders can be viewed as disregulatory diseases. The study of biochemical and neurohormonal links to brain mechanisms that control the disease process has expanded, creating this whole new definition of diseases of disregulation.

This understanding of processes of the brain indicates that the brain contains the central adaptive resources for recovery from illnesses or from stress responses. Biofeedback training offers a window into the mechanisms of the dysfunctions through physiological information. The focus of self-management interventions considers the behavioral and emotional changes that will alter psychopathophysiological processes.

Self-Management and Biofeedback

At the heart of biofeedback/self-management training is the concept that the mind/body interface is a self-regulatory system. Self-regulation is an automatic feedback system that runs effectively until negative input disrupts the cycle. A negative sign or symptom forces the body to strive for a reregulated state, sometimes at the expense of an adaptive balance, producing pathological equilibrium. The stress response is an example. Henry (1992) noted that a challenge perceived as easy to manage will elicit an initial active coping response and accompanying release of norepinephrine. Difficulties in managing the task will first change the neuroendocrine parameters, then produce other efforts at adaptation.

In Henry's animal model, the path toward pathology began with threat. As anxiety arose, the norepinephrine/epinephrine ratio decreased; as distress grew, cortisol levels rose, and a passive mode of coping was observable. The ratio of catecholamines to corticoids decreased as frustration and uncertainty grew. Finally, the model of posttraumatic stress syndrome emerged, with repression and denial expressed in impaired attachment and increased irritability. The corticoids paradoxically returned to normal, but lasting emotional trauma remained. Such pathological reregulation is abundant in our own patient populations. But the model also fits for the less traumatized conditions in which anxiety, anger, and depression are dominant features.

Personal control is the cornerstone in the goal orientation of biofeedback/self-management training. In a disregulated condition the threat of lack of control is great. In studies demonstrating a sense of loss of personal control, the predictability of adaptation on the part of the subjects is tenuous. Self-control reflects a degree of self-competence. Very early in their series of studies of somatic complaints Pennebaker, Burnam, Schaeffer, and Harper (1977) found that there is a relationship between perception of control and the incidence of physical complaints. The mechanism of symptomatology seems to be unrelated to physiological functioning but related to the subject's self-control and understanding and prediction of events (Pennebaker et al., 1977; Tetrick & LaRocco, 1987).

A signal that self-management training is a success can be seen by restoration of personal control. Indeed, an operational analysis of personal control suggests that one can measure such indicators as the following:

1. Behavioral control in ability to influence or modify events.
2. Cognitive control by processing of information so as to reduce the cost of adaptation.
3. Decision control through taking opportunities to choose from a number of courses of action.

Personal control is clearly a matter of central focus in self-management training.

Biofeedback is a basic element of our repertoire of health care offerings. We do not always label it as such, nor do we use it to its maximum. We feed back weight, temperature, and blood pressure measures to patients. How often do we think to use photos, mirrors, or audiovisual tapes to inform persons of their general appearance as a mark of health status, as could be done in eating disorders, depression, or anxiety states? The more formal field of biofeedback training, on the other hand, is oriented to the physiological and cognitive-affective processes that are integral to the disregulatory diseases being treated. It has relied on instrumentation of measures such as digital temperature, electromyograph readings, skin conductance, heart rate, and EEG activity as indicators of maladaptive responses. The field places heavy emphasis on training in consciousness as the means for making use of information in achieving self-regulation.

Much of the success in biofeedback treatment has to do with the conceptual approach to the training. The roots of biofeedback training emerged from operant conditioning theory, embracing a limited concept of physiological training without recognition of the neural, cognitive-affective components that are now critical to present-day theory. Biofeedback training is more than merely physiological training of neural pathways. Rather, it is a cognitive event, that of information processing of biological signals. Feedback enables the subject to become consciously aware of the interface between bodily status, environmental events, and internal cognitive information. It provides behavioral strategies to alter physiological activity.

Biofeedback Mechanisms

Biofeedback as an intervention modality is only as effective as the specificity of information that is offered to the patient in relation to the symptom disorder. The specificity of the information is dependent on understanding how symptoms might be generated. Because mechanisms of illness are not simple and linear, the feedback is also likely to be convoluted. Thus, much feedback cannot easily be explained to patients as it is derived from bioinstrumentation. It would be a mistake to oversimplify biological signals as if they represented the mechanisms. The clinician's skill lies in focusing on a changing signal as an approximate and representative indicator of bodily processes in a chain of disregulatory activities. The following two examples are sketched to demonstrate the difficulties of the use of biological signals to help patients to self-manage chronic symptoms.

Hypertension Self-Regulation. Information about control of heart rate is one method of training patients to control high blood pressure. This therapeutic protocol incorporates respiratory and heart rate biofeedback based on the work of Grossman (1991), who noted that control of cardiovascular system integrity by the central nervous system could be observed through the respiratory sinus arrhythmia. The coupling of respiratory and heart rate action is key, because respiration is under voluntary control and can be used as the training device. The patient is trained to breathe deeply, using abdominal muscles, and can be shown the tracing of respiratory sinus arrhythmia on the computer screen. By training to fit the excursions of respiration and respiratory sinus arrhythmia together, heart rate changes and, subsequently, blood pressure can be shown to lower.

Being taught the link of the sympathetic nervous system with blood pressure and the link of emotions and relaxation responses with sympathetic arousal, the mind/body connection is being made to help patients learn to control bouts of hypertension. At home, self-regulation of self-monitored labile hypertension can reduce the average blood pressure markedly.

Attention Deficit Disorder/Cognitive Impairment. A striking feature of many disorders in which attention is restricted and the ability to organize, plan, and concentrate is deficient is that the EEG pattern shows an inability to marshal the proper brain frequencies to allow these functions (Linden, Habib, & Radojevic, 1996; Lubar, 1991). A common EEG pattern is an excess of theta frequency, the slowest wave pattern in the spectral array of all frequencies. This is found in attention deficit/hyperactivity. It is seen in persons with mild closed head injuries, in elderly persons who are losing memory, and in any number of chronic symptom patterns such as chronic heart disease and chronic fatigue syndrome. Patients can be taught to inhibit theta brain activity and increase another dominant frequency. In this case the training must be extended over a time span long enough to reorganize the brain wave pattern and create a habitual state. Self-training can augment the laboratory feedback, using mental tasks and other stimuli to trigger the desired frequency pattern at home.

Summary

Today, self-regulating actions will go far in preventing the progress of pathology, obviating the need for more drastic medication management or surgical intervention. The role of biofeedback in nursing practice can be extensive when the time comes that nursing action is not directed by large institutions. A greater amount of autonomy of practice will be mandatory in outpatient practices caring for patients with chronic diseases. Biofeedback is an augmentation to traditional treatment and need not be seen as a replacement treatment, thus positioning persons to choose either biofeedback or another traditional therapy.

HELEN KOGAN BUDZYNSKI

See also
STRESS

CHILD AND ADOLESCENTS MENTAL HEALTH INTERVENTIONS

Traditionally, child and adolescent psychiatry has tended to narrowly focus on mental illness, that is, diagnosable mental disorders characterized by alterations in thinking, mood, or behavior associated with distress or impaired functioning. Recently, the Surgeon General's Report on Mental Health (U.S. Department of Health and Human Services [DHHS], 1999) has broadly encompassed public health to include not only mental illness but also mental health. "Mental health is a state of successful performance of mental functions, resulting in productive activities, fulfilling relationships with other people, and the ability to adapt to change and to cope with adversity" (DHHS, 1999, p. 4). The emphasis on mental health magnifies the importance on health promotion and preventative services, especially for children and adolescents. The latest research on early brain development has focused public attention on promoting the early establishment of neurological processes and structure that are related to later developmental processes, including mental health. Likewise, the emphasis on mental health in the early years is reflected in the new Taxonomy on Infant Mental Health (Zero to Three/National Center for Clinical Infant Programs, 1994) with importance placed on the early attachment process and relationship building. In 1995, The National Institute of Mental Health (Reiss & Price, 1996) and the Institute of Medicine (Munoz, Mrazek, & Haggerty, 1996) have together generated a national agenda on prevention research related to mental health within a life span developmental framework.

Nursing research has encompassed mental health and illness in child and adolescent populations through two specialty domains. Pediatric nursing research examines developmental processes and trajectories over time with an emphasis on early interventions and prevention science. Psychiatric nursing examines alterations in developmental processes with an emphasis on biopsychosocial explanations and interventions. Together, pediatric and psychiatric nursing research provide a wide angle lens for the advancement of understanding mental health and illness processes and trajectories over time, including preventative and rehabilitative interventions.

Mental health and illness research is interfaced with a growing concern about the mental health of our children and adolescents as reflected in statistical profiles on suicides, homicides, violent acts, delinquency, school suspensions and drop outs, substance abuse, depression, child abuse/neglect, and peer harassment. More and more children are living in poverty, with 20% to 30% estimated to be (DHHS, 1998). Domestic violence expressed in the home, neighborhood, and schools is on the rise. Approximately one in five children exhibit a mental health disorder (DHHS, 1999).

Biopsychosocial Model of Development: The Ultimate Synthesis

How mental health developmental trajectories become established is perplexing and complex. The individual difference question about why some children do well and others do not continues to be asked and studied. Modern neuroscience advances a rich understanding of mental health as a dynamic phenomenon that reflects the interactive process between a child's genetic inheritance and life experiences. Similarly, the current trends in child and adolescent mental health services are designed and delivered increasingly in a manner that recognizes the complex and dynamic nature of developmental processes based on the *intrapersonal* tenet that the mind and body are inseparable and the *interpersonal* tenet that nature and nurture interact within a social and cultural context. Development entails periods of transitions and reorganizations marked by age-appropriate challenges.

Range and Design of Assessment and Intervention Protocols

The integrative science of mental health and illness has generated child and adolescent assessment and intervention protocols based on a biopsychosocial developmental model that entails several common principles.

- *Family-centered interventions* acknowledge families as essential partners in the treatment process with children and adolescents. Clinical-based interventions are more likely to generalize to the home setting when families are involved in the development, implementation, and evaluation of interventions.
- *School-based intervention* increases the treatment strength and generalization to an important peer arena, where important life skills are practiced endlessly all day throughout the week.
- *Primary care, day care and schools* offer mainstream access to populations of children and adolescents and thus provide opportunities for early identification programs and preventative interventions. Innovative mental health programs are being incorporated into the normalcy of public settings and thereby minimizing stigmatization and maximizing the notion of mental health as a natural and essential component of health in general.
- *Community involvement* in mental health programs assures that the child's and adolescent's social-cultural life context will be addressed through *culturally sensitive interventions.*
- *Case management based on an integrative systems approach* to mental health services assures that multiple service sectors are collaborative and coordinated on behalf of youths and their families.
- *Coping with daily stresses and major traumatic events* are becoming essential life skills in the world of constant change, evolving technology, and exposure to public violence.
- *Pharmacological interventions* need to be based on empirically derived information about children and adolescents, especially prioritized populations who have an evident bioneurological basis to their mental disorder such as fetal alcohol syndrome, attention deficit hyperactivity disorder, obsessive-compulsive disorder, and schizophrenia as well as youths who appear to have a genetic propensity to depression and anxiety.

Empirical Evidence

Recently, more emphasis has been placed on evaluating the effects of mental health psychosocial and pharmacological interventions as evidenced through the number of professional tasks forces, clinical practice parameters, and review articles based on metaanalysis. One such evaluation effort was taken by the

American Association of Psychology (Chambless, Baker, Baucom, & Beutler, 1988; Chambless et al., 1996) who established rigorous criteria to categorize psychosocial interventions as "well-established treatments" versus "probably efficacious treatment." The review of child and adolescent interventions revealed that although most *psychosocial interventions* were evaluated as effective in comparison to no treatment, the efficacy of a given therapeutic approach for a specific diagnosis is less well known because too few well-controlled studies have been conducted (Kazdin, 1993; Lonigan, Elbert, & Johnson, 1998). Although the majority of mental interventions did not meet the highest level of empirically based criteria for "well-established treatment," including replication by two or more independent researchers, the evaluation of parent training programs for managing disruptive oppositional behaviors in youths resulted in 12 treatments identified as either "well established or probably efficacious" (DHHS, 1999, p. 16) In particular, the newer community-based multisystemic family-focused intervention holds promise, especially for adolescents who exhibit conduct disorder.

Other interventions showed promising results as a "probably efficacious treatment." For example, family-oriented interventions such as multisystemic family therapy were most effective for generational patterns of substance abuse and delinquency. Cognitive-behavioral therapies appear to have merit for treating depression and anxiety in children and adolescents, particularly school-based interventions. (Kaslow & Thompson, 1998; Ollendick & King, 1998). The cognitive-behavioral interventions entail a broad range of specific therapeutic approaches such as cognitive restructuring, recognition and clarification of thoughts and associated emotions, and behavioral skills training for social, coping, relaxation, and self-control competencies. Psychodynamic and interpersonal therapies have been studied less and thus the empirical support for these approaches is limited and unknown, although clinical case studies suggest further evaluation is warranted.

Pharmacological treatment of mental disorders in children and adolescents has primarily been extrapolated from controlled clinical trials on adults. Even though the scientific basis for the safe and effective use of pediatric psychotropic medications is very limited, the number and types of prescriptions have significantly increased in the past 10 years, which may depict an over reliance on quick biological solutions to complex mental disorders and stressful, fast-paced lifestyles. And yet, psychotropic medications used cautiously and selectively and combined with psychosocial therapies may benefit many children and adolescents, particularly psychostimulants for attention deficit/hyperactivity disorder (ADHD) and the SSRIs (selective serotonin reuptake inhibitors) for obsessive compulsive disorder (Biederman, 1991; DHHS, 1999; Strober, Freeman, Rigali, Schmidt, & Diamond, 1992). Further research would clarify the role of SSRIs, antidepressants, mood stabilizers, and newly developed antipsychotics in treating children and adolescents.

Science-Practice Synergy

The efficacy of psychosocial therapies is more evident and greater in research settings than in the real world of clinical practice, which is characterized by wide variability due to patient, therapist, contextual, and setting factors (Goldfried & Wolfe, 1996; Kazdin, 1996). Differential treatment responses may be associated with one's gender, race/ethnicity, socioeconomic status, sexual orientation, and cultural factors as well as the presence of comorbid mental and physical conditions. In addition, the issue of patient acceptability, and adherence adds to the variability as well as the inclusion of understudied and undeserved populations. A growing body of knowledge suggests that culturally sensitive psychosocial interventions are related to adherence and clinical outcomes (Sue, 1998). External validity requires clinical utility considerations such as feasibility, generalizability, and cost:benefits ratio (Barlow, 1995).

However, recent advancements promote a dialectical resolution between practice and research. Health care reform has placed emphasis on accountability in clinical practice, asking questions about the cost effectiveness of interventions, including questions about individual differences and differential treatment responses in understanding cost:benefit ratios. With an emphasis on accountability and quality practice, Child and Adolescent Clinical Practice Parameters (Dulcan & Bernet, 1998; McDermott & Dunne, 1997) and Clinical Paths (Magyary, Brandt, & Kovalesky, 1999) have been developed for clinicians as guidelines for scientific-based practice. As clinical practice standards highlight accountability, research standards for intervention design are becoming inclusive of not only controlled efficacy studies for testing internal validity but also field-based noncontrolled effectiveness studies for examining external validity. Together, both types of designs yield data on mental health programs that address accountability issues in clinical practice. When examining internal and external validity, the type and duration of clinical outcomes are important. Too few child and adolescent interventions have been examined for long-term primary and secondary effects at the individual, family, school, and community level. Variations in developmental patterns coupled with treatment-induced change patterns create unique challenges for child and adolescent research.

Finally, the recent emergence of "positive psychology" with a focus on optimal functioning expressed at the individual, family, community, and societal levels will continue to highlight the necessity for studies on protective factors and mental health promotion and prevention (Seligman & Csikszentmihalyi, 2000). A template for how to conduct preventative research is exemplified in the long-standing history of early intervention research. Despite the numerous conceptual and methodological challenges, early intervention research such as Head Start has generated a solid body of knowledge that substantiates the finding that high-risk infants and young children respond favorably to early intervention programs as evidenced by controlled efficacy studies and noncontrolled effectiveness studies (DHHS, 1999). Nursing science and practice have contributed substantially to the conceptualization and testing of early intervention programs promoting infant and child mental health. This body of knowledge on early development and interventions linked to later childhood and adolescent developmental trajectories will provide a comprehensive scientific basis promoting mental health and treating mental illness.

DIANE MAGYARY

See also

NURSE-PATIENT INTERACTION
NURSE-PATIENT RELATIONSHIP

CHILD FAILURE TO THRIVE

Classification of Failure to Thrive

Failure to thrive is a term used to describe a deceleration in the growth pattern of an infant or child. Typically, the deceleration is a growth deficit whereby the rate of the child's weight gain is below the third to fifth percentile for age, based on standardized growth charts. A deceleration in a child's growth pattern can occur for any number of physiological reasons; but when a child's lack of weight gain is attributed to psychosocial factors rather than to organic or disease-related factors, the term *nonorganic failure to thrive* (NOFTT) is used.

Traditionally, the failure to thrive syndrome has been classified into three categories: organic, nonorganic, and mixed. Although the term NOFTT frequently is used in contemporary literature, most experts agree that the classification is not so clear because all cases of failure to thrive have an organic etiology (i.e., undernutrition).

Nonorganic failure to thrive is a common problem of infancy and early childhood, and researchers have documented a dramatic increase in its incidence since the late 1970s. It accounts for 3% to 5% of the annual admissions to pediatric hospitals and about 10% of growth failure seen in outpatient pediatrics. Infants with NOFTT typically present not only with growth failure but also with developmental and cognitive delays and signs of emotional and physical deprivation, such as social unresponsiveness, a lack of interactive behaviors, rumination, anorexia, and poor hygiene.

Historical Perspective

Infant nutrition has long been the focus of pediatric research. Holt (1897) was one of the first to describe marasmus, a significant infant nutrition problem and a condition similar to the failure to thrive syndrome described in contemporary literature. It was in 1915 that the term *failure to thrive* was first used in the pediatric literature to describe rapid weight loss, listlessness, and subsequent death in institutionalized infants. In the early 1900s, the mortality rate for institutionalized infants was near 100%, and few realized the importance of environmental stimulation and social contact for infant growth and development. It was during this time that the first foster home care program for institutionalized marasmic infants was developed. The home care program involved the identification and training of families, by nurses, to care for the ill infants, and it included a significant amount of nursing intervention to monitor the progress of the infants. Unfortunately, this early work was not recognized by the pediatric community, despite a 60% drop in the mortality rate of marasmic infants cared for in the foster homes.

It was not until 1945 that the concept of failure to thrive captured the attention of the psychiatric and pediatric communities. In a classic paper, Spitz (1945) described depression, growth failure, and malnutrition in 61 foundling home infants. He used the term *hospitalism* to describe the syndrome that he observed, and he proposed that a lack of emotional stimulation and the absence of a mother figure were the main contributors to infant growth failure. Spitz postulated that with adequate love, affection, and stimulation, the infants would grow. Researchers demonstrated weight gain in infants with hospitalism when stimulation and affection were provided. Thus, these findings provided a foundation for a failure to thrive theoretical framework based on maternal deprivation in institutionalized infants.

In the mid-1950s a number of case reports were published in the psychiatric literature that documented depression, malnutrition, and growth failure in infants living in intact families. These case studies were the first to report feeding and interactional difficulties between the mothers and their infants. Feeding episodes for the mothers were anxiety-provoking, which led the mothers to decrease both the frequency of infant feedings as well as their contact with the infants. Ethnologists and child development experts began studying institutionalized and noninstitutionalized infants to further define the concepts of maternal deprivation and failure to thrive. On the basis of several studies, researchers concluded that decreased maternal contact led directly to failure to thrive in the infants. From these works the maternal deprivation framework for failure to thrive was established, and the mother's role in the infant's well-being became a central focus. Support for this framework grew as data accumulated documenting the association between maternal neglect and failure to thrive in infants.

Current Perspective

The maternal deprivation framework predominated in the literature until the late 1970s, when a transactional framework was developed to explain the psychosocial correlates of NOFTT. The transactional framework proposed that an infant's growth and development were contingent on the quality of parental care, the nature of parent and infant interactions, and the ecological conditions impinging on the family. Furthermore, the transactional model recognized that the quality of the parent-infant interaction reflected infant characteristics as well as parent characteristics. Historically, the emotional deprivation component of NOFTT has been investigated more than the nutritional deprivation component. Although experts in NOFTT would agree that malnutrition is the primary biological insult, systematic studies investigating this element are lacking.

Nutritional deprivation again became the focus of NOFTT research in the early 1970s, when some researchers disputed the hypothesis that maternal deprivation was its principal cause. More recent evidence suggests that the environmental deprivation may occur before the undernutrition. Although the primary cause of NOFTT may never be fully understood, it is apparent that nutritional deficits are dependent on the environmental context in which they occur.

The transactional model of pediatric medicine is similar to the ecological model developed by pediatric nurses and used to explain NOFTT (Barnard & Eyres, 1979; Lobo, Barnard, & Coombs, 1992). The ecological model focused on the three major interaction components of the parent-child relationship: those of the child, the parent, and the environment. These interactions are synchronous and reciprocal. Barnard and her colleagues (Barnard et al., 1989) emphasized the importance of the parent's and child's physical and emotional characteristics, as well as the supportive or nonsupportive nature of the environment in understanding the interactions. Researchers have examined parent-child interactions by means of direct, structured observations during feeding and other situations and found that NOFTT infants were less vocal and interactive with their parents and that the parents of these infants were less able to determine their infants' needs, compared to NOFTT infants and their parents. From this it is evident that interference with the reciprocal process of the parent-child relationship disturbs the opportunity to attain optimal growth and development. Because growth problems, such as NOFTT in infancy, place a child at significant risk for developmental delays as a toddler, it is important to recognize the interactional problems between parents and their infants so that interventions aimed at improving interactions can begin early in the parent-child relationship.

HEIDI VONKOSS KROWCHUK

See also
CHILD AND ADOLESCENT MENTAL HEALTH INTERVENTIONS
STRESS

COMFORT

Definition

Comfort has been conceptualized for nursing as a holistic outcome of patient care. It is defined as the experience of having the needs for relief, ease, or transcendence met in four contexts of experience. Relief, ease, and transcendence as three types of comfort were derived from a concept analysis of comfort by Kolcaba and Kolcaba (1991). The four contexts for experiencing comfort are physical, psychospiritual, environmental, and social; they were derived from the literature on holism (Kolcaba & Kolcaba, 1991).

Comfort care is nursing care that is intended to enhance a patient's comfort beyond its known baseline. Comfort care consists of goal-directed, comforting activities (process) through which enhanced comfort (product) is achieved. The process is initiated by the nurse, often in conjunction with the patient and family, after an assessment of the comfort needs of the patient. Because the specified product or goal is enhanced comfort, a successful process is evaluated by comparing comfort levels before and after nursing interventions. The process is incomplete until the product of enhanced comfort is achieved (Dretske, 1988).

Theory of Comfort

Kolcaba (1994) provides a theoretical framework for practicing comfort care and for generating nursing research about comfort. Briefly, the theory states that interventions should be designed and implemented to address unmet comfort needs of patients and their families. Patients and families are recipients of nursing care, and they perceive the effectiveness of nursing interventions in the context of existing intervening variables. Intervening variables are factors that recipients bring to the situation, such as financial status, existing social support, previous experience with health care, and religious beliefs. If recipients of nursing care perceive that their comfort is enhanced through effective nursing interventions, those interventions qualify as comfort measures. Such comfort measures strengthen patients and their families during stressful health care situations, thereby facilitating health-seeking behaviors.

Schlotfeldt (1975) discussed health-seeking behaviors in terms of those that are internal (fertility, healing), external (self-care, functional status), or leading to a peaceful death. Consistent with holism, conscious and subconscious experience influence motivation for health-seeking behaviors. Because health-seeking behaviors are constructive, they are reciprocally and positively related to comfort. In the theory of comfort, comfort is the immediate goal of nursing interventions, and health-seeking behaviors, specific to the research questions(s), are subsequent goals.

Relevance to Nursing

As a heuristic device, comfort care plans for individual patients or patient/family situations have been designed for students who are learning to apply comfort care to their patients (Kolcaba, 1995) and families (Kolcaba & Fisher, 1996). There are several advantages for teaching comfort care. First, it is theory-based nursing. Second, it is satisfying to patients because it is individualized and holistic. Third, it is satisfying to students because they become aware of and are given credit for all comfort measures that they implement for their patients. Fourth, it is appropriate for diverse settings. Fifth, it is easy to learn because students are familiar with the concept of comfort through their own experiences.

After a brief introduction to the theory, nurses are able to practice comfort care without the heuristic device of plans. When comfort care is used as a framework for organizing nursing care, that care is more efficient because many comfort measures can be implemented during one patient encounter. Nurses and patients find comfort care satisfying and productive because enhanced comfort is theoretically related to progress in physical therapy, collaboration with new health regimens, or faster healing.

Research

The content domain of comfort provides a diagram for designing interventions and problem-focused questionnaires. Holistic interventions, such as massage, music therapy, art therapy, guided imagery, therapeutic touch, and comfort care itself, can be targeted to several aspects in the grid at one time. Unmet needs of patients or families in specific health settings can be identified, and specific interventions can be designed to meet those needs. Unmet needs also can be translated into items on questionnaires to determine baseline comfort and postintervention comfort. Comfort questionnaires should have positive and negative items relevant to the research setting to represent each aspect of the domain. Although comfort is state specific, a successful intervention theoretically should demonstrate increasing comfort over time. Therefore, at least three repeated measures of comfort should be collected in an intervention study where increased comfort is a desired goal.

The theory of comfort directs research in several ways. First, it guides nurses to test relationships between particular holistic interventions and comfort; an effective intervention is positively and significantly related to an increase in comfort over time. Second, it guides nurses to test relationships between comfort and health-seeking behaviors. If the relationship is positive, nurses have a pragmatic rationale for enhancing their patients' comfort. Third, it guides nurses to construct predictive models for interventions that enhance comfort and facilitate desired health-seeking behaviors.

Observational studies have been conducted to determine what kind of comforting actions are important for patients and what the term comfort actually means to patients. These studies were about the process of comfort care; they did not define the outcome of comfort.

Quantitative comfort studies are in their infancy, primarily because comfort has been operationalized only recently. But instruments developed from the content domain of comfort were sensitive to group differences in comfort during the immobility period following cardiac catheterization for different types of restraints and to differences in comfort between community dwellers and hospital patients. Several intervention studies in which comfort is the desired outcome are in progress: effectiveness of music therapy for persons having dressing changes for burns, effectiveness of comfort care for postsurgical incontinence, and effectiveness of guided imagery for women who choose conservative therapy for early breast cancer.

Future Directions

To demonstrate that comfort is an important mission for nursing, further research is needed to determine the relationship between enhanced comfort and health-seeking behaviors. Decreased length of stay for hospitalized patients, decreased readmissions, faster progress during rehabilitation, and increased functional status related to enhanced patient comfort would interest administrators, funding agencies, and policymakers. Further research also is needed to replicate experimental studies that have demonstrated the effectiveness of holistic interventions. When nurses wish to test such interventions, they should use an outcome consistent with a holistic paradigm; comfort is such an outcome.

KATHARINE KOLCABA

See also
MUSIC THERAPY
NURSE-PATIENT INTERACTION

COMMUNITY MENTAL HEALTH

Antecedents of the Community Mental Health Movement

The ebb and flow of social policy in the United States is marked by gradual shifts in public perception and evaluation of the problems that beset the society in any given era. Thus, the convergence of major societal trends gave rise to the Community Mental Health Centers Act of 1963; the first of these trends had arisen from the earlier passage of the National Mental Health Act (Public Law 79-489) in July 1946. This act created the National Institute of Mental Health (NIMH) and appropriated significant federal monies to support innovations in training, research, and practice in the field of mental health. The act designated four core mental health disciplines: psychiatry, psychology, social work, and psychiatric nursing (Bloom,1984). Funds from this act allowed financial support for students and faculty at the undergraduate and graduate levels in psychiatric nursing.

This federal infusion of dollars into the states required that each state would have a central planning authority charged with the responsibility for planning and evaluating community-based mental health services, the first time in U.S. history that the federal government had assumed responsibility for what had for more than a century been the exclusive duty of the states. This latter fact is most often attributed to the efforts of Dorthea Lynde Dix, who sought to have the abysmal community-based mental health care of the 1840s (i.e., asylums, jails, almshouses) replaced by a system of state psychiatric hospitals.

In the decade after the passage of the Mental Health Act there was growth in the number of state mental hospitals as well as in the number of admissions. Subsequently, Congress enacted the Mental Health Study Act to examine the human and economic problems of mental illness, and the Joint Commission on Mental Illness and Health was established. At the end of a 5-year period the commission presented its report to President John F. Kennedy. Three months later the President transmitted a message to Congress in which he outlined a "bold, new approach." This message framed the substance of what was to develop as the Community Mental Health Centers Act of 1963. The act provided for federal money to be matched with local dollars for construction of community-based mental health centers. Planning grants were given to each state to inventory mental health needs and resources. The country was divided into some 1500 catchment areas, with the idea that eventually each catchment area would have its own center. The act mandated five essential services: inpatient care, partial hospitalization, emergency services, consultation, and education. Later, five additional services were added to the mandate: precare and aftercare, diagnostic services, rehabilitation, training, and research and evaluation.

In the years since 1963, Congress has extended and amended the act several times. In 1977, President Jimmy Carter and his wife, Rosalynn Carter, brought to the White House a long-standing concern for the care and treatment of persons with mental disabilities and mental illness. President Carter's first act was to establish a President's Commission on Mental Health, with Mrs. Carter serving as honorary chair. The report of this 1977 commission contained more than 100 recommendations. The major recommendations were to provide universal access to treatment at reasonable cost to all who needed it and to work toward high quality of services. Specific recommendations focused on working with the community to lessen the stigma associated with mental illness by (a) developing community supports, (b) providing for careful protection of basic rights, (c) focusing on prevention, and (d) expanding the research base to increase the available knowledge. Thus, in 1980, when the Community Mental Health Centers Act was scheduled to expire, Congress began to work on the new legislation, Public Law 96-398, the Mental Health Systems Act.

However, the mood of the country had changed. President Carter was not reelected in 1980 and was succeeded by Ronald Reagan. The Reagan administration had promised less federal government intrusion into the affairs of state governments; thus, the proposal for block grants was accepted, and the previous 20 years of categorical grant experience were negated. In 1981 the budgetary provisions for the Mental Health Systems Act were repealed, and the system of block grants was established. There are, however, legacies from this era of community mental health.

Treatment Approaches in Community Mental Health

Prior to the 1960s, long-term therapies were normative. Short-term therapy, crisis interpretation, and mental health consultation are now standard practice in the field (Bloom, 1984; Lancaster, 1980). Each modality has made a major contribution to the therapeutic armamentarium of mental health practitioners. Equally important, if not more so, intellectual work of the community mental health era yielded a set of concepts that continues to prove useful to the ongoing study of body and mind relationships. The conceptual notions of early childhood interventions, genetic risks, the importance of healthy pregnancy to future well-being, and other concepts led to an approach that examines risk factors and the incidence of mental illness. This era also sowed the seeds for the beginning work on the relationship between stress and illness. This was reflected in the emphasis on community-based mental health education as a strategy for prevention (Beisser & Rose, 1972).

An integral feature of all aspects of the community-based approach was an emphasis on citizen participation at all levels—national, state, and local. This forged an interesting alliance of lay people with professionals. However, the continued vocal and sometimes adversarial participation of consumers and their families in the planning, delivery, and evaluation of mental health services is a major strength in the struggle to achieve parity for mental health care with all other health care.

In the latter part of the 1990s, the community-based mental health delivery systems are faced with the additional challenge of managed care. How well the states can respond to these emerging mandates is yet to be seen. Some states have begun to shape new systems from older community-based systems, with evaluations yet to be completed (Inglehart, Hiebert-White, & Zuercher, 1995). What is clear is that the institutional responses to the problems of mental health and mental illness are shaped by prevailing belief systems. The decade of the 1990s has been called the "decade of the brain." It is to be expected, then, that the focus for research, treatment, and training will continue to shift away from some of the core values that have shaped community mental health programs.

GRAYCE M. SILLS

See also
MENTAL HEALTH IN PUBLIC SECTOR PRIMARY CARE
MENTAL HEALTH SERVICES RESEARCH
PSYCHOSOCIAL INTERVENTIONS

CONSULTATION-LIAISON NURSING

Consultation-liaison nursing (C/L nursing) is an advanced practice specialty area in psychiatric-mental health nursing (American Nurses Association, 1990). The C/L role was developed in the early 1960s in general hospitals to focus on the psychosocial aspects of physical illness (Lewis & Levy, 1982). C/L nurses now function in multiple settings including general hospitals, long-term care, emergency rooms, and home health agencies. C/L nurses function as members of multidisciplinary teams (Yoest, 1989), as consultants to nursing staff (Roberts, 1997), and in private practice (Schulmeister, 1999).

C/L nurses provide direct and indirect care (Lewis & Levy, 1982). Many C/L nurses use Caplan's (1970) model of consultation. In this model, a *client-centered consultation* focuses directly on the biopsychosocial needs of the hospitalized client. A *consultee-centered consultation* focuses indirectly on the patient by targeting the health care providers' needs for knowledge, skill, confidence, or objectivity (Caplan, 1970).

A review of C/L nursing literature reveals an abundance of published articles. However, most are theoretical or clinical papers. There are few systematic studies.

The role of the C/L nurse is diverse, and C/L interventions draw from multiple frameworks (i.e., developmental, social roles, systems theory, grieving, and others). This may be one reason why it has been difficult for C/L nurses to conduct outcome-based research. Another reason for the research shortage is the historical tendency for C/L nurses to function as members of C/L teams. While this role may work well in practice (Yoest, 1989), findings related to nurses seem to be embedded in the medical literature.

There is growing evidence that psychiatric problems are common among the physically ill (Mallory, Lyons, Scherubel, & Reichelt, 1993; Mayou & Hawton, 1986). And medical patients with psychiatric comorbidity appear to require longer lengths of stay and increased nursing time (Mallory et al., 1993). C/L nurses have long served significant roles in addressing these issues. However, C/L nurses have recently been vulnerable to cost-cutting measures, and research is warranted.

The Role of the Consultation-Liaison Nurse

Studies aiming to delineate the role and functions of the C/L nurse were characteristic of the research conducted in the late 1970s and early 1980s. C/L nurses and C/L physicians were compared by Stickney (1981), who differentiated referrals made to the nurse versus those made to the psychiatrist. Findings indicated that the nurse was more likely to see the nursing staff alone or for behavioral reasons, while the psychiatrist was more likely to see the client for psychiatric reasons. Wolff (1978) studied the problems that led medical-surgical nurses to make referrals to a C/L nurse. Referrals were more likely when the client evidenced psychopathology or when the patient elicited negative emotional responses in the nurse.

More recently, Roberts (1998) conducted a qualitative study to explore staff perceptions of the role of a C/L nurse on a hematology unit. A single focus group interview was used. Open coding was used to analyze data. Findings indicated that nursing staff valued the following: the C/L nurse's availability and visibility, objectivity, counseling skills, and ability to distinguish normal patient reactions from mental illness. The nursing staff perceived themselves to lack the confidence and skills required to address patients' psychosocial needs. Finally, the C/L nurse was valued for providing support to staff. A strength of this study is the depth of the findings. A weakness acknowledged by the author is the small sample size (N = 3). This study should be continued with larger and more diverse samples.

General Medical Units

Consultation-liaison nursing arose when psychiatric units were established in general hospitals. Medical-surgical staff called on psychiatric nurses for assistance in understanding patients psychosocial needs (Simmons, 1982). Some studies have since examined the degree to which C/L services impact on the care of medical patients.

Lyons and associates (1986) studied 419 cases referred from general hospital units to a C/L service (psychiatrist and nurses). The authors sought to determine the relationship between *timing of the consultation* and *length of hospital stay.* Findings indicated a positive relationship between early referrals to C/L and shorter lengths of stay. However, this study did not specifically focus on the contributions made by C/L nurses.

The relationship between *consultations* and overall *nursing care hours* was examined on general medical units by Mallory et al. (1993). This retrospective study examined 1734 C/L referrals in a major medical center. Data were obtained from charts, from a C/L database, and from fiscal files. C/L referrals were divided into three groups based on the hours of C/L services delivered: low, medium, and high intensity. Findings suggested significant differences between subgroups that call for separate examination in this and future studies. The high intensity group appeared a more complex and difficult subgroup, and nursing care hours decreased the least among this subgroup after C/L service. The medium intensity group was the largest group and the group had the greatest decrease in nursing care hours after the C/L service. A positive correlation was also found in this group between *timing of the C/L referral* and *length of stay.* The low intensity group was comprised of clients with primary psychiatric disorders and those referred late in the hospital stay for a psychological aspect of their physical illness. Within this low intensity group, the C/L physician more often saw those with primary psychiatric diagnoses while the nurse was more likely to see those coping with a psychological aspect of a physical illness.

The effect of C/L nursing interventions on the care of medical-surgical clients needing constant observation (termed "sitters") was studied by Talley, Davis, Goicoechea, Brown, and Barber (1990). A randomized, experimental design was used to test the hypotheses that clients with "sitters" who receive C/L nursing consultation would require fewer sitter shifts, have more charted nursing observations, have fewer incidents, have fewer sitter walkouts, and have fewer days of hospitalizations. The sample size was adequate (N = 107). Findings did not support the hypotheses. The authors note that the absence of a correlation between C/L nursing and the outcome variables was disappointing but not surprising given the wide range of variability on outcome measures. They also recommend that future studies focus on smaller units of C/L intervention and more homogeneous groups of subjects with similar behavioral problems.

Future studies need to continue this quest for differentiation among subgroups of medical clients referred for C/L services. Outcome studies could then focus on target interventions, measuring outcomes of specific approaches derived from psychiatric nursing theory.

Subspecialization Within C/L Nursing

There is a recent trend toward *subspecialization* within C/L nursing (Moschler & Fincannon, 1992). While C/L nursing originated in the general medical setting, C/L nurses now specialize in oncology, geriatrics, emergency nursing, and AIDS. This trend may ultimately make it more feasible for the C/L nurse to conduct outcome-based research.

C/L nurses caring for hospitalized persons with AIDS were the focus of a report authored by Kurlowicz (1991). The author used a retrospective review and analysis of consultation records from C/L experience over a 6-year period. Several themes categorized the work done by the C/L nurse, including: management of nurses' emotional reactions, assistance with reducing staff stress, managing disruptive clients, clarifying psychological needs of clients, evaluating mental status, offering clients support, and making community referrals.

Oncology units are also utilizing C/L nurses. Fincannon (1995) conducted a retrospective chart review to examine the nurse-generated referrals made from a cancer center to C/L nurses. The sample included 102 psychiatric consults documented in the charts. Findings revealed that five major psychiatric problems constituted reasons for referral: depression, anxiety, adjustment disorder, "difficult to care for," and dementia.

The geriatric population is another subgroup benefiting from the services of C/L nurses (Pajarillo, Sers, Ryan, Headley, & Nalven, 1997). This will increasingly become the case as the number of elderly persons in the United States is rapidly growing. Geriatric C/L nurses have specifically made advances in the literature in terms of describing their unique, subspecialty role (Pajarillo et al., 1997; Smith et al., 1990). However, systematic research studies are limited, and studies are warranted.

Recommendations for Future Research

C/L nurses have advanced this specialty area of psychiatric nursing practice through the publication of theoretical and clinical papers. However, systematic studies are very limited and outcome-based studies are clearly in order. Future studies could benefit from the growing trend toward subspecialization by focusing on more homogeneous subgroups and outcome variables and by focusing on specific C/L interventions that target clients, families, or staff.

MARIANNE MILES

See also

NURSE-PATIENT RELATIONSHIP

PRIMARY AND MENTAL HEALTH SERVICES INTEGRATION

CREATIVE ARTS AS NURSING INTERVENTION

"Giving form to feeling is perhaps the ultimate empowerment, and acts of artistic expression, in and of themselves, carry their own healing" (MacKay, 1989, p. 300).

For children and for adults who have difficulty verbalizing experiences, the playful arts and drama offer an opportunity to access thoughts and feelings unavailable to them through words alone (Blatner & Blatner, 1997). This may be particularly important for those who have experienced or witnessed the trauma of abuse or domestic violence (who score significantly higher in anxiety, muscle tension, and cognitive disorganization (Cornman, 1997)) and who need to symbolize and rework those events to master them (Gil, 1998). Because of the importance of creating a relationship and establishing self-care and functioning prior to dealing with trauma (Chu, 1991), professional nurses are in an ideal position to assist clients to use creative expression for healing.

For children up to age 11, play is the primary, dynamic form of communication that matches their inner psychic structure and is used until they are able to verbalize abstract concepts (Ginott, 1961; Landreth, Homeyer, Glover, & Sweeney, 1996). For adults who have childhood play deficits as a result of having been required to move into adult responsibility while still in childhood, there is an "act hunger" (Blatner & Blatner, 1997), a desire to act out roles unavailable to them as children. "Playing it out" (Erikson, 1963) is healing for these individuals.

The purpose of this article is to encourage nursing personnel to use the power and pleasure of the creative arts and play as healing modalities pertinent to the complexities of today's health care problems. The following are examples of professional nursing studies using creative arts for the health of clients.

Creative Expression Used with Child Survivors of Abuse

In a study of play and self-expression in 11 school-aged children who had experienced a sexual trauma (Emerson, 1992), children expressed anger, and attitudes toward males/perpetrators/father, toward mother, being good, being ugly/messing up, food/eating, hiding, and safety in four sessions with the nurse investigator. The sessions focused on play, and there was no mention of abuse by the investigator. The children demonstrated the effects of abuse in lack of interactional skills and the tendency to take the roles of abuser or victim. All showed signals of comfort during the process of play and subsequent relaxation and fuller self-expression, especially when in the pretense of fantasy play. The findings of this study had implications for children and for nursing practice, theory, research, and education.

> "Play/the arts provide a distancing process by which children can identify with objects (ed: e.g., puppets, dolls), and project and process their feelings. . . . When

> changes occur in play, the child takes an active role on his or her own behalf, . . . to compensate . . . for real losses. When children go from passive and helpless victims to agents of change in play, reparation begins" (Gil, 1998, p. 9).

Riddle (1997) developed an adolescent inpatient sexual abuse group based on Lewin's Model of Change that used art activities and role-play along with journaling and personal storytelling for treatment of the sequelae of abuse. The pilot group was labeled "educational-supportive" (p. 20) and nonpsychotic, affectively stable male and female adolescent inpatients took part. Lewin's three steps necessary for change to occur, (1) unfreezing of present situation, (2) movement to a new level, and (3) refreezing at the new level, took place. The group became an established part of the unit treatment schedule.

These three steps parallel the three stages of recovery from trauma described by Ellensweig-Tepper (2000) in her study of trauma group psychotherapy for female adolescents with posttraumatic stress disorder (PTSD) from abuse. The stages of (a) focus on safety, (b) remembrance and mourning, and (c) reconnection with ordinary life (Herman, 1992) were accomplished through weekly brief, solution-focused therapy focusing on strengths and times when the trauma was *not* affecting the participants.

Creative Expression for Children Housed in a Domestic Violence Shelter

Emerson and three nursing students replicated a study by Morris (1994), who used a short-term structured group therapy intervention called Superkids for psychiatrically hospitalized children with a history of abuse. The intervention was applied to the preschool and school-aged children housed in a domestic violence shelter. Through skits and drawings, the children were able to express feelings of shame/blame, anger, fear, trust, and love, and to create multiple responses to abusive situations they had experienced. They showed more positive affect with adults, and reduced aggressive behavior over the 5-week cycle of meetings. They experienced a sense of belonging and hope like those in a study of 2- to 6-year-olds in a shelter by Gilbert (1988). Future research would focus on application of standardized measurement tools to demonstrate empirically the positive short- and long-term effects on the children of creative role-play to transform experiences of violence.

Adult Women Abused as Children

Adult women who have been abused as children often seek counseling because they have difficulties maintaining healthy relationships. They may appear to function well in their daily lives, but live with high levels of fear, anxiety, and depression (Cornman, 1997).

In a group therapy situation with four women 30 to 40 years old, the expressive arts served as an enjoyable icebreaker in initiating treatment. Dramatic role-play and the arts gave the women the distance from real-life events to permit them to acknowledge past abusive experiences while finding new ways of relating comfortably. Therapeutic play served as a buffer against stressful life events by allowing for practice to reduce fears, and development of a more playful attitude was inoculation against stress (Schaefer, 1998).

The difficulty releasing past ways of relating among group participants demonstrated the need to teach problem solving, conflict management, and specific self-esteem enhancers such as releasing negative self-talk and using positive affirmations. This combination of creative arts with cognitive-behavioral techniques was developed for use with the adolescent population detained in juvenile justice.

Creative Arts for Adolescent Girls Detained in Juvenile Justice

Studies have shown that an increased rate of violence and adult criminality occurs among youth with childhood experiences of physical and sexual abuse, neglect, and exposure to domestic violence (Shelton, 2000; Widom, 1995). Adolescents detained in a youth facility in one mid-Atlantic state were identified with a 60% rate of mental disorders; 68% rate of child abuse history; and 80% subsequent unhealthy responses such as substance abuse, promiscuity, and violent activity. Exposure to violence and abuse, "alters a child's cognitive and emotional orientation to the world and causes trauma by distorting the child's self-concept, world view, or affective capacities" (Finkelhor & Browne, 1985, p. 354). Children who attempt to cope with the world through the distortions developed in relationships with trusted but abusing adults develop severe behavioral and relational problems. Based on the outcomes of a similar curriculum designed and tested with a male youthful offender population (Shelton, 2000), an 18-session psychoeducational Break the Cycle program was developed for a pilot with female offenders (Emerson & Shelton, 2000). The intervention was designed to incorporate use of playful creative arts for role exploration in relation to self, family, and society; and cognitive-behavioral education to increase coping skills to reduce risk of domestic violence. Outcomes in this female offender population will determine revisions of this gender-specific curriculum and its application to a larger population.

Opportunities for Prevention Through Developing Coping Skills

Advanced practice mental health nurses used a 10-session intervention called Teaching Kids to Cope (TKC) with 40 (nonoffending) high school students with depressive symptoms. Specific strategies were used to encourage group cohesion, correct distortions, and encourage experimentation with problem solving in the here and now. Outcomes were less depression and new coping behaviors (Puskar, Lamb, & Tusaie-Mumford, 1997).

Creative Expression for Adults in Community Care

Creative expression of feelings and attitudes is a pathway to the achievement of psychological health and insight (Johnson, 1987). Two groups of posthospitalized psychiatric patients in community day treatment participated in a weekly creative arts activity with nursing students in a rural Southeastern state. One activity involved the patients' use of varied arts and crafts materials to create a mask or other symbol of their experience of themselves in relation to nondisabled people around them and share it with peers. The result of the activity was that patients learned something about themselves, and made connections with student caregivers (as nondisabled people).

Conclusion

Creative expression of experiences provides expansion into the affective and psychomotor realms that words may not reach. Spontaneity as experienced in the expressive arts is a tool for finding the playful, creative, more accepting whole self needed for coping with a complex history of trauma (Blatner & Blatner, 1997; Emerson, 1997; Schaefer, 1998). Using creative, nonnarrative expression empowers patients to explore and master overwhelming experiences, increase interpersonal skills, and bridge communication gaps. Professional nurses are in a position to facilitate growth and healing with the playful creative arts.

ELISSA EMERSON

See also
CHILD ABUSE
VIOLENCE

CULTURAL ASPECTS OF PSYCHIATRIC MENTAL HEALTH NURSING AND RESEARCH

Psychiatric and mental health problems arise in every culture and their innumerable real-life combinations. Culture encompasses shared and learned patterns of beliefs, customs, emotions, and knowledge that shape conduct. Generalized beliefs about health generally include ideas about the mind and the interactive self and keeping those in good order through such social and moral recommendations as overall balance in living, avoiding excessive emotional stress, and maintaining positive personal and social interrelationships (Loustaunau & Sobo, 1997). Among peoples not limited to scientific interpretations, mental illness is typically viewed as situated in social interaction, related to magical or supernatural intervention, and integrated both with physical health/illness and with other problems of living. The present trends toward reintegrating the mind and spirituality into biomedical health care fit well with holistic, traditional orientations of bio-psycho-social-spiritual healing. The mind is increasingly recognized as a major factor in healing both within and between persons and as extending beyond conventional ideas about space and time (DiLima & Painter, 1998). However, the inextricable intertwining of physical and mental health, until recently, more accurately characterized traditional ethnopsychiatric and ethnomedical belief systems than that of scientific medicine.

Psychiatric Mental Health Assessment

How problems are expressed, recognized, and managed vary widely. Assessment is challenged by the behavioral nature of psychiatric symptoms, embedded as they are within varying patterns of communication, social organization, relationships with time and space, worldviews, and living environments. Transformation of mechanical biomedicine to providing care congruent with the needs of diverse peoples requires new ways of assessing, understanding, and describing. Accuracy and fairness in assessing depend on sensitivity to and awareness of the culture-specific definitions of normality and abnormality; knowledge of expectable patterns of thinking and behavior, and of the implications of labeling and intervention; and skill in communication and recognition of culturally diverse, culturally shaped, and culturally acknowledged patterns of deviant thinking and behavior (Kavanagh, 1999).

Normalcy Throughout the Lifespan

Although every society labels some behaviors as abnormal, dichotomizing illnesses into physical and mental is a Western concept that is increasingly criticized (Goleman & Gurin, 1993). What is considered "normal" and "abnormal" is always shaped by cultural perspectives (McElroy & Townsend, 1996). With increased attention to the natural healing abilities (and reactions against conventional biomedicine as too far removed from nature and too focused on technology), there is more emphasis on healing than curing. All aspects of the nursing process must reflect flexibility adequate to recognize culture-specific patterns of normality and abnormality (that is, from the perspectives that clients hold) and as they relate to rapid social change; the facts of managed care; and a considerable repertoire of traditional (folk), conventional, alternative, and complementary (combined) approaches to health care.

Health Promotion and Risk Reduction

Mental health promotion and risk reduction are tied to improving psychosocial and environmental and physical conditions. Increased risk for mental illness is associated with living in poverty; sexual and physical abuse; and disruptive and inadequate family and personal relationships. While social dynamics tied to racism, sexism, classism, ageism, and ethnocentrism undermine mental health, interactive processes that facilitate positive intercultural encounters and communication are both the first line of defense and, along with the appropriate therapeutic drugs when needed, the most effective intervention. A critical perspective must be maintained for health care providers to recognize the difference between natural biases (some things being noticed and not others) and negative bias (some views and strengths getting left out); and between generalizations (changeable starting places for comparing typical behavior patterns with the facts, i.e., what is actually observed) and stereotypes (seeing what is expected and missing what is not expected). Whereas open, mutual relationships increase chances of understanding clients' views and providing culturally appropriate care, negative stereotyping leads to prejudicial attitudes (negative expectations about a group that are applied to individual situations) and discriminatory behaviors (treating people unfairly and the "isms") (Kavanagh, 1999).

Emotional Health

Biomedical psychiatry tends to locate disorders within individuals, while cross-cultural and anthropological research shows that disorder can be rooted in society. In contemporary culture, numerous forms of social disconnectedness and unhealthy personal expectations encourage a wide range of stress and distress responses. Many people develop mental health problems within the matrix of genetic predisposition, learning that is not confluent with lived experiences, social expectations, and stressful life circumstances (McElroy & Townsend, 1996). Culture plays a significant role in shaping expressions of distress, as well as coping strategies. For instance, in North America, where family environments are often stressful, overly individuated, and overstimulating, abuse and neglect of personal relationships are common. Crime, drug use, and suicide are prevalent problems that may be related to limited perceived hope and connectedness (Harrison, 1997). Addictive behaviors employ rituals and idioms that both communicate emotional distress and provide buffers against emotional pain, feelings of helplessness and futurelessness, and anxiety.

Issues in Environments of Care

Every society has a traditional herbal ethnopharmacology, and it is crucial to know what preparations clients may be using in addition to (or instead of) those medically prescribed. Meanwhile, biomedical drugs tend to be tested on European American populations with too little known about racial and ethnic variability among pharmacokinetics (metabolism rates and actions of drugs) and pharmacodynamics (affects of drugs on the body). Of particular concern are time required for absorption, duration of action, distribution in the body, and method of excretion. For example, a granulocyte count is important before administering clozapine because about 20% of Jewish Americans of Ashkenazi descent develop agranulocytosis when the drug is used to treat schizophrenia (Andrews & Herberg, 1999). Many Asian Americans and Arab Americans require relatively low dosages of neuroleptics and psychotropics, and about 20% of African Americans metabolize diazapam poorly. African Americans are also generally at increased risk for extrapyramidal side effects from tricyclic antidepressants.

Pathologic Conditions in Psychiatric Mental Health Nursing

While psychopathologies such as schizophrenia, depression, somatoform disorders, and anxiety reactions occur in all cultures (Dana, 1998), there are both similarities and differences between *Diagnostic and Statistical manual of mental disorders* disorders and those problems described as "culture-bound." All require cultural formulations to understand, assess, and intervene because of marked variation in forms of expression in symptomatology with moral, religious, political, social, and ethnic differences. Problems-in-living exist in all cultural groups but differ in prevalence and response to intervention. There is no consensus on classifying such problems, but their labeling has become less of an issue with increased understanding of the importance of complementary and alternative fields of practice that are less concerned with diagnostic categorization than is conventional biomedical psychiatry. Many nurses are involved with modalities such as relaxation techniques, meditation, imagery, support groups, various psychotherapies, hypnosis, yoga, biofeedback, dance and movement therapies, music therapy, massage and bodywork, art therapy, spirituality-focused approaches, with other culture-specific interventions recommended for relief of problems (DiLima & Painter, 1998).

Neurological and Cognitive Issues

With the Western penchant for innovation, composites of Eastern and Western techniques are increasingly employed in management of neurological and psychiatric problems. Acupuncture is used for relief of a variety of health conditions and has few adverse side effects (DiLima & Painter, 1998). Energy-based therapeutic approaches (e.g., healing touch, therapeutic touch, polarity, reiki, jin shin jyutsu, reflexology, acupressure, and shiatsu massage) provide natural potential for nursing intervention in pain and other problems (Kelly & Ludwig, 1995).

New treatments for cognitive distortions (inaccurate, defective thinking, and irrational thoughts) emphasize examination and reframing interpretations of meanings of events (DiLima & Painter, 1998). Addressing relationships among thoughts, feeling, beliefs, behaviors, and physiology, cognitive therapies can reduce depression and anxiety and reduce health-risking behaviors and physical symptoms.

Priority Research Areas in Psychiatric Mental Health Nursing

With the globalization of biomedical paradigms, culture-oriented nursing research prioritizes both topics that are inadequately understood and methods that emphasize inductive and interpretive research involving clinical narratives and meanings (e.g., Kleinman & Seeman, 2000). A prime example is research to identify concernful practices grounded in lived experience for providing appropriate care (Diekelmann, 1994–1999; Kavanagh, Absalom, Beil, & Schliessmann, 1999). Other research emphasizes understanding and legitimizing of religion and spirituality and interrelationships between spirituality and healing (Brown, 1999; Shorto, 1999). Ethnographic studies of relationships between cultural contexts and emotional distress, with emphasis on dynamics that influence, make sense of, and heal distress and pain are increasingly available and useful (e.g., Desjarlais, 1992; Sobo, 1995). Research emphasizing mind-body interventions, complementary therapies, community mental health, and providing mental health services to multicultural populations fit well with nursing's holistic paradigm.

KATHRYN HOPKINS KAVANAGH

See also
STRESS

EMPATHY

The concept of empathy in nursing has received considerable attention as a central "helping" component in the nurse-patient relationship. Although there is some evidence that empathy was prevalent in nursing interactions as early as the late 1800s (Sutherland, 1993), it was not until Carl Rogers's 1957 address to the American Nurse's Association on the essential characteristics of a therapeutic relationship that nurses began to examine seriously the concept of empathy and its application to nursing practice. Early nursing authors called for increased awareness of empathy and its therapeutic value. Since that time there has been an uncritical and overwhelming acceptance of the importance of empathy in nursing. Nevertheless, after years of use and a growing body of literature related to empathy, conceptualization of the term remains incomplete, studies of nurses' empathetic ability appear contradictory, and evidence of the beneficial effects of empathy on health care outcomes is inconclusive (Bennett, 1995; Morse et al., 1992; Pike, 1990; Sutherland, 1993). Recently some authors have begun to question the usefulness and appropriateness of empathy in nursing practice (Morse et al., 1992; Pike, 1990).

Empathy has been described as a complex "bi-directional interpersonal" phenomenon, and as such it has eluded simple definition (Bennett, 1995, p. 37). A cursory review of the literature reveals a wide range of definitions, including descriptions of empathy as a trait, a state, an interpersonal process, a feeling, a sensitivity, an attitude, and an ability. In many cases authors struggle to offer clear definitions. There have been several attempts to clarify meaning and components of empathy and to determine areas of consensus. An analysis of the concept of empathy, based on a review of psychological and nursing literature, revealed four components of empathy: moral, emotive, cognitive, and behavioral (Morse et al., 1992). For example, emotional empathy is the arousal or responsive component resulting in empathic insight and followed by an emotional response. The empathetic responsc is felt by the caregiver on perception of the emotional distress within the other.

Although nurses have not focused on all components of empathy, Bennett (1995) indicates that there is consensus that empathy involves both cognition and affect in a multistage, cyclical process. However, models used in nursing to illustrate the process of empathetic communication have been simplistic. One exception to this is the model proposed by Morse, Bottorff, Anderson, O'Brien, and Solberg (1992). Attempts to differentiate empathy from related concepts, such as intuition and inference, is an important step toward conceptual clarity (Morse, Miles, Clark, & Doberneck, 1994). In summary, nurses' dependence on definitions from research on empathy in other fields such as counseling psychology has precluded description of how empathy may exist in nurse-patient interactions. A strong conceptualization would be particularly useful to nurses, but this remains a continuing challenge (Gagan, 1983; Morse et al., 1994).

Empathy has been a central concept in a large number of research investigations over the past two decades. Nurse researchers have attempted to measure levels of empathy, identify characteristics of empathetic nurses, describe factors that influence ability to empathize in nursing, describe functional levels of empathy as they are demonstrated in nursing, evaluate the effectiveness of educational programs on empathy, and document patient outcomes. Most studies focusing on empathy have been descriptive, using questionnaires or interviews. Evaluations of educational programs have been based on quasiexperimental designs.

Despite the amount of time and energy devoted to investigating empathy and its uses in nursing practice, our understanding of empathy has expanded very little. Several authors have concluded that knowledge development has been hampered by methodological problems, including the inadequacies of instruments used to measure empathy, use of small samples, cross-sectional designs, and inadequate analytical methods (Bennett, 1995; Morse et al., 1992). Progress also has been hampered by a lack of empathy research in nursing focused on the development or testing of theory about empathy and its uses in nursing as well as the lack of attention to other aspects of therapeutic rapport (genuineness, warmth, trust) so that the specific contribution of empathy is clearly delineated (Bennett, 1995). Others have noted the exclusive attention of researchers to measuring the observable, objective components of empathy (i.e., cognitive and behavioral) while ignoring the subjective, nonmeasurable components (i.e., moral and emotive) as an important obstacle to understanding empathy (Morse et al., 1992).

There are many questions that remain unanswered in relation to empathy. Readers may want to refer to the extensive list of key questions that Bennett (1995) has developed. Of fundamental importance will be delineation of how empathy is practiced in the various clinical settings, when and where empathy should be used, and the patient outcomes (positive and negative) that can result when nurses use empathy. If multidimensional conceptualizations of empathy are to be used as a basis for research, this will have direct implications for the selection of appropriate measures and designs to reflect this complexity. Finally, it is important that nurses remain open to the possibility that other concepts, yet to be identified and described, may represent significant components of the nurse-patient relationship better than concepts borrowed from other disciplines, such as empathy (Morse et al., 1994).

JOAN L. BOTTORFF

See also
NURSE-PATIENT INTERACTION
NURSE-PATIENT RELATIONSHIP

FAMILY CAREGIVING OF THE MENTALLY ILL

Family caregiving of the mentally ill is defined as the family of a mentally ill member providing guidance, assisting with educational and vocational goals, creating a sense of self and belonging, and providing basic physical and psychological needs for the mentally ill member (Kempe, 1994). Psychiatric care has increasingly become community focused since the 1960s, with families assuming more of the primary care role (Johnson, 1990). Recent policy changes in providing care to the mentally ill in public and private hospitals resulted in most clients being discharged to their families and receiving their care in the community (Tucker, Barker, & Gregoire, 1998).

As family caregivers assume more of the care for their deinstitutionalized mentally ill members there has been an increasing awareness of the many difficulties experienced by family caregivers (Maurin & Boyd, 1990). The contemporary deinstitutionalization policy attempts to unite the mentally ill with their families as a means of providing community care. This approach often places family caregivers into a role for which they are unprepared and from which they were often excluded in the past. In contrast to other types of chronic illness, the mental health professionals have been involved in a limited way with families of the mentally ill. The family caregiver has a need for increased assistance from the professional if successful integration of the ill member into the community is to occur.

Alliances

Professionals are beginning to recognize the need for building a strong alliance with the family caregiver of the mentally ill if quality care is to occur for the mentally ill member (Foreman & Marmar, 1985). Alliance building is defined as a close association that develops between the psychiatric nurse and the family caregiver to work together collaboratively based on mutual respect, trust, and commitment (Kempe, 1994). Building an alliance between the professional nurse and the family caregiver was found to be an important strategy in the provision of perceived satisfaction with the care provided for the mentally ill member by the family caregivers (Kempe). Family-focused care, defined as mental health care including the entire family, has long been requested by families and reported by the National Alliance for the Mentally Ill Organization, an advocacy group for families with a mentally ill member formed in 1979.

A chronic mental illness effects the family in many ways, including changes in roles, changes in the subsystems within the family, with a possible isolation of family members from each other as well as from outside influences. Families who seem to successfully handle a chronic illness of a family member without major disruption are characterized as having varied intrafamily interactions, utilizing a variety of social support networks within the community, encouraging autonomy among family members, utilizing a variety of problem solving skills, and adjusting with flexibility to family role changes (Lefley, 1996).

Burden

The difficulties experienced by families are commonly defined as caregiver burden or the negative impact of living with a mentally ill member. Research in the area of burden has become more complex as a wide range of variables have been studied (Maurin & Boyd, 1990). There is generally a consensus that the patient's level of functioning, symptom control, and related behaviors are key in the degree of burden experienced by family caregivers (Loukissa, 1995).

Early studies on family burden classified burden as objective (referring to practical problems such as financial and work issues) and subjective (refers to issues such as depression, loss, and embarrassment experienced by the family) (Hoenig & Hamilton, 1966). Recent studies have identified other variables that contribute to burden such as: the caregiver's perceptions of the situation, the type of coping strategies used by the caregiver to manage the situation, and the social supports available to the caregiver (Webb et al., 1998). Coping strategies are the usual ways that individuals handle stress (Lazarus & Folkman, 1984). Those caregivers who use problem solving techniques to cope with the behaviors of their mentally ill member experience less burden and better adjustment (Bentelspacher, Chitran, & Rahman, 1994).

Social support has been described as important to families and linked to better family adjustment to issues related to caring for the mentally ill member (Magliano et al., 1997). The social support described as most helpful is a large affirming social network of support that also participates in the care (Solomon & Driane, 1995).

The effects of feelings of burden on well-being have also been studied (Friedman & King, 1994). Friedman and King found that there was greater well-being with greater emotional support. The concepts of well-being and burden were further studied by Webb et al. (1998) who found that a greater burden was experienced by family members when there was a higher frequency of positive and negative symptom behavior. Well-being was found to be higher when there were more positive symptom behaviors and when problem-solving techniques were used with related social support.

A study done by Tucker et al. (1998) found that caregivers were more distressed by depressed behaviors than any other behaviors displayed by their ill members, including acute psychotic episodes. As needs of the mentally ill increased, so did the distress experienced by the caregiver. An earlier work (Jones, 1996) supported that the number of tasks required of the caregivers increased distress as well as the lack of independence of the patient and severity of the illness.

Coping Strategies

Coping strategies related to family caregiving are defined as those methods used by the family caregiver to manage events related to the care of the mentally ill member. Coping strategies selected by families were influenced by the amount of social and professional support they receive. Participation in support groups and psychoeducational groups was related to successful problem-oriented coping and feeling less burden. Emotional-focused coping is related to feeling high levels of family burden by family caregivers due to their lack of use of problem-solving skills (Solomon & Draine, 1995).

A variety of tools have been identified to measure the experience of caregiving. The Experience of Caregiving Inventory (ECI) is one of the more recent and is a self-report measure of the experience of caring for a relative with serious mental illness (Szmukler et al., 1996). The Camberwell Assessment of Need (Phelan et al., 1995) is used to establish perceptions of need in 22 areas from the mentally ill and asks how much help they receive from caregivers and other related services. Coping styles are measured frequently by the Way of Coping Questionnaire (Folkman & Lazarus, 1980). The Way of Coping Questionnaire is a 67-item checklist measuring the use of behavioral and cognitive strategies to manage stressful behaviors of the mentally ill. Items were classified into problem-focused coping (developing a plan aimed at altering the situation) and emotion-focused coping (changing one's response to a behavior).

Conclusion

Improving relationships of health professionals with family caregivers of the mentally ill is key to providing quality care to families with a mentally ill member. Professional attitudes and approaches are changing based on the success of research in the areas of burden, family coping strategies, the need for alliances between family caregivers, and the decreasing stigma toward the family due to a research-supported biological basis of major mental illnesses. The National Alliance for the Mentally Ill has also been instrumental in building a strong grass roots advocacy group for family caregivers of the mentally ill at the local community level.

In reviewing the research to date, it is suggested that further research needs to be done, and new measurement tools need be developed, especially in the area of ways to successfully assist families to provide the required caregiving for the mentally ill member. Several directions include looking further at coping strategies used by family caregivers measuring the techniques they actually use to cope with the ill member versus the coping strategies they think they may use in a particular situation. To date there are limited qualitative studies in caregiving. Therefore, both qualitative approaches may provide a new direction in further understanding such issues as: the effects of family interpretation of mental illness and their choice of coping strategies; coping strategies of different family members within the same family system; the effects of coping strategies of family caregivers; how professionals can best assist both family and ill members; and the social and clinical outcomes of the illness.

Research in the area of family burdens is also needed. The effects of a burden felt by different family members and the links of family burden, coping strategies, and psychiatric symptoms in the mentally ill member need further exploration. Measuring the levels of burdens felt by the primary providers of care and their related health compared to those involved in the family system but not providing the care also needs further study.

Identifying additional community resources that are especially helpful to family caregivers is key to providing quality care for the family who then can better assist the ill member. Currently there are efforts to reassure families that person with mental illness will be adequately served with managed care. Unfortunately, most managed care is focused on management of short-term illness rather than on chronic conditions. Also, managed care unfortunately tends to focus on cost-cutting more than fully meeting the needs of the chronically mentally ill person and family caregiver. The usual care offered is a brief hospitalization with psychotherapy follow-up rather than with long-term rehabilitation with medications being offered as the primary solution. It is predicted that the politically active organization, the National Alliance for the Mentally ill, will continue to be instrumental in moving legislation, research, managed care, and family-focused care forward to help families with a mentally ill member to get the needed health care. Psychiatric mental health nurses and related health professionals need to expand their political activities and partner with family caregivers and organizations such as the National Alliance for the Mentally Ill to improve care available to families and their mentally ill members.

ALICE R. KEMPE

See also
EMPATHY
STRESS

FORENSIC PSYCHIATRIC CARE AND JUVENILE JUSTICE

The problems surrounding the care and control of the socially undesirable—the criminal, the dangerous, and the mentally ill—have plagued society for a long time (Peternelj-Taylor, 1999). Challenges of contemporary clinical psychiatric practice in institutional or community corrections settings are emerging as the new and unique specialty of forensics. Forensic psychiatric care specific to the juvenile justice system refers to the application of principles and practices of the mental health care specialty to assist individuals involved in the criminal justice system (Kent-Wilkinson, 2000). McNamara (1987) further differentiates the meaning of forensics as "living forensics," that part of forensic sciences dealing with the application of science to the resolution of legal issues in cases involving living victims, as opposed to forensic pathology, which focuses upon deceased victims. Living forensics, applied to the juvenile justice sector, concerns itself with victims and perpetrators of physical and sexual abuse, neglect, drug and alcohol addiction, domestic violence, antisocial and violent behaviors, nonfatal assaults, accidents and injuries, suicide attempts, medical malpractice, police and corrections custody abuse, drug trafficking, weapons, and community violence. In general, it is the application of science to the resolution of legal issues involving youth (American Academy of Forensic Sciences, 1989).

Traditionally, forensic psychiatry focused on those individuals with highly dangerous behavior in need of maximum-security treatment environments. Offenders with mental disorders found by the courts as "not guilty by reason of insanity" are mandated to receive treatment. In this context, "not guilty" does not mean the person did not commit the criminal act for which he is charged. It means that when the person committed the crime, he could not tell right from wrong or could not control his behavior because of a mental illness. Such a person, the law holds, should not be held criminally responsible for his behavior, but be placed in an environment where the act will not be repeated.

This issue is only made more complicated when the individual is a child or adolescent. How does development of moral and ethical behavior in youth influence a determination of "not guilty"? A recent case of a 6-year old shooting a classmate with a gun he found highlights the difficulty (Sleven & Claiborne, 2000). When should children understand right from wrong? When do they understand the finality of death? Who should be held responsible—the child, or their parent or guardian? Examining youth violence on a broader level—where does societal responsibility lie? The struggle with such questions is demonstrated in the changing laws specific to "waivers," whereby youth, as young as 14 in some states, are housed with adult inmates.

In the United States, there are over 100,000 youth are placed in juvenile detention and correctional facilities each year (Office of Juvenile Justice and Delinquency Prevention, 2000). Of these, 50% to 80% are estimated to experience some level of mental health or substance abuse problems (Cocozza, 1991; Shelton, 1998). The focus of forensic psychiatric care of juvenile offenders is on caring for youth (up to 22 years of age) with severe challenging behaviors. Managing these behaviors can be difficult. Behaviors such as assault, weapon-making, and severe property damage are all too frequent within forensic settings. Providing effective interventions for such behaviors require good multidisciplinary team work that is consistent and well thought out. New efforts toward collaboration between justice and treatment professionals enable the main focus of care to be spent on proactive interventions rather than reactive strategies.

Forensic Psychiatric Treatment

Mental health care services implemented in the juvenile justice system can be provided in detention centers, residential treatment centers, special schools, or in the home. Clinicians are more frequently being called on to screen less violent offenders and divert them to community treatment. More traditional roles have been to assess risk and predict dangerousness and to treat individuals with antisocial and aggressive behaviors.

The focus of research related to the care and treatment of the mentally disordered juvenile offender is not much different than research completed on other institutionalized populations with mental disorders. Seclusion and restraint, detailed assessments, milieu therapy, and suicide prevention in justice settings are commonly studied (Birk, 1992; Byrt & Reece, 1997; Inch, Rowlands, & Soliman, 1995; McMurran, 1996). Use of medications in juvenile justice settings is less common, in part due to the limited number of physicians and nurses in these settings. The application of psychiatric interventions in these settings is changed, however, because of the security focus of these treatment environments. Touch, for example, is minimized, and self-disclosure by professionals of even seemingly insignificant information is discouraged.

Strong programmatic emphasis is placed on growth and development, development of self-esteem, anger management, and rational decision-making. Youth histories of abuse and neglect, chaotic family environments, and violence-condoning communities have led these youth to be alienated from normative childhood experiences that foster mental health. Children without safe and secure emotional and physical environments have low self-esteem. The damaged psyche manifests itself through depression, character disorders, and narcissistic rage (Allen, Arber, & Leadbeater, 1990).

A Focus on Rehabilitation and Recovery

Rehabilitation is an acceptable objective for both justice and treatment professionals. Inherent in the term "rehabilitation" is the idea of recovery and optimism for the future (Pratt, Gill, Barrett, & Roberts, 1999). Deegan (1988) believes that to achieve an effective recovery the individual has to develop a "new world view." Helping someone achieve this kind of fundamental change in self-concept is of great importance. From a justice perspective, the approach has been on the individual, traditionally focused on playing "catch-up" with regard to education and skills training. Outcomes of importance to juvenile justice systems examine rates of reoffending and recidivism. The clinical perspective is less linear and includes the family in the process of recovery. Outcomes are considered unique to the individual and include overcoming barriers and pursuit of goals.

Rehabilitation requires individual motivation to pursue some aspect of rehabilitation for success. Cohen and Mynks (1993) point out that rehabilitation must be done *with* a person, never *to* a person. This hallmark of working with the individual is a point of divergence for justice and treatment professionals. Youth coming to the juvenile justice system are most likely not ready for change. Most youth enter the juvenile justice system through police referral (85%), indicating that their readiness to change is low (OJJDP, 2000).

To examine this point, a reexamination of Health Belief Models (Prochaska, DiClemente, & Norcross, 1992) is useful. When treatment (or incarceration) is seen as a better option for the condition (behavior or situation), the individual is more likely ready for change. Youth rarely welcome entry to the juvenile justice system, putting themselves and any therapeutic effort at odds. Long periods of incarceration might wear the young offender down, but it does not necessarily indicate that changes are internalized. At best the juvenile justice system services target developing the youthful offender's readiness.

Cohen, Farkas, and Cohen (1992) suggest that five distinct factors are necessary for change—recognizing the need for change, commitment to change, environmental awareness, self-awareness, and closeness to the practitioner. Shortened lengths of stay in both the justice and mental health treatment sectors, the fragmented child care services, lack of coordination and ownership for youth, and lack of funding prioritization for effective rehabilitation programming indicate that the entire child care system is not "ready." Outcomes of punitive programming are poor long term when compared to treatment and rehabilitation programming. The only outcome acceptable for the youth is one that results in the maximum health and productivity possible in adulthood.

Conclusion

Forensics represents a new era of psychiatric practice that is evolving in direct response to the sequalae of criminal and interpersonal violence. Sharing and development of good practice is a major issue facing what might be termed a multisystem professional. Divergent viewpoints, ethical concerns, and power struggles hamper good intentions. The price of productive adulthood for the increasing number of incarcerated youth is just too high. Evidence-based practice is even more important to justify the services for these underserved (or misserved) youth. Justice and mental health have been challenged to develop a model of therapeutic custody.

DEBORAH SHELTON

See also
DRUG ABUSE
SUICIDE

GRANDMOTHER CAREGIVERS

In 1997, nearly 2.3 million grandmothers had a grandchild under 18 years of age living in their home (Bryson & Casper, 1998). Most provided care to their live-in grandchildren either as a primary, custodial caregiver or as a supplemental caregiver in a multigenerational home. The number of children in the United States under the age of 18 living in the home of a grandparent has increased from 2.3 million in 1980 (3.6% of all children) to 3.9 million in 1997 (5.5% of all children). Grandparent-maintained homes with grandchildren are more common among minorities. Nationally, the percentage of homes with a grandmother (with or without a spouse) and a grandchild are 47% White, 34% Black, 15.4% Hispanic, and 3.6% other racial-ethnic. For homes with a grandmother (with or without a spouse), a grandchild and one or more parents, 48% are White, 29% are Black, 16.8% Hispanic, and 5.3% other racial-ethnic (Bryson & Casper).

Data from studies of grandmothers having either primary/custodial or partial/supplemental care responsibilities to grandchildren show that these caregivers encounter some unique stresses that may be associated with greater psychological distress and worse health than other women (Kelley, 1993; Minkler, Fuller-Thompson, Miller, & Driver, 1997; Musil, 1998; Strawbridge, Wallhagen, Shema, & Kaplan, 1997). Nurses and other health professionals may encounter grandmothers involved with raising their grandchildren in a variety of settings, including community-based support groups, mental health programs serving women and children, school systems, and primary care settings, among others. Although the phenomenon of grandmother caregivers has received much media attention recently, how caregiving and related factors affect the mental and physical health of these women and their families is not yet well documented.

Most studies to date have focused on the .75 million grandmothers with primary/custodial responsibility for daily caregiving to a grandchild. Primary caregiver grandmothers frequently accept this role due to child neglect secondary to drug, alcohol, or psychological problems in the parents (Jendrek, 1994; Kelley,

1993). Primary caregivers, whether they have legal custody of grandchildren, fulfill a parenting role with their grandchildren, often while concurrently dealing with additional issues in the family system. Although the grandchild's parent is usually absent from the home, the parent may remain a part of the larger family constellation. In the role of a primary caregiver, grandmothers must modify their lives to accommodate their new responsibilities. Many subsequently feel isolated and restricted and also experience financial stresses (Kelley, 1993). Grandchildren with emotional or physical health problems compound the stress and needs for care in these families.

The 1.4 million grandmothers who provide partial/supplemental care to a grandchild living in their home with the child's parent(s) generally provide emotional, instrumental, and financial help to both generations. The well-being of these women has been studied to a lesser extent. Unlike primary caregiver grandmothers, the involvement of supplemental caregiver grandmothers may be of shorter duration. Because the role of grandmothers who maintain a multigenerational home with a grandchild and their parents is often not clearly delineated, some report ambivalence about their partial caregiving responsibilities (Jendrek, 1994). Little research has examined the degree of conflict in such homes. Musil found that the primary and supplemental caregivers did not differ from each other in the level of overall stress but did differ in the sources and types of stress experienced (Musil, 2000b).

Health Status of Grandmothers

A number of studies have concluded that primary caregiver grandmothers in particular may be at greater risk of experiencing depressive and somatic symptoms than noncaregivers or other types of caregivers, such as adult children or spousal caregivers of the elderly (Kelley, 1993; Minkler et al., 1997; Strawbridge et al., 1997). Using National Survey of Families and Household (NSFH) data, Minkler et al. found that grandparents who became their grandchild's primary caregiver for 6 months or longer had more depressive symptoms both before and after initiating caregiving than those who did not assume this role. Data from the Alameda County Study also indicated that full-time grandparent caregivers in 1994 reported less happiness, worse self-rated health, and somewhat more depressive symptoms in 1974 and 1994 compared with noncaregivers and more financial and marital problems than those who eventually became caregivers to their spouses or parents (Strawbridge et al., 1997). Szinovacz, DeViney, and Atkinson (1999), also using NSFH data, reported that grandchildren moving into the grandparents' home, with or without their parents, was associated with increased depressive symptoms in grandmothers. There has been little work examining the long-term effects of grandmother caregiving, although Musil

(2000a) reported a trend toward primary caregivers reporting more depressive symptoms over 10 months time.

Caregiver grandmothers may have more health risks if they are minorities, poor, or unmarried (Pearson, Hunter, Ensminger, & Kellam, 1990; Strawbridge et al.; Sands & Goldberg-Glen, 1998). National data show that while 57% of grandmother-grandchild families with no spouse and no parents in the home are poor, only 14% of those with a grandmother-grandfather-grandchild are (Bryson & Casper, 1999). Solomon and Marx (1999) found that the health of married grandmothers raising grandchildren was similar to older married women without dependents in that they had better health than older women living alone or grandmothers raising grandchildren alone. Further, the age of the grandchildren, the number of grandchildren cared for, and length of time caregiving may influence health outcomes, but there has been little research about these factors (Musil, 1998; Musil, in press).

Modifying Factors of Resources and Coping

The effects of modifying factors such as support and coping on the health of grandmothers or their families have been relatively unexplored, although the data from Musil's study with grandmother caregivers show that more subjective support and problem-solving coping were associated with fewer depressive symptoms and better self-assessed health (Musil, 2000). Adequacy of informal supports may be an issue for grandmother caregivers, especially if they have less time to engage in activities outside the home or to maintain social contacts. Burnette (1997) studied informal social supports of Latino grandmothers rearing grandchildren and found that 19% lacked a confidant and 14% had no help in caregiving. Formal support through community-based initiatives, such as grandparent support groups and respite care to grandparent caregivers, is available to many grandparent caregivers.

Although there have been recent advances in our understanding of caregiving by grandmothers to their grandchildren, the longitudinal effects on the grandmother, grandchildren, and family require further research. Studies about the effectiveness of interventions that support grandmothers and their families has been minimal to date but is essential for designing effective programs of care.

CAROL M. MUSIL

See also
FAMILY CAREGIVING
STRESS

GRIEF

Definitions

Grief is the characteristic pattern of psychological and physiological responses a person experiences after the loss of a significant person, object, belief, relationship, body part, or body function. Grief includes the entire range of physical, psychological, cognitive, and behavioral responses to a loss. It is characterized by intense mental anguish and varies in duration from a few weeks to many years. Two major types of normal grief have been identified: conventional grief, which occurs after a loss, and anticipatory grief, which occurs in anticipation of a loss. Anticipatory grief is the characteristic pattern of psychological and physiological responses a person makes to an impending loss. Although there is little agreement on the exact nature of anticipatory grief, there is general agreement that anticipatory grief facilitates coping with a loss when the loss actually occurs.

Three terms related to grief should be defined: *loss*, *bereavement*, and *mourning*. Loss is defined as the experience of parting with an object, person, belief, or relationship that is valued; the loss necessitates a reorganization of one or more aspects of the person's life. Losses range from minor ones, such as the loss of a wallet, which necessitates only minor adjustments, to major ones, such as the death of a loved one, which necessitates major adjustments. Bereavement is the state of having experienced a loss, particularly the death of a significant other. Bereavement is usually but not always accompanied by grief. Mourning encompasses the socially prescribed behaviors after the death of a significant other. Such behaviors vary from culturc to culture. Mourning behaviors are symbols or conventional outward signs of grief that are socially constructed and do not necessarily indicate the presence or absence of grief. Examples include wearing black clothing or a black veil or armband.

Throughout time nurses have had key roles in dealing with grief. Nurses in diverse settings are especially involved in dealing with anticipatory grief; however, little nursing research was conducted on grief until the late 1980s.

Researchers and Major Studies

Jeanne Quint Benoliel (1983) presented a review of nursing research on death, dying, and terminal illness at a time when few nurses were conducting research in those areas. Since then research on grief and bereavement has proliferated. Demi and Miles (1986) published a review of research on bereavement, and subsequently Opie (1992) published one on childhood and adolescent bereavement. Nursing interest in grief and bereavement flourished during the 1980s and

1990s and extended to grief and anticipatory grief related to hospice care. Martinson (1995) reviewed research on pediatric hospice care and addressed both anticipatory grief and grief following the death of a pediatric hospice patient; Corless (1994) in her critique of research on symptom control within hospice care reviewed research on coping with dying, strategies, and needs. All these reviews can be located in the specific *Annual Review of Nursing Research* volume, edited by J. J. Fitzpatrick et al. and published by Springer Publishing. A number of nurses developed research programs focused on grief, including J.Q. Benoliel, R. Constantino, A. Demi, M. Diamond, M. Miles, J. Saunders, and M. Vachon.

Researchers have used both quantitative and qualitative approaches to study grief. Standardized instruments such as the Texas Inventory of Grief, the Grief Experience Inventory, and the Bereavement Experience Questionnaire have been used to assess grief manifestations. The emotional distress that accompanies grief was often measured with instruments such as the Brief Symptom Inventory, the Profile of Mood States, the Impact of Events Questionnaire, or a depression scale such as the Beck's or Hamilton's. Children's and adolescents' grief was often measured by the Child Behavior Checklist.

Much nursing research on bereavement has been directed at describing the manifestations of grief among diverse samples: bereaved parents, children, siblings, and widows; suicide survivors; and people facing a life-threatening or terminal illness. Other researchers have described bereaved persons' responses to events such as the loss of a home by fire and a spontaneous or elective abortion. Still other researchers have focused on describing nurses' responses to caring for the dying or the bereaved. These descriptive studies have used diverse methods, including grounded theory, phenomenology, participant observation, semistructured interviews, survey questionnaires, structured instruments, and q-sort techniques. For example, Jacobs (1996) used grounded theory to describe the grief experience of older women whose husbands received hospice care during their final illness; Grossman, Clark, Gross, Halstead, and Pennington (1995) used interviews to describe children's bereavement process after paternal suicide; Feldstein and Gemma (1995) used the Grief Experience Inventory to describe oncology nurses' responses to caring for dying patients; McCowan and Davies (1995) used the Child Behavior Checklist to assess patterns of grief in young children following the death of a sibling; and Kerr (1994) used a qualitative approach to assess the meanings adult daughters attach to a parent's death.

Some nursing research on bereavement has focused on comparing different modes of bereavement (suicide vs. accident, expected vs. unexpected) or comparing bereaved persons with a nonbereaved group. For example, Kovarsky (1989) compared loneliness and grief manifestations of parents whose child died by suicide with those whose chid died accidentally.

A number of nursing studies have investigated variables related to bereavement outcomes. For example: self-blame was associated with poorer outcomes after the death of a loved one (Weinberg, 1995); coping process was related to social support and adaptational outcomes in widows (Robinson, 1995); and a significant relationship was found between effective grief resolution and hope, coping styles, and death within a hospice setting among the elderly widowed (Herth, 1990).

A few studies have used quasiexperimental designs to investigate the effects of specific interventions to help the bereaved or to help nurses to better meet the needs of the bereaved. For example, researchers have studied the effect of a support group on bereaved parents whose child died from cancer, the effect of a support group on bereaved children and adolescents, and the effect of a grief workshop for pediatric oncology nurses.

Strengths and Limitations of the Studies

The descriptive studies have contributed greatly to our understanding of the grief process and the many forms it may take. The comparative and correlational studies have provided insight into variables related to good and poor bereavement outcomes. However, very little research has been done to assess the effects of bereavement interventions. More attention needs to be paid to intervention studies that address what helps people deal with anticipatory grief and grief due to a loss that has already occurred. Further, most of the participants in the studies reviewed were White Americans. With increasing cultural diversity in the United States, it is important that research address bereavement responses among diverse cultural groups. In addition, researchers should work on developing culturally relevant instruments to assess bereavement outcomes.

Ethical Issues

Grieving people are vulnerable and need special attention to protect them from studies that could increase their vulnerability. Although many grieving people find that participating in research that focuses on their grief provides them an opportunity to express their thoughts and feelings to a nonjudgmental researcher, there is the potential of increasing the participant's pain and distress. The researcher must have the skills to provide immediate support if this occurs and also should be prepared to refer participants for counseling if they need further support at a later time.

ALICE S. DEMI

See also
SUICIDE
TERMINAL ILLNESS

INDIVIDUAL NURSING THERAPY

Nursing practice is becoming increasingly complex and diverse in the twenty-first century for the psychiatric mental health nurse. Increasingly mental health services are taking place in the community rather than in inpatient settings. This trend began with the community centers established in the 1960s and was reinforced as managed care began to exert a stronger influence on health care (Caplan & Caplan, 2000). As a result, contact time between nurses and clients has become limited. In discussing individual nursing therapy and nursing interventions on a one-to-one basis, one must move beyond the traditional parameters of individual therapy as first described by Peplau and consider brief psychotherapy and crisis intervention, case management, and even family interventions, as crucial aspects of the nurse-client relationships today.

Interpersonal Paradigm

The cornerstone of psychiatric mental health nursing today is the therapeutic relationship (Gelazis & Coombe-Moore, 1993). The therapeutic nurse-client relationship is defined as the interpersonal process between a professional nurse and the client (Peplau, 1952). The nurse needs to establish trust, strive toward mutually established goals of the relationship, and focus the movement of the interpersonal process toward growth for the client (Gelazis & Coombe-Moore). Peplau (1952) described the nurse as the basic tool or resource for the betterment of the client.

Peplau's theoretical framework has become the basis for psychiatric nursing. She highlighted the nurse-client relationship as the therapeutic nursing process (Peplau, 1952). Peplau pointed out that the "nurse-patient relationship is always unique as to process and outcome" (Peplau, 1991, p. 167), and "it is the primary context in which nurses assist patients in the work they need to do in order to regain health and well-being" (p. 167). She also viewed her interpersonal relationship theory as a "framework of concepts relevant to nursing practice" (p. 167). Her explications about concepts such as anxiety, anger, and others remain relevant and useful today (Reynolds, 1986). Peplau defined the phases of the nurse-patient relationship to provide nurses with a systematic way of approaching each patient's individual needs. Both nursing psychotherapy (Simpson, 1991) and psychiatric nursing interventions (O'Toole & Welt, 1980) were based on Peplau's theoretical works.

Researchers have studied various aspects of Peplau's theory, including the phases of the nurse-client relationship (Forchuk, 1991), the various roles of the nurse studied by Morrison (Peplau, 1992), and concepts and constructs identified as important to nurses by Peplau (O'Toole & Welt, 1980). Forchuk (1991) has studied Peplau's theory and has clarified many aspects of the theory, including the assumptions, basic definitions, and the relationships between the concepts. Future researchers need to continue the study of Peplau's interpersonal paradigm for it is a rich source of knowledge about the therapeutic nurse-patient relationship and the interpersonal process as it is used and is relevant today.

Other nurse theorists have based their own ideas and frameworks on Peplau's nurse-client relationship theory (Orlando, 1961; Travelbee, 1972). Still others, such as King, have developed different theories, but communication and interpersonal aspects remain central to the theory (King, 1992). Some authors have developed scales as ways of measuring aspects of the interpersonal process (Aiken & Aiken, 1973; Clay, 1984; Layton, 1979; Mathews, 1962; Methven, 1962). Individual one-to-one nurse-client relationships continue to be highly important in psychiatric mental health nursing. Much of nursing, both inpatient and outpatient, involves the nurse's ability to engage the client in interpersonal interactions. In recent years, however, as care is more profit-driven, the nurse-client relationship has undergone some changes. The fact that the client has much shorter contact with the nurse in inpatient settings due to short hospital stays means that the phases of the nurse-client relationship, which in the past had more time to develop, now must solidify within brief periods of time. Sometimes there are only a few days available and at times only a matter of hours for contact between nurse and patients (Vaugh, Webster, Orahood, & Young, 1995).

Brief Therapy

Forchuk studied the phases of the nurse-patient relationship and developed an instrument to help nurses identify the phase of their patient relationship over time (Forchuk & Brown, 1989). Further study should be undertaken to determine the effects of briefer nurse-patient interaction. To date, outcome studies have been done, but the nature of the brief interactions that now occur in the health-care system have not been extensively researched (Lazarus, 1995; Parson, 1998). Future nurse researchers need to demonstrate that the brief encounters nurses now have with clients can also be effective.

Brief therapies or short-term psychotherapies are time limited, have limited goals, and generally cost less than longer forms of therapy (Phillips, 1985). Psychiatric nurses and particularly psychiatric nurse clinical specialists are well suited and prepared to use a brief psychotherapy model because their education and clinical experience prepares them well to use this form of therapy (Shires & Tappan, 1992). Assessment can be made by using the mental status exam and clients with acute symptoms of anxiety, thought disorder, or severe depression can be given medication (Shires & Tappan, 1992). Brief therapy usually lasts from six to twelve sessions, but for clients with chronic problems the sessions may be spaced over a 3- to 6-month period (Wells & Gionnetti, 1990). Visits tend to be shorter and may be from 15 to 30 minutes (Budman & Gurman, 1988).

In brief therapy the therapist is usually quite active and can use techniques such as homework assignments to extend treatment (Shires & Tappan, 1992). Frequently therapeutic experiences occur in the community setting (Budmen & Gurman, 1988). Nurses are usually knowledgeable regarding community resources and may work for community based agencies.

Crisis Intervention

An even briefer form of therapy and a logical extension of brief psychotherapy is crisis intervention (Aquilera, 1998). Caplan (2000) notes that a crisis usually lasts from 4 to 6 weeks and is self-limiting. The goal of crisis intervention is the positive resolution of the immediate crisis; its focus is on the present and the restoration of the client's precrisis level of functioning; its duration is usually from one to six sessions (Aquilera, 1998). Since the basis of crisis theory is reaching out to people in crisis as soon as possible to prevent dysfunction, a logical arena for crisis intervention is the community (Leighton, 2000). The psychiatric mental health nurse and clinical specialist are frequently in positions to use crisis intervention techniques, particularly in community settings.

The psychiatric mental health nurse practicing in the community setting deals with chronically mentally ill clients both in long-term therapeutic relationships and in crisis situations. In this setting communication skills are even more important because trust needs to be established in a relatively short period of time. The nurse applying crisis intervention uses her assessment skills to the utmost and builds trust to have clients confide important information. For example, if the client is suicidal, trust is a highly important element to buy time for the client so that emergency services can be sent (Wheeler, 1993).

Another nurse using crisis intervention is the triage nurse in community mental health nursing who frequently deals with suicidal clients or clients who may be dangerous or threatening to others due to exacerbation of psychiatric symptoms (Wheeler, 1993). Not only must the nurse communicate therapeutically with clients, but also with distraught families. The principles of individual therapy as outlined by Peplau must therefore be expanded to include family members and clients, all of whom may be in crisis at the time of contact (Forchuk & Dorsay, 1995; Gilliss, 1991; Wright & Leahy, 1994). Some work has been done in this area, but nurse researchers need to systematically study how the interpersonal process can be expanded to include family and others and how this process is therapeutic.

Case Management

The psychiatric mental health nurse is part of the community mental health system and is able to help coordinate care of clients through the use of case management. Often the criticism of the care of the chronically mentally ill in the community is that care is fragmented and uncoordinated (Anthony et al., 2000). Research has shown that case management services may be available to clients in the community, but that clients rarely take advantage of such services due to lack of knowledge or other reasons (Parson, 1999). Some researchers pointed out that case management can be the key to adjusting to the community for the chronically mentally ill because it provides a link for the client to the support services she needs (Forchuk et al., 1989). Forchuk (1989) recommends that an essential component of a case management model is the establishment of a one-to-one relationship, which can be the basis for continued long-term care in the community. Thus Peplau's theory comes into play through its use in case management. The Peplau case management model provides a framework for delivering nursing care and comprehensive care for the chronically mentally ill client (Forchuk et al., 1987). Further research can document the effectiveness of nurses in case management.

Conclusion

In the demanding environment in which psychiatric mental health nursing takes place today, the nurse must use basic skills in new applications. The individual therapy that nurses use is based on Peplau's interpersonal framework. This theory is still relevant and can be used in various forms of individual therapy, which includes brief psychotherapy, crisis intervention, and case management. All of these frequently occur in community settings. Nurse researchers need to study the therapeutic process in various settings and time frames to establish the effectiveness of the nurse's interactions and interventions. The interpersonal framework and theory itself also would benefit from continued study and research.

RAUDA GELAZIS

See also
INTERPERSONAL RELATIONSHIP
PEPLAU

INTERPERSONAL COMMUNICATION

The focus of this entry is on interpersonal communication in psychiatric mental health nursing. The authors conducted a computerized literature search of the CINAHL database for the years from 1990 through 1999 using the suggested subject headings for interpersonal communication. The search was limited to research and articles written in English. The resultant abstracts were reviewed for studies that focused on nurses' interpersonal communication with patients diagnosed with any type of psychiatric disorder and with other patients dealing with mental health issues. Studies also were included if they involved interaction between ill persons particularly vulnerable to emotional distress and other caregivers, such as family members. Studies were excluded if they focused on nonverbal communication or teaching nurses, nursing students, or patients. A large number of studies were located on the topic of caring, which generally included interpersonal communication; however, these studies also were excluded because the concept was broadly defined and not focused specifically on interpersonal communication. This process produced a final sample of 18 studies.

Interpersonal communication, particularly in the area of psychiatric mental health nursing, is of major importance to nursing practice and research. It is through interpersonal communication that psychiatric nurses deliver psychotherapy, and it is the way that all nurses teach patients, explain treatments, and provide patients with emotional support.

Review of Major Studies

Three predominate clusters of work were identified that met inclusion criteria. A small group of studies focused on interpersonal communication with psychiatric patients, another cluster focused on communicating with patients with Alzheimer's disease, and another cluster revolved around communication with seriously ill patients with physical health problems.

Communication with Psychiatric Patients. Only two studies were conducted that focused on communication with psychiatric clients. Pollack (1996) conducted interviews and reviewed the medical records of 33 patients with manic-depressive disorder in an acute inpatient hospital. The data were used to guide a beginning descriptive theory of information-seeking states. Patients were categorized as information seekers, information receivers, and information rejecters. Although information states were not necessarily constant, this knowledge could be used to guide patient education. Fredriksson (1998) audiotaped interviews with psychiatric inpatients to elicit their perceptions of caring conversations when talking with nurses about suffering. The third study in this category was an analysis of interviews with mental health practitioners who were asked to talk about their experiences when meeting with people they felt were lying to them (Reed, 1996). The author concluded that lying and secrecy often occur as response to an experience of powerlessness by service-users.

Communicating with Patients with Dementia. Five studies reported on interpersonal communication between caregivers and people with Alzheimer's disease. Two studies assessed communication that occurred between nurses and individuals with Alzheimer's disease (England, O'Neill, & Simpson, 1996; Tappen, Williams-Burgess, Edelstein, Toughy, & Fishman, 1997). Two other studies examined interventions with Alzheimer's patients. Using a quasiexperimental design, Swedish researchers trained nursing home staff in integrity-promoting care (Kihlgren et al., 1993). They used videotapes of morning care to compare staff and patient behavior before and after the training and with a control ward. Following training, the most prominent differences were that staff gave patients increased opportunities to take part in decisions and activities, patients were more cooperative, and there was increased verbal contact by patients and staff. Another team of investigators audiotaped focus groups (23 family caregivers and 22 certified nursing assistants) to identify successful strategies used by caregivers in communicating with persons with Alzheimer's disease (Richter, Roberto, & Bottenberg, 1995). Two themes emerged from the focus groups: environmental adjustments and reassurance. The researchers suggested that interventions must be individualized and that enhancing skills to manage disruptive behavior may prolong the family members' ability to provide in-home care. The health of caregivers of people with Alzheimer's disease has been the focus of recent research across many disciplines. Gallagher-Thompson, Dal Canto, Darnley, Basilio, Whelan, and Jacobs (1997) studied the relationship between distress in wives who were the caregivers for husbands with Alzheimer's disease and their interaction style. Fifteen couples were videotaped interacting during mealtime and during a planning task. A significant correlation was found between level of conflict in the marriage and indicators of distress.

Communicating with Nonpsychiatric Patients Vulnerable to Emotional Distress. There was a group of studies that focused on communication with seriously ill patients and their families. Some of these studies described nurse-patient communication (Chen, 1990; Elliot & Wright, 1999; McClement & Degner, 1995; Rundell, 1991). Communication of nurses with family members with a relative in intensive care was described in other studies (Jamerson et al., 1996; Murphy, Forrester, Price, & Monaghan, 1992). There is no general agreement in the research about the assessment by nurses of their communication ability or ability to accurately assess patients' communication needs (Moore & Schwartz, 1993; Fitch, Remus, & Slade, 1998). Two studies related to family communication with cancer patients (Hilton, 1994; Hinton, 1998.) The findings of these studies indicate that families need assistance from nurses in openly communicating.

Methods

No programs of research were evident, and the majority of studies were descriptive. All studies were characterized by small, convenience samples that do not permit generalization to other groups. In a change from previous reviews, most researchers used tested instruments with good reliability and validity. This body of research could be strengthened if researchers would agree on priority areas of focus, if there could be widely agreed on constitutional and operational definitions of concepts, if more comparison studies were conducted, and if studies were replicated.

Researchers

European and Canadian nurse researchers are currently conducting many studies on interpersonal communication. These are mostly qualitative studies focusing on older adult care and reflect the philosophy of nursing and relatively newer research history in these countries. Nurses from the United States have focused their work on describing communication with patients with critical or terminal illnesses.

Conclusions

Similar to the conclusions following our report in 1990 (Garvin & Kennedy), we found the state of the science in interpersonal communication to be descriptive, fragmented, and primarily reflective of single studies by multiple researchers. Although studies could be clustered around a few topics, there was no evidence that any systematic programs of research were being developed. Interestingly, psychiatric nurses are not studying interpersonal communication with psychiatric patients. More research on communication is being conducted in medical-surgical areas and in nursing homes than in psychiatric settings.

Our review revealed, however, that psychiatric nurses are doing a commendable job of examining the effect of various psychiatric interventions that require the use of interpersonal communication on patient outcomes, such as, the effect of cognitive therapy on depressed persons and examining variables that influence informational needs of patients.

Future Directions

Despite years of application of research findings from other disciplines and nursing, there still exists a discrepancy between nurses' perceptions of what patients and families need and what patients and families report they need. This seems to suggest that the small convenience samples used in the past are perhaps too heterogeneous for accurate conclusions. Future research might better be focused on identifying specific variables, such as, psychological profiles, ethnicity, and phases of adaptation to different diseases, that influence the type and amount of communication that patients need.

Psychiatric nurses have been criticized for focusing too much attention on nonpsychiatric populations and not paying more attention to clients with mental illnesses. Given the paucity of studies on communication with psychiatric patients, it might seem reasonable to conclude that psychiatric nurses are still not focusing on the needs of clients in their discipline. However, if one conceptualizes the work that psychiatric nurses are doing in looking at the effectiveness of specific interventions on patients with psychiatric disorders, then it appears that the criticism may be misplaced. By necessity, these therapies are using interpersonal communication, but they are not being classified under this term. Focused reviews of specific therapies would be useful to convey progress in these areas.

Finally, in reviewing this literature, the authors noted an emerging trend. Several studies not included in this review revealed an increased use of technology to deliver nursing care. For example, computers are being used to conduct group therapy and support groups to provide education to patients. It is expected that this trend will become even more prevalent in the future. Studies are needed of factors that enhance the effectiveness of computer-mediated interpersonal communication. Psychiatric mental health nurses can play an important role in leading this research.

CAROL W. KENNEDY
BONNIE J. GARVIN

See also
NURSE-PATIENT COMMUNICATION
NURSE-PATIENT INTERACTION
NURSE-PATIENT RELATIONSHIP

MENTAL DISORDERS PREVENTION

The prevention of mental disorders is defined by the Institute of Medicine (IOM, 1994) as interventions that reduce the occurrences of mental disorders or delay their onset. The assumption underlying the science of prevention is that many mental disorders result from environmental stressors. Moreover, dysfunctional intra- and interpersonal patterns that evolve from social inequities also contribute to the development of mental disorders (Albee, 1996).

The goal of preventive intervention is to reduce malleable risk factors or enhance protective processes. Risk factors are those attributes or circumstances that contribute to an individual's vulnerability (Rutter, 1987). The likelihood of developing a mental disorder increases for adults with each additional risk factor that they possess or encounter. Among children, each additional risk exponentially raises their susceptibility to mental disorders (Reiss & Price, 1996). Protective processes, on the other hand, are the compensatory resources that moderate or even mollify the negative consequences of adversity (Rutter, 1987). Protective factors include individual attributes such as an easy temperament, high IQ, and environmental supports (Coie et al., 1993). Effective parenting or other caring adults are two environmental supports that increase the resiliency of children, thus, reduce the likelihood of developing mental disorders (McClowry, 1998). For adults, a supportive marital relationship can be protective (IOM, 1994).

Preventive science also includes epidemiological and other descriptive studies that identify how risk factors and protective processes are related to mental disorders. The results from such studies inform interventionists on program design and clinical applications. Preventive intervention can be integrated within a clinical practice. Or it can be a standardized protocol that is, or is not, tested empirically. In any case, a partnership with the community in which the intervention occurs is necessary to assess the cultural appropriateness of the program (McClowry & Galehouse, 2000).

Two major classification of preventive intervention exist. The first evolved from a public health perspective (IOM, 1994). Primary prevention is intended for individuals who do not have mental health problems, but who wish to gain greater competence. Secondary prevention is intended for individuals and families who are at risk for developing mental disorders because they live in communities with more than one environmental stressor. Appropriate participants in secondary preventive intervention include those individuals who are experiencing mild or moderate psychological symptoms, but who are not in crisis. Tertiary prevention is directed at those who are in crisis. The goal of such intervention is to prevent psychiatric hospitalization or incarceration. Once the crisis is past, such individuals and families should be directed to primary or secondary intervention programs to sustain or enhance their adaptational outcomes.

The more current classification put forth by the Institute of Mental Health (IOM, 1994) considers prevention appropriate only in the absence of a diagnosable mental disorder. Universal preventive interventions are directed at populations of individuals. Kellam and Rebok (1992) described a universal intervention that was offered in the Baltimore public schools to prevent academic failure.

Selective prevention is intended for individuals, families, and communities who are at risk for the development of mental disorders. McClowry and Galehouse (1998) explained how they developed INSIGHTS into children's temperament for innercity children and their caretakers. Williams et al. (1997) provided intervention for the siblings of chronically ill children.

Indicated interventions are for those high-risk individuals who have biological markers or who have experiencing early psychological symptoms of a mental disorder that has not reached a *Diagnostic and statistical manual of mental disorders-IV* diagnostic level. Schepp et al. (1999) reported on an indicated intervention for adolescents who are diagnosed with schizophrenia.

Preventive intervention can be directed at any mental disorder. The Institute of Mental Health (1994) focused on five: conduct disorder, depressive disorders, alcohol abuse and dependence, schizophrenia, and Alzheimer's disease. The same prevention principles can, however, be applied to other disorders such as anxiety, obsessive-compulsive, and posttraumatic stress reactions. Nurses in a variety of settings have engaged in clinical intervention programs that are preventive in nature such as suicide prevention, HIV education, pregnancy prevention, bereavement support, parenting programs aimed at reducing child neglect or abuse, domestic violence, and drug abuse. Other examples of prevention programs are those aimed at foster parents, children of divorced parents, support for chronically ill family members and their caretakers, and children of incarcerated parents.

Preventive intervention programs often lack standardization and, too seldom, are tested to see whether they are achieving their intended outcomes. Like all new sciences, the field needs to test the effectiveness of structured research protocols to increase its credibility and to enhance its knowledge base.

When planning prevention programs, interventionists need to understand the mechanisms that are related to the disorder that they are trying to prevent. They also need to be aware of the developmental implications. The timing of prevention programs is critical for maximizing effectiveness. The optimal time is before dysfunctional behaviors are established (Coie et al., 1993). Transitional times that occur during the life course are particular periods during which individuals and families are vulnerable. The birth of a child or the death of a family member are just two examples of such normative experiences that are transitional and, thus, appropriate for preventive intervention.

Future Directions

A current controversy within the prevention field is whether mental health promotion is part of prevention. Using the Institute of Mental Health (1994) definition, it is not. Albee (1996) argues that it should be because individuals and families that have enhanced their protective processes by participating in programs or services that enhance social competence or self-esteem are more stress resistant. A broader orientation such as the one offered by Albee (1996) is consistent with a nursing perspective that views mental health and disorder as a continuum rather than as distinct entities.

Prevention science is also consistent with a nursing perspective in another way. Nurses have a history of being engaged in such clinical interventions, often labeling them "anticipatory guidance" (McClowry & Galehouse, 2000).

Unfortunately, nurses engaged in such preventive services are experiencing the same challenges that face other disciplines in health care settings. The time restraints imposed by the current health care system compromise the amount of time many health care providers can spend with their clients. Since most types of preventive services, whether called anticipatory guidance or by other names, are not reimbursable from third-party payers, there is the danger that preventive intervention will be regarded as inconsequential compared to other health needs. As patient advocates, nurses will need to work diligently to make sure preventive services remain a priority.

The Institute of Mental Health (1994) report cited three major components that are critical for building an adequate infrastructure to support prevention intervention. A higher level of funding dedicated to preventive intervention and the related basic prevention science topics is necessary. In turn, the demonstration of the effectiveness of prevention programs will support that this type of research is valuable and worthy of further funding.

Coordination across federal, state, and private agencies will be difficult to achieve, but necessary to assure that duplication of services is avoided and that the highest quality of programs are offered. Dissemination of findings should be conducted so that constituents and the multiple funding agencies are kept informed of the developments of the field.

Highly qualified researchers and interventionists are also needed to advance the field. The limited number of nurse researchers conducting prevention intervention research is apparent. The way to prepare nurses to engage in such research and to be interventionists is the same as for other professions. Interdisciplinary courses and training provide the ideal model.

SANDRA GRAHAM MCCLOWRY

See also
MENTAL HEALTH IN PUBLIC SECTOR
MENTAL HEALTH POLICY
STRESS

MENTAL HEALTH IN PUBLIC SECTOR PRIMARY CARE

In the then Soviet community of Alma Alta in 1978, primary health care was delimited by the World Health Organization to meet the challenge of low life expectancy and high childhood mortality in many countries. Primary health care was determined to be low-cost, universally accessible, essential health care. This definition of primary care has been adopted throughout the international community, but in the United States primary care has become synonymous with service delivery because of the capitalist economic system that underlies health care. Unfortunately, community-based health status goals often are lost when emphasis is placed on service over care.

Primary care service delivery is housed in multiple organizational types that offer diverse services. Organizational structures mostly can be differentiated along the lines of the ability of the client to pay for services. Public sector clients, those who are publicly insured or uninsured, typically are cared for in tax revenue–supported agencies that must care for all who present themselves for health care. The effect of this dual primary care system is a real inequity in health care.

Disadvantaged persons clustered in low-income communities often have more immediate and pressing needs than obtaining formal health services. These include substandard housing, poor nutrition, environmental exposure, and crime. When they do use primary care services, public sector clients often find them to be inaccessible, not easy to use, and culturally insensitive. Many of these clients do not have a regular primary care physician, and they often delay seeking needed health care. Public sector clients are more likely to be hospitalized, for longer periods and for otherwise easily treated health care problems, than are privately insured individuals. The health of individuals within these relatively impoverished communities would be better served through public health modalities of intervention.

How primary care services evolved in this country is relevant to the provision of public sector mental health care. There is a growing movement in this country to reintegrate physical and mental health care within primary care. One factor motivating the move to integrated care is high prevalence rates of psychiatric disorders, estimated at 20% or more of primary care clients. Reintegration of physical and mental health care into primary care also is motivated by inadequate detection and treatment of psychiatric disorders by primary care physicians.

The service-based definition of primary care has led to two service-based models of psychiatric care. In for-profit settings serving the privately insured, the consultation-liaison model of psychiatric care has emerged: the primary care provider assumes responsibility for clients' mental health care. Staff psychiatrists and psychologists support primary care physicians in provision of mental health care. The specialty model of psychiatric care has been implemented in primary care clinics associated with tertiary care settings that serve many public sector clients. Specialty mental health providers assume responsibility for individual clients either collaboratively or as a referral from the primary care physician.

The efficacy of these models for mental health outcomes has been evaluated in randomized clinical trials. Results show that mental health services offered in primary care can be effective in detecting and treating depressive disorders under controlled conditions. Intervention seems less successful for persons with comorbid anxiety disorders or those who show symptoms of personality disorder. Findings demonstrated some support for integrating mental health with primary care.

Despite three generations of controlled studies of mental health care in primary care, including several randomized clinical trials, there are few findings that are applicable to public sector primary care. One reason is that there are few investigators examining mental health service delivery in primary care, and those tend to be clustered in a few sites. Because of this, most trials of mental health treatment have been limited to urban settings with samples containing mostly middle-class, middle-aged women. In many such studies treatment subjects fared no better in mental health outcomes than did controls. Attrition of subjects was high in many studies, especially among public sector clients. These findings have led some investigators to speculate about the cost-effectiveness of detection and intervention programs for psychiatric disorder in primary care.

With one notable exception there has been little evaluation of the efficacy of mental health interventions in the context of the organization in which they are provided (Katon & Gonzales, 1994). Research designs do not account for the pattern of heath services use by disadvantaged groups, nor do they acknowledge that patterns of mental health services use are different from those for more conventional primary care services. Because the constituencies of public sector clients and the mentally ill overlap, mental health services delivery in primary care must be designed to encourage the use of services by these related disenfranchised groups.

There is growing recognition that the public health definition of primary health care chosen at Alma Alta must be adopted here if there is to be a significant impact on the health of the most vulnerable Americans (Barnes et al., 1995; Fowler & Padgett, 1994). This is especially true for those with psychiatric disorders, who appropriately fear the consequences of being labeled mentally ill (Neighbors & Jackson, 1996). Stigma, coupled with cultural insensitivity, often combines with monetary and resource concerns to keep disadvantaged public sector patients from accessing care until well into an illness episode. Models of mental health identification and detection must move into the community, be combined with other kinds of health care services, and be based in homes and community facilities. In these settings disadvantaged persons can seek health care without fear of being labeled "crazy," attend to multiple health care needs within the confines of one visit, and not expend significant personal resources in obtaining care.

Herein lies the test for nursing research and practice. Nursing already has provided considerable leadership in implementing public health models of care, as both practice and research evaluation models (Olds & Kitzman, 1990). Many of these models targeted at-risk, pregnant, adolescent and young women and had improved child outcomes as the primary intervention target (Hauenstein, 1992).

There is little evidence that these intervention research and practice programs have integrated mental health care into their treatment paradigm. This is a crucial omission, often cited by the researchers as a reason for less than optimal outcomes in their studies.

Many university-based schools of nursing have begun to initiate academic-community partnerships that aim to increase clinical training sites, provide settings for community-based research, and improve the health care of selected disadvantaged populations, with care provided in community settings. These linkages form an ideal setting for testing integrated models of health care that simultaneously and systematically address physical and mental health concerns. It is crucial, however, that they be designed and evaluated so that mental health care is within the mainstream of the client's physical health care. In this type of intervention model, health status outcomes for well-child care include the reduction of depression and anxiety in the mother and enhanced parenting. Outcomes for young men with abdominal pain include reduction in alcohol and nicotine abuse.

Process outcomes evaluated in these public health models include the degree to which services are actually used by the community, what settings are most effective, and the extent to which services are provided in a holistic fashion. This latter point would include the degree to which psychiatric and physical health care are integrated within and across settings of care. Outcomes measured by research evaluation designs accompanying these intervention paradigms must include measures of both physical and mental health, cost-effectiveness of services, and determination of what interventions are most effective in achieving health status goals.

Primary care nursing interventions aimed at reducing documented psychiatric disorders in specific communities and integrating mental and physical health care will need significant research attention to document their utility. Because they represent a variation in health care, careful documentation of their impact on community health status goals must be evaluated. Moreover, because public health models of primary care generally, and mental health in primary care specifically, are new, they will have to be modified and reevaluated in a variety of primary care organizational types and community settings. Nursing research has much to contribute to this process of returning holistic, truly primary health care to the community.

EMILY J. HAUENSTEIN

See also
COMMUNITY MENTAL HEALTH
MENTAL HEALTH SERVICES RESEARCH

MENTAL HEALTH POLICY: RELEVANCE FOR PSYCHIATRIC NURSING RESEARCH

> When one is describing and analyzing mental health policy . . . The absence of knowledge rarely inhibits individuals from advancing allegations that have but little basis in fact. On the contrary, policy innovations based on theory and hope rather than fact are debated (although always with the rationalization that they are justified by empirical data). Under such circumstances, it is hardly surprising that the outcomes of innovation often have little to do with initial expectations. Nowhere is the accuracy of this generalization better illustrated than in the evolution of mental health policy. (Grob, 1992, p. 29)

Introduction

The Surgeon General's *Report on Mental Health,* released in December of 1999, provides a synthesis of the state of the art of research in the field. Although the report falls short of making evidence-based policy recommendations, it does provide guidelines to future research that could serve to inform mental health policy decisions. To become an integral part of the scientific community that can influence policy development, psychiatric nurse researchers must be aware of ways in which policy has influenced practice (and hence research) in the field, some current policy developments, and potential for designing programs of research that are policy relevant.

Policy Development and Influence

Public policy is formed in a social and political context and owes its shape to prevailing concepts of economics and cultural and political values that are influenced by special interest groups. Over the past five decades, mental health policy has been shaped by its close linkage with the public welfare system, the zealous advocacy of a variety of mental health commissions, both state and federal, as well as beliefs of professionals rooted more in philosophy and ideology than in empirical science (Grob, 1992; Mechanic, 1987). Ties to the public welfare system have made mental health policy vulnerable to the increasingly conservative attitude of the electorate toward entitlement programs and the "re-moralizing of poverty" (Grob, 1992; Mauch, 1998). The impact of this conservative attitude is visible in benefit restrictions, in the increasing numbers of persons with serious mental disabilities who are in jails and prisons (Petrila, 1998), in decreasing state funds for mental health in many states, and in resistance to parity legislation in the private sector. In fact, a primary significance of the *Report on Mental Health* is that it comes from the office of the Surgeon General, thus enfolding mental health in the general rubric of the public's health and into the shadow of primary care and health care policy. Adding to mental health policy woes is the imperative, created by the advent of managed care, to provide cost-effective treatment, as well as that created by increasingly organized and vocal consumer and family member groups to improve the quality of that care.

In a fascinating treatise, Hadley (1997) described the impact of funding on mental health policy from 1950 to 1990 and the four "semi-autonomous operating public mental health systems" that resulted, each of which "only add[ed] a new layer of administrative demand and new incentives to a system in which the incentives were already quite complicated" (p. 404). None of these new incentives encouraged either cost-effective services or evidence-based treatment. What did develop was a proliferation of regulations and administrative procedures, fragmentation of care, increased cost, and, in some states, an increase in numbers of services to fewer people (Hadley, 1997; Roth, Lauber, Crane-Ross, & Clark, 1997). The policies that created the complex, unwieldy multiplicity of systems described by Hadley were all based on "testable assumptions but they were mostly accepted on faith" (Mechanic, 1987, p. 81).

Current Developments

In the past decade, advances in science and technology and increasingly sophisticated methods of field research have enhanced an expanding body of knowledge in the field of mental health (Rose, 1996; Solomon, 1997). This knowledge has the potential to shape the development of mental health policies based on evidence of best practices. Such policies could promote the establishment of a continuum of appropriate and effective services relevant to the needs of the people served. Research studies that would aid in policy formation would demonstrate that of the multitude of services, settings, and providers that have proliferated since the 1950s, which have been shown to be efficacious as defined through empirical science and effective, as defined not only by researchers and clinicians but, more importantly, by consumers and family members? And, what new systems and innovative programs are needed to improve quality and promote recovery[1] as opposed to maintenance in the community and systems dependence (Clement, 1997)?

The Surgeon General's report points the way for clinicians and researchers to continue to develop empirical evidence that can influence the formation of policies that will promote standards and practices that are evidenced-based. To

[1]The concept of recovery as it is currently used in the mental health field applies primarily to adult consumers.

bring greater standardization to care and treatment, researchers must work together to link structure, process, and outcome, thus, reducing "overlapping activities [in some areas, leaving] gaps in others" (Bickman & Salzer, 1997, p. 288). "The knowledge base that presently exists is a shaky foundation on which to base an intervention-outcome research agenda" (Mohr & Fantuzzo, 1998, p. 9).

The charge to link structure, process and outcome presents a challenge to psychiatric nursing researchers. In their review of psychiatric nursing outcome research, Merwin and Mauck (1995) used Donabedian's paradigm for quality of care, (linking of structure, process, and outcome) and classified 77 (of 1247) articles as outcome studies or studies that could influence the development of an outcome. Only two of the 77 studies included all three of the clinical domains as defined by Donabedian. The first of these, a study by Killeen (1993) examined parental self-image in disadvantaged families (structure), the processes by which that influence is exerted and the relationship of children's evaluations of themselves in areas important to their families to measures of their own self-esteem (outcomes). The second study, connected setting (structure), program provided to treat anxiety disorders (process) and treatment outcomes (Waddell & Demi, 1993).[2] Additionally, Merwin and Mauck point out that few of the studies were replications, and most did not build on prior research or utilized similar conceptual models, methods, or measurement tools. With some notable exceptions, Morrison, 1992; Farrell, Koch, & Blank, 1999; Murphy & Moller, 1993, to name a few, this finding seems characteristic of research in mental health in general, particularly that conducted in disciplinary isolation (Bickman & Salzer, 1997).

One example of research focused on influencing mental health policy is that being conducted at the University of Virginia School of Nursing in the Rural Mental Health Project. For example, the studies by Farrell et al. (1999) looked at factors that predict whether mental health consumers released from state hospitals experience continuity of care, and the processes that promote such. Further, they demonstrate the critical role played by psychiatric nursing as bridges from hospital to community settings

Future Potential

The future potential for psychiatric nursing research to influence the development of mental health policy requires that researchers link structure, process, and

[2]As an interesting aside, none of the studies analyzed by Merwin & Mauck are found in the references in the Surgeon General's report. However the first author of one study, Hamera (1993) is the first author of a 1992 article entitled *Symptom monitoring in schizophrenia: Potential for enhancing self-care* that does serve as one of two nursing articles appearing in that report in Chapter 4 and four nursing articles in Chapter 5. (Although not done as a nursing study, the principal investigator for the well known Vermont longitudinal studies also cited in Chapter 5 is Courtney Harding whose basic preparation is in nursing.)

outcomes. To do so in light of the complex nature of these research problems, both inter- and intradisciplinary programs of research need to be developed that include persons that receive services as well as those that provide services in all phases of the process. For this to occur, meaningful discourse must be established between researchers, clinicians, and persons and families who are the recipients of programs and services. Discourse between the three groups can "redress the balance of power between users [of services] and professionals" (Tilley, Pollock, & Tait, 1999, p. 56) to allow the "little stories" of consumers and clinicians to "influence the 'Big Story' of policy" (p. 53). Without active discourse, outcome studies will continue to find that effective outcomes are related more to consumer perceptions than to mix of services, provider or personal and system characteristics, and that consumer and provider perceptions differ (ODMH, 1999).

The ability of psychiatric nursing researchers to impact policy development can be enhanced by partnering with our colleagues in community health, epidemeology, and evaluation research, particularly in analysis and application of large data sets. Collaborative, interdisciplinary, multisite research projects increasing the development of studies that build on work already done are needed (Merwin & Mauck, 1995). The Director of the Department Mental Health in Ohio (Hogan, 2000) recently explained the lack of interest in mental health on the part of legislators "We are neither a priority or a problem" (Hogan, 2000). Psychiatric nurse researchers, joining with consumers, families, clinicians, and other researchers can help to demonstrate that mental health is integral to total health for all people.

JEANNE A. CLEMENT

See also

MENTAL HEALTH IN PUBLIC SECTOR
MENTAL HEALTH SERVICES RESEARCH

MENTAL HEALTH SERVICES RESEARCH

Mental health services research (MHSR) is a relatively new body of research that focuses on issues of access to care, quality of care, outcomes of care, and cost of care. This field of research has gained recognition and increased federal grant funding in the past 10 years, sparked by the nation's interest in accountability and cost-effectiveness of health care. Mental health services research is a specialty area of health services' research and gains methodological strength from the growing knowledge base created by general health services research.

Mental health services research, as interdisciplinary research, benefits from the integration of disciplinary knowledge from clinical, administrative, and social sciences disciplines. Researchers from the clinical fields of psychiatric nursing, psychiatry, psychology, and social work and counselors and primary care providers often join with scientists from the fields of sociology, economics, statistics, business/health administration, and public health to combine clinical knowledge and methodological expertise in order to design the complex studies necessary to measure access, quality, and cost of care. Collectively, the results of MHSR are used to influence and improve the mental health delivery system.

The National Institute of Mental Health (NIMH; 1991) recognized the need to prepare more researchers as mental health service researchers and suggested that researchers need solid research training in their primary discipline (usually obtained through doctoral education) and proposed MHSR training through a postdoctoral fellowship program. Psychiatric nursing's contribution to outcome research provided a building block for the profession's contribution to interdisciplinary MHSR. Merwin and Mauck (1995) determined that most psychiatric nursing outcome research focused on clinical outcomes, but studies also addressed provider outcomes and rehabilitation public welfare and humanitarian outcomes based on NIMH's classification of mental health outcomes.

Increased numbers of doctorally prepared nurse researchers with postdoctoral training in MHSR are needed in order to include a nursing perspective within the rapidly developing interdisciplinary MHSR arena. Only one of the NIMH-funded MHSR centers is housed in a school of nursing (University of Virginia) and directed by a nurse. Examples of MHSR conducted by nurses includes the work of Hauenstein (1996b) on in-home intervention with depressed women, Merwin (1995) and Merwin, Goldsmith, and Manderscheid (1995) on rural mental health human resources, and Fox, Merwin, and Blank (1995) on rural mental health services.

JEANNE C. FOX

See also

CHRONIC MENTAL ILLNESS
COMMUNITY MENTAL HEALTH
MENTAL HEALTH IN PUBLIC SECTOR PRIMARY CARE
SCHIZOPHRENIA NURSING RESEARCH

MINORITY ISSUES IN MENTAL HEALTH

A focus on the mental health needs and clinical presentation of psychiatric disorders in persons from ethnic minorities is fairly recent. Historically, discussions paralleled the civil rights movement of the 1960s, continuing into the 1970s and 1980s. Not only were service needs a part of the discussion, but also the need to develop culturally competent professionals including mental health care providers from minority groups. Concurrently, federal regulations began to require inclusion of ethnic minority persons and women in funded research programs. However, this did not result in broad changes in the mental health system to provide culturally appropriate services to ethnic minority group members. In addition, knowledge based on systematic research continued to lag for several reasons. Often ethnic minority groups were not represented or underrepresented in samples. In some samples, there was proportional representation of a specific minority group, but there were often inadequate numbers to really examine inter- and intragroup similarities and differences. In addition, many scientists interpreted findings based on a comparative model that defined the dominant group as 'normal' and the minority group as 'deviant.'

In the Surgeon General's report on mental health (US Department of Health and Human Services [USDHHS], 1999), the point is made that persons from racial and ethnic minority groups continue to be underserved (Center for Mental Health Services [CMHS], 1998) by a mental health system that is ill prepared to meet their needs. Further, there is empirical evidence that minority group persons continue to face multiple barriers in the mental health system that prevent them from seeking and participating in treatment. This occurs despite the fact that research as well as anecdotal clinical observations support the need for linguistically and culturally competent care (USDHHS, 1999).

In the last decade, there has been an increase in data-based publications addressing health issues for ethnic minority groups both in nursing and other disciplines. This has included research related to mental health and psychiatric disorders. Much of the work has focused on epidemiological surveys and service utilization. In addition, psychometric studies have been carried out to further evaluate the use of instruments that measure psychiatric phenomena such as depression and depressive symptomatology. More recently, with the advent of genome research and clinical trials on the newer psychoactive agents, there is a new impetus to explore similarities and differences in ethnic groups. Even with the current research, scientists and clinicians lag behind in addressing the mental health and psychiatric care needs of ethnic minority persons. Further, as often occurs, advances in scientific knowledge do not necessarily result in desired changes in clinical practice and service delivery systems.

If one examines the nursing literature on minority mental health, one discovers there is much work still to be done. It appears that there are an increasing number of doctoral dissertations that focus on minority mental health. However, dissertations by doctoral nursing students that address minority mental health issues are not readily available to students, clinicians, and policy makers. A greater proportion of the literature is descriptive, anecdotal information that includes literature reviews of extant literature. For example, de Leon Siantz (1994) addresses Mexican American migrant families, Tabora and Flaskerud (1994) describe depression in Chinese Americans, and Warren (1994) discusses depression in African American women. The nursing literature also includes literature that addresses models for cultural competence (Campinha-Bacoate, 1994a) and an application of cultural assessment (Giger & Davidhizar, 1995) in Mexican Americans (Becthel, Davidhazer, & Tiller, 1994). One can also find nurse authors addressing minority mental health needs in the gerontological literature, again often anecdotal and reviews of multidisciplinary sources. Examples include Louie's discussion of mental health needs of Asian elderly (1999) and Torres (1999) description of barriers to mental health services for Hispanic elders. The research literature that is cited most often comes from other disciplines or multidisciplinary teams that include a nurse researcher (Baker, Espino, Robinson, & Stewart, 1993), and there is an expanding body of empirical work in the gerontological literature. Therefore, to address minority mental health issues, literature addressed in the remainder of this section will include not only sources from nursing authors but other disciplines as well. This is necessary to address particular mental health issues for ethnic minority groups. Specific information regarding each of the four recognized ethnic minority groups in the United States are overviewed. This is followed by a description of barriers to mental health services experienced by minorities. A brief discussion of the emerging area of ethnopsychopharmacology is presented, followed by conclusions.

Ethnic Minority Groups

The federal government recognizes four ethnic minority groups: African American (Black), Asian/Pacific Islander, Hispanic American (Latino), and Native American/American Indian/Alaska Native/Hawaiian Native (CMHS, 1998). It is important to remember that the governmental definition of ethnic groups does not include all ethnic or racial minority groups. Further, such classification clearly does not represent in any way the diversity within groups. Therefore, any description of and research findings reported for any one of the four identified groups should be viewed with caution. To assume that all members of a group "fit" general descriptions and aggregate group data can result in the same type of erroneous stereotyping that often occurs when a minority group is compared to the dominant cultural group. Much of the research needed to address intragroup differences has not yet been done. Thus, what follows is generalized information about a particular ethnic minority group and related mental health issues. Not all subgroups are represented individually, so one must expect that with a particular subpopulation of clients there may be differences as well as some similarities.

African Americans

African Americans currently comprise the largest ethnic minority group at 12.5% of the US population (US Department of Commerce, Census Bureau [USDC-CB], 1999). According to the Surgeon General's report on mental health (1999), African Americans (AA) continue to have higher prevalence rates for mental disorders than Whites. Of particular note is a 105% increase in suicide among AA males age 15 to 19 from 1908 to 1996 (Centers for Disease Control [CDC], 1998). Reiger et al. (1993) suggested that African Americans are more at risk due to lower socioeconomic status. However, there continues to be evidence of misdiagnosis that may reflect misinterpretation of symptoms (Mohr, 1998). African Americans are more likely to be diagnosed with schizophrenia than affective disorders (Jeste, 1996; Lawson, 1996a) or generalized anxiety disorders (Turner & Cooley-Quille, 1996).

The clinical presentation of depression in African Americans differs from that of their White counterparts. One is more likely to observe somatic complaints (Turner & Cooley-Quille, 1996) and paranoid symptoms (Lawson, 1996b) in depressed AA clients. Lawson (1996a) reports that irritability may be the presenting symptom for mania in this group. Some AA clients with obsessive-compulsive disorder (Lawson, 1996b) or posttraumatic stress disorder (Lawson, 1996a) may be diagnosed with psychosis. Campinha-Bacoate (1994b) proposes that some African Americans and Black Caribbean clients may be suffering from culture-bound illnesses (Leff, 1981) such as voodoo illness. As a result of misdiagnosis, socioeconomic status, type or lack of health insurance, and barriers such as mistrust of the health care system, African Americans are overrepresented in acute psychiatric settings and underrepresented in outpatients settings (Snowden & Cheung, 1990). The disparity in representation is even more marked in private settings, although Snowden (1998, cited in USDHHS, 1999) proposes that economics alone cannot explain this difference in service use. Snowden notes that underrepresentation in outpatient settings frequently occurs in working, middle class, privately insured African Americans. The narrowest gap in the disparity in service utilization is seen in community-based, publicly financed mental health programs (Snowden, 1998 cited in USDHHS, 1999) and among older adults (Padgett, Patrick, Burns, & Schlesinger, 1995).

Of even greater concern is data that suggest that African Americans are more likely to be committed involuntarily (Jeste, 1996; Lawson, 1996b); placed in seclusion (Lawson, 1996b); ordered higher doses of medication and given depot medications (Jeste, 1996); and to use emergency rooms for mental health care (USDHHS, 1999). Once in treatment, African Americans tend to leave treatment sooner and be less likely to adhere to treatment regimes than other groups (Lawson, 1998b).

Asian Americans/Pacific Islanders

Asian Americans/Pacific Islanders represent a diverse group of persons culturally that are the fastest growing minority group in the United States (Herrick & Brown, 1999). At present they comprise only 4% of the population (US Census Bureau, 1999). As a whole, this ethnic population is less likely than any other group to use mental health services (Leong & Lau, 1998, cited in USDHHS, 1999). A pattern of underutilization appears to be even greater in newer immigrants (Sue, Zane, & Young, 1994). Although the need for mental health services in the Asian community is recognized, there is a lack of systematic knowledge regarding mental health patterns in Asian American/Pacific Islanders, particularly in ethnic subgroups. Despite the paucity of data, it is thought that several factors affect acknowledgement of the need for mental health services and help-seeking in this population. It is known that persons from Asian cultural traditions may be more likely to present with somatic symptoms for psychiatric disorders such as depression (Herrick & Brown, 1999). Thus, Asians/Pacific Islanders may be more likely to present in primary health setting when experiencing a mental health problem. Thus, a depressed Asian person may present with headaches and stomachaches rather than with depressed affect (Kim, 1995; Stewart, 1995). Also, Asian American clients may present with a culture-bound illness that may be psychiatric in nature. For example, Hwa-Byung (anger disease) is an illness that may present in Korean Americans (Kim, 1995), and may meet criteria for major depression (Lin et al., 1997).

Service utilization may also be explained by cultural definitions of illness that include explanation for etiology. Mental illness may be explained as a person having a lack of harmony and balance (Sue & Sue, 1990). So mental health is the result of avoiding bad thoughts (Stewart, 1995). In addition, sharing one's emotions may be seen as unacceptable (Kuo & Kavanagh, 1994), resulting in a "loss of face" and concomitant stigmatization. Kim (1995) notes that Asians more often will seek support from their families and traditional healers. If one does enter treatment, Asian clients are more likely to drop out because of the lack of culturally sensitive care, including language differences, and conflict about treatment regimes (Cheung & Snowden, 1990; Jung, 1998; Stewart, 1995).

Hispanic Americans

Hispanic Americans make up 11.4% of the US population, and are expected to be the predominant minority group by 2050, representing 24.5% of the population (US Census Bureau, 1999). Data suggest that there are minimal differences in lifetime rates of mental illness between Hispanic Americans and Whites (Vega & Kolody, 1998 cited in USDHHS, 1999). However, there is a paucity of research on mental health issues in adequate samples of Hispanic subgroups. Methodologically sound studies of prevalence, service use, and treatment are sorely needed. Extant work has identified multiple cultural barriers to mental health services for subgroups that have been identified (Ruiz, 1995). The situation is further complicated by discrimination by providers (Arroyo, 1996; Ruiz, 1997), and a lack of Hispanic care providers (Garza-Trevino, Ruiz, & Venegas-Samuels, 1997).

Much literature continues to be clinical in nature, such as Bechtel and colleagues' (1998) discussion of patterns of mental care among Mexican Americans. Epidemiological work by Vega and Kolody (1998 cited in USDHHS, 1999) indicates lower rates of mental disorders in immigrants compared to native-born Mexican Americans. Underutilization of mental health services has been reported in female Puerto Rican and Mexican Americans, while women with depressive symptoms are overrepresented in medical surgical settings (Duran, 1995; Jimenez, Alegria, Pena, & Vera, 1997). In addition, the difference in depressive symptomatology between Hispanic females (46%) and males (20%), which may be different in subgroups and affected by factors other than gender, needs further examination. Greater knowledge of diagnosis of symptoms of mental disorders within a cultural context and use of traditional practitioners and medicines is needed to provide culturally competent services specific to Hispanic subgroups' values, beliefs, health seeking, and language.

Native Americans/American Indian/Alaska Native/Native Hawaiian

The Native American group is only documented to be 0.9% of the population (US Census Bureau, 1999). Little data are available on the incidence and prevalence of mental disorders in Native Americans (USDHHS, 1999). Alarmingly high rates of suicide have been reported (Indian Health Service, 1997; Wallace, Calhoun, Powell, O'Neil, & James, 1996). Depression is described as a significant problem in native populations (Kinzie et al., 1992; Nelson, McCoy, Stetter, & Vanderwagen, 1992). It is believed that substance abuse and dependence, including alcohol addiction, occurs at twice the rate of any other group in the United States (USDHHS, 1998). Manson (1998 cited in USDHHS, 1999) reports that posttraumatic stress in Native American veterans is more prevalent than in Whites. Like African Americans, Native Americans are overrepresented in nonprofit, acute psychiatric settings (Snowden & Cheung, 1990). Now that more tribal councils have taken over supervision and management of health services, research is need to explore mental health and disorders, treatment, and outcomes in a culturally specific system of care.

Barriers to Care

Several financial, organizational, and diagnostic factors are thought to be relevant to patterns of mental health service utilization by ethnic minority persons in

(USDHHS, 1999). Specifically, the system still does not provide services that are perceived to be culturally sensitive and competent. Exactly to what degree certain factors may contribute to utilization, including the accuracy of ethnic minority clients' perceptions of the system, remains unclear. Five specific barriers are discussed in the Surgeon General's report on mental illness. It should be noted that the following barriers probably do not function independently but interact with one another simultaneously.

The first barrier to care is the particular health-seeking behavior of an ethnic group. Several authors report that minorities are less likely to use outpatient mental health services (Gallo, Marino, Ford, & Anthony, 1995; Zhang, Snowden, & Sue, 1998). It is suggested that the lack of availability of providers with specific language skills may contribute to lack of help-seeking by some minority persons (Taylor, 1989). In addition, some ethnic minority persons may be more comfortable seeking help from traditional healers and care providers.

Another barrier to care is mistrust of the health care system and governmental programs. For example, African Americans have a long history of experiences with racism, segregation, and discrimination in this country (Priest, 1991). This includes dealing with a mental health system that has reflected institutional racism resulting in some instances in misdiagnosis and subsequent inappropriate treatment. Other ethnic minority persons, such as Latino immigrants, may mistrust any governmentally run program because of past experiences with their native governments (Garcia & Rodriguez, 1989) or fear of scrutiny by immigration officials.

A third barrier is the stigma that many Americans feel regarding mental illness (USDHHS, 1999). For many African Americans, stigma and embarrassment occur because the cultural expectation is that they be self-reliant and resolve through personal determination (Snowden, 1998 cited in DHHS, 1999). Asian Americans may need to save face and prevent family embarrassment.

Costs of services can be a major barrier for some ethnic minority persons. Availability of insurance may play a role in financial barriers to service, though the exact role is not clear (USDHHS, 1999). Minority group members are less likely to have private insurance, but even those who do are underrepresented in certain types of mental health treatment (Snowden, 1998 cited in DHHS, 1999). However, patterns of mental health service use by minority groups are not explained by cost alone (USDHHS, 1999).

Finally, clinician bias is a very real barrier to the mental health care of ethnic minorities. Patterns of overdiagnosis and misdiagnosis of psychiatric disorders (e.g., schizophrenia) in African Americans continue to be reported (USDHHS, 1999). Underdiagnosis (e.g., no problem) appears to be operant when evaluating the clinical presentation of Asian Americans (Takeucchi & Uehara, 1996). In mental health care, the diagnosis of psychiatric disorders is based on evaluation of clinical behavior, including thought patterns expressed through linguistic patterns.

Behavioral and linguistic pattern norms are expressions of one's cultural experience and context. Thus, a clinician's ethnocentric orientation and experience, no matter how good one's intentions, can obscure one's ability to observe and interpret the behavior and language of someone who is different culturally. This results in inaccurate diagnosis and subsequently the development of inappropriate treatment plans. In addition, there is a lack of data on clinicians' use of the Culturally Bound Syndromes identified in the *Diagnostic and statistical manual of mental disorders-IV* manual (American Psychiatric Association, 1994) and related treatment regimes.

Ethnopsychopharmacology

Ethnopsychopharmacology is a relatively new area of research and clinical interest. It includes a focus on genetic, cultural, and psychosocial factors that affect the pharmacokinetics, pharmacogenetics, and pharmacodynamics of psychoactive medications (USDHHS, 1999; Mohr, 1998). It is important to note that many health professionals, including psychiatric mental health nurses and nurse researchers, have not been exposed to this new area of inquiry. Further, empirical evidence remains scant because of the lack of inclusion of ethnic minority subject in clinical trials (Mohr, 1998). Even if ethnic minority subjects are included in studies, the number of persons from ethnic subgroups is often too small to evaluate similarities and differences in pharmacological responses and compliance behaviors.

There is, however, growing evidence that there are ethnic variations in enzymatic activity that can affect the absorption and metabolism of psychoactive drugs. It is suggested, for example, that 33% of African Americans and 37% of Asians are "slow metabolizers" of certain types of antipsychotics and antidepressants (USDHHS, 1999; Lin et al., 1997). On the other hand, some ethnic subgroups may have patterns of "extensive," or fast, metabolism (Mohr, 1980). For example, a small percentage (5%) of persons of Spanish heritage seem to be "extensive," or fast, metabolizers resulting in low drug plasma levels at what is considered a therapeutic dose (Lin et al., 1997; Mohr, 1998).

Other dimensions of ethnopsychopharmacology is the exploration of cultural, psychosocial, and environmental factors that may affect the use of and response to psychoactive medications in ethnic groups. This includes examination of misdiagnosis and misinterpretations of symptoms by mental health professionals (Mohr, 1998), particularly, but not exclusively, by professionals who are not from the ethnic minority group of the client they are treating. Additional factors can include communication difficulties, including language barriers, and mistrust of the health care systems and the providers who represent it. Further, folk beliefs and use of traditional healers and medications may have indirect or direct effects on responses of ethnic minority clients to treatment with psychoactive agents.

The advent of genetic and biochemical studies of psychiatric disorders may have been an impetus to examine ethnic variations in responses to psychoactive drugs. The genetic and biological differences seem to follow a pattern in persons who are ancestrally and culturally connected (Mohr, 1998). Knowledge about cultural and psychosocial factors remains speculative, largely based on clinical observation and descriptive data. The challenge is to develop meaningful research studies that adequately sample ethnic minorities. This requires not just aggregating data within particular groups such as African Americans and Asian Americans, but requires looking within the four governmentally defined ethnic minority populations to identify variations in ethnic subgroups as well.

Conclusions

The main message is that although progress has been made in addressing minority mental health, there is much work to be done. For example, some of the data cited appears in yet unpublished manuscripts. In addition, research needs to move beyond descriptive work and service utilization studies. Questions need to be asked that address factors related to barriers to obtaining service for various ethnic minority groups. Additional work is needed to examine clinical presentations of psychiatric phenomena in diverse cultural groups. Further, psychometric work to test and norm measures of symptoms in ethnic minority subgroups is needed. In addition, scientists must develop knowledge of culturally bound syndromes and related interventions. In newer areas of inquiry such as ethnopsychopharmacology, it is necessary to develop models and theory that explain the effect of culture, environment, and psychosocial factors on adherence to and efficacy of drug treatment regimens. There is also a lack of midrange intervention theory regarding the provision of culturally competent diagnosis, management, and treatment. Any of these areas are appropriate areas of inquiry for nurse researchers with expertise in psychiatric mental health care. What is needed is greater awareness of knowledge gaps followed by a commitment to address minority mental health issues when conducting research.

DIANA LYNN MORRIS

See also

AMERICAN INDIAN AND ALASKA NATIVE YOUTH SUICIDE
MENTAL HEALTH POLICY
MENTAL HEALTH SERVICES RESEARCH

MUSIC THERAPY

Music therapy is the use of a musical intervention to improve physiological and psychological health and well-being. For music to be therapeutic, there must be an interaction between the music and the person who desires a health outcome (Meyer, 1956). Music therapy may be provided by a registered music therapist; however, any member of the health care team may suggest to patients that music can be helpful for stress, pain, mood, or exercise. Nurses can assess musical preferences, offer a choice of selections, and encourage patient involvement in the music with the goal of achieving specific health outcomes.

Throughout history, music has been used for a variety of therapeutic purposes by primitive people—ancient Egyptians, Persians, Hebrews, Greeks, and Romans. Music has been used to ward off evil spirits, prevent or cure illnesses, relieve depression, modify emotions, and achieve inner harmony. Early cultures had little means to treat disease, so music and spirituality were used to provide comfort and help people cope. During the Renaissance, physicians became interested in the scientific basis of healing. Because many physicians were also musicians, they believed in the therapeutic value of music and incorporated it in their training and practice. From the 17th century onward, physicians studied the effect of music on physiology and psychology. During this time there was debate over the need to focus on what type of music was effective versus what type of person responded positively to music. At the beginning of the 20th century, the first laboratory studies of the physiological effects of music were conducted on animals and humans. These experiments demonstrated changes in vital signs and body secretions related to various types of music, but they are rejected by most investigators today because of the poor quality of measurement, analysis, and control. In the 1930s music began to be used in patients' hospital rooms, in surgery prior to general anesthesia, and during local anesthesia. It was used in obstetrics and gynecology to reduce the side effects of inhalation anesthetics. During the past 50 years music has been used to (a) reduce acute, chronic, and cancer pain; (b) reduce stress and anxiety; (c) potentiate the effects of analgesic medications in patients during and after surgery and during labor and delivery; and (d) promote exercise.

Music can stimulate, soothe, encourage, or give pleasure to patients. Music has been found to reduce muscle tension, reduce pain and anxiety, raise levels of beta-endorphins, and lower adrenocorticotropic stress hormones. Nursing reviews of research on the effect of music on health outcomes can be found in chapters by Buckwalter, Hartsock, and Gaffney (1985), Cook (1981), Guzzetta (1988), and Chlan (1998). The *Journal of Music Therapy* is another resource. Music has been found to improve the immune system, salivary cortisol, and cardiac autonomic balance. It has also been investigated for its effect on sleep disturbances, cancer pain, and acute and chronic pain during stressful or painful procedures (e.g., injections and lumbar punctures). Music has been generally found to reduce anxiety before and during surgery, with injections, in chronically ill patients, in intensive care patients, and after myocardial infarction. It has been studied in agitated elderly or psychiatric patients, in critically ill patients, and in those who are comatose or dying.

Music has been categorized into stimulative and sedative types. Stimulative music has strong rhythms, volume, dissonance, and disconnected notes, whereas sedative music has a sustained melody without strong rhythmic or percussive elements. Stimulative music enhances bodily action and stimulates skeletal muscles, emotions, and subcortical reactions in humans. Sedative music results in physical sedation and responses of an intellectual and contemplative nature (Gaston, 1951). Precategorization by the nurse, however, does not consider the kind of subject response.

To choose music that is therapeutic, the nurse should consider the nature of the music, the patient preferences and the health state. Variations in the music include the type of music and the intensity, tempo, rhythm, pitch, tone, timbre, blending, complexity, melody, familiarity, length, variety, and novelty. Variations in the patient include age, sex, cultural background, musical preferences, music training, participation in music, degree of auditory discrepancy, time available, and most of all, degree of liking for the music under consideration. Variations in the nature of the health state determine whether music is needed to cheer, encourage, and soothe or will be used to relax, distract the mind, stimulate exercise, or evoke emotions of joy, triumph, resolve, or peace.

Music is economical for patient use. Tapes, compact discs., and players are relatively inexpensive, and a small library can be maintained on any nursing unit. Music piped into patients' rooms also may be available. Nurses can suggest that patients and their families bring in favorite music from home that is likely to invoke healthy responses. They can refer patients to a music therapist if one is available.

Future research in music may include studies that determine the kinds of music that are effective for health outcomes in countries around the world, between cultures in each country. More work on comparing symptomatic response with physiological response is needed to generate theories of conditions in which music is effective, how it affects body processes, and what effect it has on recovery, immune function, and health.

Music brings an air of normalcy, entertainment, pleasure, and escape into a world where illness is often the enemy and both patients and caregivers are fighting back. Music is an integral part of most people's normal lives and should not be forgotten when they go to hospitals and other health care facilities. With the increased reliance on technology in health care today, music can add a humanistic touch. But beyond the humanistic value of music is the therapeutic value in reducing stress, pain, anxiety, and depression and promoting movement, socialization, and sleep.

MARION GOOD

See also
STRESS
STRESS MANAGEMENT

NO-SUICIDE CONTRACTS

A contract is simply an agreement between two or more parties. Treatment contracts have been used in healthcare settings to achieve a variety of goals. Contracts represent a partnership between a client and a healthcare professional to support treatment adherence (Laidlaw, Beeken, Whitney, & Reyes, 1999; Newell, 1997), to enhance the learning and practice of health-promoting behaviors (Hart & Westin, 1996; Zandee & Oermann, 1996), and to reduce recurrence of unhealthy behaviors (Dyckoff, Goldstein, & Schacht-Levine, 1996). Some contracts specify rewards, or contingencies, to reward positive behavior, reflecting their origin in behavioral theory.

Other treatment contracts, however, do not rely on contingencies for reinforcement of a desired behavior, but presumably capitalize on both the strength of the therapeutic alliance and on the motivation of the client for change. This is generally the case with no-suicide contracts. No-suicide contracts (also called safety or no-harm contracts) are used when the client has a history of self-harm behavior or is experiencing thoughts about self-harm.

First described in the literature within the framework of transactional analysis, the no-suicide contract was defined as a statement by the adult ego state of the client to take responsibility to remain safe (Drye, Goulding, & Goulding, 1973). As with all types of contracts, no-suicide contracts may vary in the degree of explicitness with which they are negotiated and endorsed by each party. Written contracts may include formal statements of treatment goals and responsibilities of each party, a time frame that specifies the life of the contract, and signatures of both parties. Alternatively, a contract may consist of a note handwritten and signed by the client that asserts his or her intent to remain safe. Contracts may also be verbally negotiated.

There are many possible motives for the negotiation of a no-suicide contract. These may include promoting the autonomy of patients who are assessed to be competent, openly communicating caring by the professional to the client, invoking the expectation that cultural norms regarding honoring one's word will be upheld, providing time for the client to work out specific problems, and reducing client and staff anxiety (Assey, 1985; Drye et al., 1973; Fremouw, Perczel, & Ellis, 1990; Loomis, 1985). No-suicide contracts do not, however, protect the healthcare provider from legal action should the client later commit suicide (Simon, 1998).

Relevance to Nursing Research

No-suicide contracting is identified as a suicide prevention measure in the literature of psychology (Bongar, 1991; Fremouw et al., 1990), medicine (Depression Guideline Panel, 1993; Pary, Lippmann, & Tobias, 1988), and nursing (Fontaine, 1999; Varcarolis, 1998). Individuals who are at high risk for suicide are often hospitalized. In the hospital, nursing is the professional group that has the most direct, ongoing contact with and responsibility for the client. Consequently, among the health care disciplines, nursing has a particular duty to evaluate the outcome of suicide prevention interventions such a contracting. This is particularly true since contracting is often used as an assessment strategy. If the client is willing to contract for safety, staff may become less vigilant in observing the client's behavior or in restricting access to potentially harmful objects.

Review of Major Studies

There is very little research regarding no-suicide contracts. Relevant studies cluster into two broad categories. The first set of studies examines contracting from the perspective of the mental health professional. The second category of research explores the relationship between no-suicide contracts and self-harm or suicidal behavior.

Davidson and colleagues surveyed the attitudes of licensed psychologists regarding no-suicide agreements. The return rate of 35% was low. The psychologists agreed that no-suicide contracting was appropriate with adults and adolescents, but not with children. The clinicians believed that individuals who were moderately suicidal construed more benefit from contracting than did clients with mild or severe suicidality. The report did not clearly describe the percentage of psychologists that routinely use contracts, stating only that most respondents "often" use the agreements with adults (Davidson, Wagner, & Range, 1995).

Drew (1999a) surveyed all licensed psychiatric inpatient facilities in Ohio. No-suicide contracts were used by staff in 79% (n = 66) of the responding hospitals (response rate was 82%). Contracts were negotiated with every admitted patient in only one hospital. In the other hospitals they were used after suicidal ideation was expressed (83% of those hospitals that used contracts), after self-harm (79%), or after a patient was admitted because of self-harm behavior (65%). Nurses negotiated contracts with patients in all of the hospitals except one. The exception was a state hospital. Contracts were usually verbal (74%) or handwritten (72%) rather than standardized and preprinted (15%).

This descriptive research suggests that no-suicide contracting is commonly practiced. Psychologists considered contracting appropriate and effective with moderately suicidal adolescents and adults. In inpatient settings, nurses were among the professional groups who contracted with clients. Contracts were not used indiscriminately but were negotiated when high suicide risk was assessed. The attitudes of hospital staffs toward contracting were not elicited in the latter study.

With respect to the correlational research, Jones and colleagues examined the use of contracts with children to reduce a wide range of acting-out behaviors including aggression, sexual behavior, and suicidal behavior in a psychiatric inpatient setting (Jones & O'Brien, 1990; Jones, O'Brien, & McMahon, 1993). These were contingency contracts in that staff decisions regarding privileges were explicitly based on the child's willingness to meet the terms of a behavioral agreement. In the first study, a questionnaire was administered to a small sample of hospitalized children (Jones & O'Brien, 1990). The subjects rated several treatments including contracting for a change in privileges. The children ranked contracting as "very high" in helping them change their behaviors. Subsequently, Jones et al. (1993) compared the incidence of acting-out behaviors before and after contracting was implemented through a retrospective review of incident sheets. Two percent of children engaged in suicidal behavior before contracts compared to 0.2% of children after contracting was in effect.

Drew (1999b) conducted a retrospective review of 650 charts of adults who were inpatients on the psychiatric units of two hospitals. Controlling for level of restriction and degree of nursing consistency, patients with no-suicide contracts were at higher risk for self-harm behavior (OR = 7.43, 95% CI = 3.26–16.92). Contracting appeared to be an indicator of high risk-for-suicide status rather than having a causal role in self-harm behavior. Nonetheless, there was no evidence that no-suicide contracting served to protect against self-harm behavior.

In summary, the three studies that examined the relationship between no-suicide contracting and self-harm behaviors addressed two populations, children and adults. While they, along with the descriptive studies, do lay a foundation for further research, they suffer from the limitations of retrospective reviews of medical records including threats to internal validity and concerns regarding the reliability of record keeping. Additionally, their findings were inconsistent.

Directions for Future Research

While the occurrence of self-harm behavior or suicide is clinically significant, it is, statistically, a rare event. As a result, the evaluation of suicide prevention techniques is quite difficult. Prospective designs that compare the outcomes of treatment with and without the negotiation of a no-suicide contract would have the most potential. However, a very large sample of high-risk individuals would be required to yield enough cases of persons who harmed themselves (Robins & Kulbok, 1986). Additionally, the intervention (contract) would have to be carefully designed and distinguished from standard care. A more efficient, but less robust, method would be a retrospective case-control design. A difficulty with this method lies with the identification of cases (Cohen, 1986). This problem could, though, be addressed if data were collected immediately after an occurrence of self-harm behavior. Additional information could be obtained via a client interview. This would allow for assessment of the client's perspective on the nature and effect of suicide prevention measures on behavior. Data would also be collected on clients who are matched controls.

Conclusion

The evidence suggests that no-suicide contracts are frequently used but inadequately evaluated. Contracting may have therapeutic value. But until the practice is more thoroughly evaluated, modifications in suicide prevention measures must be based on a thorough, ongoing assessment of suicidal risk, rather than on the client's willingness to contract for safety.

BARBARA L. DREW

See also
MENTAL DISORDERS PREVENTION
SUICIDE

NURSE-PATIENT COMMUNICATION

Communication is an essential component of nursing intervention, and in some cases it is the intervention itself. As a result, there has been considerable focus on understanding communication as it occurs between nurses and patients. Although communication has been defined in many ways, common features include the transfer or sharing of information in a dynamic process that involves a common set of rules. Depictions of this process typically illustrate messages being sent back and forth between two separate and discrete entities—the sender and the receiver using both verbal and nonverbal channels of communication. This conceptualization of communication has dominated discussion, theorizing, and research on nurse-patient communication, with few exceptions. However, with the emergence of caring theory in nursing, the assumption that communication takes place from a position of distance and from within discrete boundaries has been questioned. Montgomery (1993) suggested that overlapping circles may represent a more appropriate communication model, reflecting nurses' incorporation of the other's subjective experience during caring encounters.

The terms *nurse-patient communication* and *nurse-patient interaction* have sometimes been used interchangeably in the literature. However, it appears that nurse-patient interaction is increasingly being used to refer to the complex dynamics that occur between nurses and patients, of which communication is a key component. The study of communication between nurses and patients appears to be increasingly reserved for the examination of specific verbal or nonverbal behaviors that may be important in nurse-patient encounters.

In the study of nurse-patient communication, most attention has been focused on nurse-initiated verbal and nonverbal behaviors, such as touch, empathetic verbal responses, and blocking statements. Researchers have attempted to describe how nurses use specific communication behaviors, factors that influence the use and interpretation of these behaviors, and their effect on desired patient outcomes. However, research efforts have been hampered by inadequate conceptualizations of the communication behaviors under study. Touch, for example, has been the topic of much research. Primarily viewed as a channel of communication that can function independently of others, it has been studied in isolation from other verbal and nonverbal behaviors. Recent investigations of touch have indicated that a broader concept may be necessary. Eye contact, tone of voice, body position, and purpose of the interaction may all influence the meaning of a touch gesture. The potential value of inductive approaches, such as grounded theory, ethnoscience, and qualitative ethology in developing a more complex understanding of specific communication behaviors such as touch (Bottorff, 1993; Estabrooks, 1989) and in identifying new patterns of communication, such as the comfort talk register (Proctor, Morse, & Khonsari, 1996), has been demonstrated. Using these approaches, the situated nature of communication is taken into account.

The effect of nurses' communication behavior on patients has been a subject of considerable study. Dependent variables have been measured in a number of ways, including investigator-developed questionnaires, standardized questionnaires, interviews, observational measures, and physiological indices. Yet methodological problems associated with lack of clear or consistent communication interventions, small sample sizes, inadequate attention to reliability and validity of measurements, and lack of adequate control of extraneous variables, in addition to the use of a wide variety of settings, patients, and dependent measures, make it difficult to identify areas of coherence among findings. Inadequate control of other forms of communication that may be associated with the behavior that is the focus of investigation may influence outcomes and explain inconclusive findings. It may be that the most fruitful avenue for future research is to study specific communication behaviors of interest in the context in which they occur, rather than as isolated behaviors in contrived settings. Paying more attention to the perceptions of patients may also assist in determining which effects of nurses' communication behaviors should be addressed.

Recently, researchers have begun to focus on patient verbal and nonverbal behaviors in an attempt to identify behaviors that have particular significance for nursing practice. The underlying assumption is that patient behaviors communicate important information that can be used to guide clinical decision making. For example, detailed analysis of videotaped behaviors of postsurgical neonates has lead to the identification of observable pain responses (Coté, Morse, & James, 1991). Using similar methods of analyses, the examination of maternal sounds and verbalizations during second-stage labor revealed differences between adaptive and nonadaptive sounds, providing important cues to guide caregiver behavior (McKay & Roberts, 1990). Moreover, these findings are important because they indicate that evoking a "no noise" rule during second-stage labor is contraindicated.

Although expert nurses often intuitively recognized the meaning of behavioral cues, they were not able to clearly identify the behaviors they were responding to. Microanalysis of videotaped patient behaviors, using approaches like ethology help to explicate clinically relevant patterns of behaviors that can be used as a basis for enhancing the nurse's sensitivity to subtle changes in patient behavior or appearance. In addition, identification of clinically significant behavior patterns also can provide a foundation for the development of outcome measures to evaluate the efficacy of particular nursing interventions. By observing patients in the emergency room, behavioral indicators of escalating levels of distress were identified and provided researchers with the outcome measures to evaluate the efficacy of nurse-initiated interventions such as those aimed at comforting patients (Intrieri, Cerdas, & Morse, 1994). If the interventions are effective, changes in levels of patient distress in the hypothesized direction should be observed.

Methods of data collection that record the actual communication behaviors of nurses and patients, such as audiotape and videotape recordings, are essential to expanding our understanding of communication behaviors although they are time-consuming, expensive, and often intrusive. Taking advantage of advancing technologies to record and analyze physiological indices and communication behaviors simultaneously is an important future direction. Much work remains in identifying and describing important communication concepts that are the foundation of effective nursing interactions and interventions.

JOAN L. BOTTORFF

See also
COMFORT

NURSE-PATIENT INTERACTION
NURSE-PATIENT RELATIONSHIP

NURSE-PATIENT INTERACTION

Nurse-patient interaction refers to the dyadic reciprocal interactions that occur between nurses and patients in the context of providing and receiving nursing care. Early nursing theorists such as Peplau, Orlando, Travelbee, and Widenbach, who drew attention to the process of interaction in nursing practice, prompted researchers to describe, operationalize, and measure the efficacy of nursing interactions. In 1977, Diers and Schmidt classified the rapidly expanding research on nurse-patient interaction as descriptive or correlational studies, studies that measure the indices of nursing by using hypothetical interactions, and studies that describe or evaluate nursing interactions using conception or interaction frameworks borrowed from other disciplines (e.g., counseling psychology). These initial research efforts were largely focused on single channels of communication (e.g., nurse conversation or touch) and produced only partial information about the interaction. Resulting failures to capture relevant clinical data prompted the redesign of instruments and studies specifically for examining nurse-patient interactions. As one example, the Nurse Orientation System developed by Diers was used by researchers to examine the effect of nursing on patient experiences of pain (Diers, Schmidt, McBride, & Davis, 1972).

Researchers continued to study those aspects of the nurse-patient interaction that were quantifiable, using predominantly deductive approaches; and despite the use of increasingly sophisticated techniques, the results of many studies raised concern about the quality of nurse-patient interactions. Some researchers attempted to explain their findings in terms of nurses' lack of communication skills or their busy workloads; others pointed to problems inherent in the research, citing a lack of attention to the patient's role in nurse-patient interaction, unsubstantiated assumptions about the nature of nurse-patient interactions, and failure to take into consideration important contextual factors that influence nurse-patient interactions as major issues (Jarrett & Payne, 1995; May, 1990). In addition, in the absence of adequate definitions of nurse-patient interaction or its components (e.g., touch) researchers used narrow and simplistic conceptualizations. As a result, in deciding a priori what behaviors were important to study, researchers risked missing important behaviors or focusing on insignificant behaviors; as a consequence, they ended up with incomplete or invalid descriptions.

As support for "caring" in nursing developed in the 1980s, theorists drew attention to the complexities inherent in the process of providing nursing care, stimulating a resurgence of interest in examining nurse-patient interactions with a variety of new approaches, such as grounded theory, conversational analysis, ethology, and discourse analysis. By using inductive approaches, researchers identified nurse and patient behaviors that were important to study (rather than deciding this a priori), explored interaction patterns from the perspective of the nurse and patients, and considered important factors of context and relationship. Studies completed by researchers such as Carl May, Maura Hunt, Jocalyn Lawler, and Janice Morse are representative examples. Using these new approaches, researchers identified exceptional nursing interaction skills, such as "tactics," "comfort talk," "minifisms," and other previously unrecognized interaction strategies that nurses typically used in clinical settings—skills that were rarely part of communication courses and often devalued.

One of the most important developments in the study of nurse-patient interactions is the use of video technology. Videotaping observations preserves the observational context, verbal content, nonverbal behaviors, and interactive processes for analysis and coding. Of particular advantage is the ability to repeatedly review videotapes, both in real time and in slow motion. This facilitates in-depth study of a wide range of simultaneous behaviors, including rarely occurring events and subtle or rapid changes in behavior. Videotaped observations are particularly useful when studying interactions with patients who are preverbal, unconscious, or otherwise unable to recall interactions with sufficient detail.

When videotaped observations of naturally occurring nurse-patient interactions are used as data for qualitative studies, new patterns of interaction have been revealed. For example, by use of qualitative ethology (Morse & Bottorff, 1990), an analysis of videotaped interactions of cancer patients and their nurses led Bottorff and Morse (1994) to suggest alternative ways of looking at and structuring nurse-patient interactions to capture the unique styles of interaction that are characteristic of nursing practice. The four types of attending identified in this study captured the dynamic nature of interaction between nurses and patients from a more global perspective than did previous sentence-by-sentence analysis. This facilitated the identification of subtle changes between and within interactions that were not possible using previous dichotomous descriptions of interactions (e.g., therapeutic/nontherapeutic) and took into account more than just the component of verbal communication.

Although these new lines of research show promise and appear to be unraveling some of the unique complexities inherent in nurse-patient interaction, much work remains to understand nursing interactions as they occur in health care settings, including patients' homes or other community settings. Far more attention has been given to identifying and describing components and patterns of nurse-patient interaction than studying the efficacy of different types of interactions in relation to patient outcomes. It appears that some patterns of interaction may be powerful therapeutic tools, yet more systematic investigation is needed to demonstrate these effects. Furthermore, negative or undesirable psychological and physiological sequalae associated with interaction patterns should be documented.

Although the definition of nurse-patient interaction has not received careful attention, the focus has been on the verbal and nonverbal behaviors of the nurse. Yet increasingly, patients are being encouraged to take an active role in decision making and their nursing care. To develop innovative and supportive strategies to foster collaboration in care and involvement in decision making, a sound understanding of the nature of interactions between nurses and patient, with a strong focus on the role of patient behavior in these interactions, is necessary. In addition, the links between nurse-patient interaction and types of nurse-patient relationships must be explored.

JOAN L. BOTTORFF

See also
NURSE-PATIENT COMMUNICATION
NURSE-PATIENT RELATIONSHIP
PEPLAU'S THEORETICAL MODEL

NURSE-PATIENT RELATIONSHIP

The interpersonal relationship between nurses and patients has become an important subject of discussion, theorizing, and research since Peplau and Orlando introduced the concept of the nurse-patient relationship as an essential component of nursing practice. Recognition of the need for individualized nursing care, the introduction of new approaches to care delivery (e.g., primary nursing), increasing concerns about dehumanization related to advances in technology, and the emergence of theories delineating caring as a pivotal concept in nursing have reinforced the centrality of the nurse-patient relationship in contemporary practice. The nurse-patient relationship is now viewed as essential content in nursing curricula, and clinicians value the development of therapeutic relationships with patients as a significant part of their work. Yet despite the overwhelming endorsement of the importance of the nurse-patient relationship, the practical difficulties associated with developing relationships remain unresolved. Of importance are issues related to balancing personal involvement and professional detachment. Other important issues concern building relationships in contexts where the organization of nurses' work limits involvement or where reporting practices undermine the development of trust. Issues also arise from challenges related to renegotiating relationships in response to changes in patient dependence and vulnerability.

Nurses have attempted to identify the unique characteristics of the nurse-patient relationship through their conceptualizations, although to date there is little evidence to support this assumption. The nurse-patient relationship has been described as a therapeutic instrument with levels or types of involvement and as an interactive process requiring the active participation of both patients and nurses. Important components of the nurse-patient relationship include concepts such as empathy, trust, respect, knowing the patient, commitment, advocacy, and social control. Nursing writers critiquing current conceptualizations of the nurse-patient relationship have pointed out the failure to consider the collective nature of nursing work and other realities of everyday practice such as the provision of bodily comforts (May, 1990; May & Purkis, 1995). Theorists such as Sally Gadow and Jean Watson have attempted to explain the nature of the links between nurse-patient relationships and positive health care outcomes, and there is some empirical evidence that supports these assertions.

Although researchers have begun to explore the complex dynamics involved in nurse-patient interactions and their therapeutic potential, there is relatively little empirical data related to what takes place in everyday clinical settings to support current conceptualizations of the nurse-patient relationship. Early investigations of nurse-patient relationships were influenced by definitions from the social sciences and the traditions of logical positivism. However, explanations of the relationship proved difficult to quantify. With increasing acceptance of qualitative research methods in nursing, researchers have turned to a variety of new approaches to examine patterns of relationships in nursing, including grounded theory and narrative analysis. For representative examples, see Carl May (1991), Janice Morse (1991), and Joan Liaschenko (1997). These studies have revealed important new information about nurse-patient relationships, some of which has contradicted professional rhetoric surrounding the development of these relationships. For example, Morse's (1991) grounded theory analysis revealed that nurses used several strategies to increase the level of involvement, including sharing personal information. This strategy often is not condoned in nursing textbooks.

The complexities inherent in the nurse-patient relationship demand that the research agenda be augmented by micro-level approaches (such as sociolinguistics, ethnomethodology, and in-depth videotape analysis), advances in interpretive methodology (e.g., using a feminist perspective), and triangulation (e.g., triangulating conversational analysis with data from ethnographic research), as well as by taking advantage of constructionist, critical, and postmodern theory to understand the dynamics of nurse-patient relationships (Lowenberg, 1994; May, 1990; May & Purkis, 1995). For example, observational studies of the development of nurse-patient relationships as they occur in everyday clinical settings would augment nurses' narratives of memorable relationships. Some researchers are exploring the potential value of using video recorders to capture the development of relationships over time. Detailed analysis of videotaped patient and nurse behaviors at the interaction level have produced some encouraging results.

For the most part, researchers have focused on the affective dimensions of nurse-patient relationships by interviewing nurses, particularly those who were able to provide exemplar cases. Other dimensions of the nurse-patient relationship should be examined, as well as outcomes, as they relate to different phases and types of relationships. Attention must be given to the patient's perspective and role in shaping relationships. Morse's (1991) research was a beginning step in unraveling the strategies that patients used to increase or decrease the rate and level of the developing relationship. Finally, assumptions related to the consistency of nurse-patient relationships across clinical settings require empirical examination. Most research efforts have been concentrated in acute care settings. Nurse-patient relationships in other contexts also should be studied, including community health and home care nursing.

JOAN L. BOTTORFF

See also
NURSE-PATIENT COMMUNICATION
NURSE-PATIENT INTERACTION
PEPLAU'S THEORETICAL MODEL

PEPLAU'S THEORETICAL MODEL

Peplau's theoretical ideas about interpersonal relations in nursing were formulated in the 1940s and published in 1952 after a lengthy dispute with publishers about the ability of a nurse to author a book. At a time when nurses were "doers" for patients and "followers" of physicians' orders, Peplau's theoretical work and teachings helped catapult nursing from an occupation to a profession. This precipitated a need for nurses to understand and establish interpersonal relations with patients, as the significant context in which nurses facilitate patients' health.

Through Peplau's therapeutic relationship, the patient develops inner resources for healthy behaviors by actively participating with the nurse in the change process. Peplau's interpersonal relationship is also a process through which nursing knowledge is developed and validated (Reed, 1996b). Peplau (1992) purposefully linked her theory to practice and research, as evidenced in her basic assumption that "what goes on between people can be noticed, studied, explained, understood, and, if detrimental, changed" (p. 14).

Overview of the Model

Peplau's theoretical model was based on study, observation, and analyses of nurses and patients and derived from the work of Harry Stack Sullivan and other psychodynamic perspectives. Peplau's (1952) classic descriptions of nursing express the nature and goals of the interpersonal process: "Nursing is a human relationship between an individual, who is sick, or in need of health services, and a nurse especially educated to recognize and to respond to the need for help" (pp. 5–6). Nursing is an "educative instrument, a maturing force, that aims to promote forward movement of personality in the direction of creative, constructive, productive, personal, and community living" (p. 16). Consistent with her earlier statements, Peplau (1988) described nursing as an "enabling, empowering, or transforming art" (p. 9). The interpersonal relationship was how nurses assessed and assisted people to attain healthy levels of anxiety and resume mental health and development. The components necessary for an interpersonal relationship were the nurse, patient, professional expertise of the nurse, and needs of the patient.

Peplau's (1952) four phases of the nurse-client relationship are orientation, identification, exploitation, and resolution. Throughout these phases the nurse functions cooperatively with the patient in the roles of stranger, resource person, counselor, leader, surrogate, and teacher. The nurse's range of focus includes patient, family, and community (Peplau, 1952).

During the phase of orientation, the patient has a "felt need" and seeks professional assistance (Peplau, 1952, p. 18). This is the first step in the personal growth of the patient. The nurse and patient initially experience the role of stranger as the patient seeks assistance from the nurse. During this phase the nurse gathers observable data, recognizing that the power to accomplish the tasks at hand always resides within the patient (Peplau, 1952). The nurse and patient collaborate on a plan, with consideration of the educative needs of the patient.

The focus during the identification phase is to assist the patient to incorporate personal power to address the problem. The relationship is flexible enough for the patient to function dependently, independently, or interdependently with the nurse, based on the patient's developmental capacity, level of anxiety, and other needs. The nurse may assume the role of surrogate, counselor, resource person, and leader during this phase (Peplau, 1952).

The exploitation phase marks the time when patients have identified their own resources and strengths. They are enabled to derive full benefits of the interpersonal relationship and other services offered by the nurse to the patient (Forchuk, 1994; Peplau, 1952).

The final phase in the interpersonal relationship is that of resolution. Patients move beyond the initial identification with the helping professional and engage their own strengths to foster health, outside the therapeutic relationship.

According to Peplau (1952), health is a "word symbol that implies forward movement of personality and other ongoing human processes in the direction of creative, constructive, productive, personal and community living" (p. 12). Health is linked closely to successful management of anxiety, which ranges from pure euphoria to pure anxiety. Between these anxiety extremes, as determined by nurse and patient, is an optimal level of anxiety for healthy functioning. The nurse uses a complex set of strategies to assist the patient in using energy provided by the anxiety to identify and grow from a problematic situation (O'Toole & Welt, 1989; Reed, 1996a). Illness forces a "stock-taking by the sick person, which nurses can use to promote learning, growth and improved competencies for living" (Peplau, 1992, p. 13).

Research, Practice, and Education

Peplau's theoretical model can be categorized as a middle-range theory. It is narrower in scope than a conceptual model or grand theory. The model addresses a limited number of measurable concepts (e.g., therapeutic relationship, anxiety). The theory has a specific focus on the characteristics and process of the therapeutic relationship as a nursing method to help manage anxiety and foster healthy development. As such, the model is directly applicable to research and practice.

Peplau was explicit in promoting theory-based nursing practice and research-based theory. Research based on Peplau's theoretical model has addressed a variety of nursing problems, including (a) the work roles and practices of psychiatric–mental health nurses, (b) understanding specific phases and roles in the nurse-patient relationship, (c) recovery from depression, (d) working with patients infected with HIV, and (e) family systems nursing.

A major strength in Peplau's theory of interpersonal relations is its application to psychiatric–mental health nursing practice and to nursing wherein the nurse-patient relationship is relevant. Examples of this theory's application can be found throughout the literature on nursing research and practice.

Peplau's theory permeates all areas of nursing education. A philosophy of nursing curricula is belief in the value of a therapeutic nurse-patient relationship that focuses on needs, resources, and active participation of patients and supports collaboration between nurse and patient.

Future Directions

Peplau's theoretical model continues to be used by nurses who desire to advance nursing's knowledge base. Peplau's original contributions have become knowledge in the public domain and are not always acknowledged by researchers, clinicians, and educators. Nevertheless, the interpersonal relations theory continues to influence nursing theories, education, and practice (O'Toole & Welt, 1989). Peplau's philosophy of nursing and approach to knowledge development connect theory, practice, and research in creative ways (Reed, 1996b).

The reawakening of nursing by Peplau's ideas in the 1950s continues today through exploration, study, and use of the science-based practice of interpersonal relations in nursing. Through research and practice applications the theoretical model will continue to be refined and enhanced to meet contemporary needs of society. Peplau's theoretical ideas are expected to withstand the current health care crisis and to provide future nursing research for the cost-effective resources for health that exist within patient-nurse relationships.

NELMA B. SHEARER
PAMELA G. REED

See also
MENTAL HEALTH IN PUBLIC SECTOR PRIMARY CARE
NURSE-PATIENT RELATIONSHIP

PREGNANCY: ANXIETY AND CONFLICT

This paper focuses on research reports from 1987 to 1999 on maternal anxiety in pregnancy, including childbirth and postpartum outcomes. Also refer to the author's extensive two-part review of the literature on anxiety in pregnancy published in *Behavioral Medicine* (Lederman, 1995). Most research literature has focused on assessing prenatal stress and anxiety and predicting pregnancy or birth outcomes. This paper and the two-part review also consider intervention studies and their effectiveness.

Major Studies, Results, and Future Directions

Studies of maternal anxiety cite psychosocial factors as the most frequent and significant influences on pregnancy adaptation, birth outcomes, and subsequent postpartal maternal/infant adaptation. These psychosocial factors include social support, wantedness and acceptance of pregnancy, the number and kind of prenatal stressors and life events, and personality factors.

Trimester Differences in Anxiety Levels. In general, pregnant women have higher anxiety than nonpregnant women in all trimesters of pregnancy (Lederman, 1996; Singh & Saxena, 1991). However, investigators differ in their reports of when anxiety is highest. Singh and Saxena (1991) report that anxiety peaks in the fifth month, then declines, and rises again in the eighth and ninth month, and decreases once more postpartum, reaching normal at 6 months. Sailaja and

Swaminathan (1992) reported that maternal anxiety was highest in third trimester of pregnancy. Yet, in another study (Dorn, Susman, & Petersen, 1993) anxiety and depression at 20 weeks gestation versus a measure at 34 to 36 weeks predicted more strongly to maternal postpartum anxiety and depression than prior measures of life optimism, self-worth, age, or cortisol reactivity. Lederman (1996) reported significant correlations between state of anxiety and anxiety and conflict pertaining to developmental dimensions in all trimesters of pregnancy. Other investigators also show that depression and anxiety in the first 20 weeks of pregnancy were consistent and strong predictors of postpartal depression and anxiety (Dorn et al., 1993), and that first trimester depression and other psychosocial factors were predictive of low birthweight (Paarlberg et al., 1999). Early first or second trimester anxiety measures appear to be stable predictors of later levels of anxiety and can target women who would benefit from early counseling assistance.

Planning, Wantedness, and Acceptance of Pregnancy. Higher anxiety (Kalil, Gruber, Conley, & Sytniac, 1993; Najman, Morrison, Williams, Andersen, & Keeping, 1991) and depression (Najman et al., 1991) have been reported for mothers with an unplanned and unwanted pregnancy, while few mothers with wanted children experienced such feelings. Assessments of the mother can determine the wantedness or acceptance of a pregnancy. Criteria for acceptance include whether the mother: (a) planned, wants, and accepts the pregnancy; (b) is predominantly happy versus depressed; (c) accepts bodily changes; (d) tolerates discomforts and responds to recommendations for relief; and (e) in late pregnancy, has resolved conflicts associated with early ambivalence (Lederman, 1996). Decisions regarding wantedness of pregnancy almost always remain stable or constant (Lederman, 1996). Thus, counseling intervention for a mother with an unwanted pregnancy may require different maternal plans and caretaking goals than when the mother desires a child and wishes to be a parent. Prenatal developmental and adaptation variables such as: (a) acceptance of pregnancy; (b) readiness and preparedness for parenthood; and (c) relationships with significant others may be stronger correlates and predictors of prenatal adaptation and outcome than general personality and stress measures. This is because these measures assess factors that are unique and particularly relevant to the maternal experience of pregnancy. Another reviewer (Lobel, 1994) similarly notes that conceptualization and measurement of stress specific to pregnancy may need further examination.

Stressful Life Events. In recent literature, perceived stress and life event stress are more consistently associated with birth outcomes, including preterm birth, low birth weight, and gestational age at birth. In a prospective study of 90 women, maternal prenatal stress factors were significantly related to infant birthweight and gestational age at birth, after controlling for biomedical risk factors (Wadhwa, Sandman, Porto, Dunkel-Shetter, & Garite, 1993). Greater specificity in the identification and prediction of gravidas at risk for low birthweight occurred with biopsychosocial risk assessment versus biomedical risk alone. (Herrera, Salmeron, & Hurtado, 1997). Others (Vartianen, Suonio, Halonen, & Rimon, 1994) report similar results and provide support for a biopsychosocial model of maternal neuroendocrine and psychosocial responses to stress that are related to birth outcomes. Also, evidence exists that suggests that prenatal stress factors predict the quality of parent-infant interactions (Noppe, Noppe, & Hughes, 1991) and childhood psychopathology (Ward, 1991).

Social Support. Social support attenuates anxiety, but not always. Kalil et al. (1993) reported that both state and trait anxiety were lower when emotional support was offered by the husband or a confidante. Norbeck and Anderson (1989a) found that the combination of high life stress and low partner support was associated with the highest subject anxiety. A sample of low-income Hispanic mothers reported that a support network of families and formal institutional services was extremely helpful in decreasing the effects of psychosocial problems and the physical demands of pregnancy (Zayas & Busch-Rossnagel, 1992). Others report similar findings of support in low-income African American subjects, which also were associated with improved infant gestational age (Edwards et al., 1994). However, in another study younger subjects reported benefits from spousal support, but experienced greater, not less anxiety from extended family support (Hobfoll & Leiberman, 1989). The impact of support was greater for subjects with a poorer sense of anxiety mastery; those with greater mastery were more resistant to environmental and social stressors. A high level of mutual spousal affection has been associated with lower levels of maternal anxiety symptoms (Zimmerman-Tansella, Bertagni, Siani, & Micciolo, 1994), while a partner's underestimation of maternal prenatal stress is associated with depression and feelings of being unsupported (Chapman, Hobfoll, & Ritter, 1997). The significance of a good marital relationship is widely acknowledged and is a stable predictor of postpartal marital satisfaction (Tomlinson & Irwin, 1993).

Cultural Differences. Norbeck and Anderson (1989b) reported differences based on ethnic background. For Blacks, social support from the woman's partner or mother accounted for 35% of the variance in gestation complications and 14% of the variance in prolonged labor or the need for cesarean section. For Whites, high rather than low support accounted for pregnancy outcomes, while none of these variables were significant for Hispanics, who had low complication rates. Thus, the effects of social support are moderated by age, ability to master anxiety, cultural factors, and the nature and source of support.

Levin (1991) used a confirmatory factor analysis with a sample of Black and Hispanic mothers to model the sources of anxiety in pregnancy. The first factors revealed were anxiety about being pregnant, childbirth, and hospitalization. Second order factors included age, marital status, and worry about health. Arizmendi and Affonso (1987) also found that the most intense stressors for both pregnancy and early postpartum in a middle class Caucasian sample were internal concerns. These concerns centered on: (a) physical symptoms, (b) body image, (c) fetal/newborn welfare, (d) labor and delivery, and (e) changes in living patterns. However, in a replication (Green, 1990) of the Arizmendi and Affonso study (1987) with indigent African American mothers, external, rather than internal events, such as mate and spouse issues (communication, support), lack of money, family stressors, job and career problems were cited more frequently and with higher stress intensity. In this study the investigators noted no differences in frequency and intensity across trimesters for these socioeconomic and relational variables. Yet, several trimester differences for psychosocial and developmental variables and for different ethnic or cultural groups have been reported (Lederman & Miller, 1998).

The majority of studies to date report low or only moderate relationships of psychosocial and personality variables with pregnancy outcomes. This may be due to homogeneity of samples (lower stress and less variability in middle class samples), lack of measurement sensitivity to cultural differences, and the use of single versus multidimensional measures of anxiety. Studies need to be guided by theoretical and empirical criteria (Lobel, 1994) and their usefulness and specificity for designing intervention studies.

Psychophysiologic Responses to Anxiety. Anxiety may be expressed through a number of neuroendocrine pathways. The sympathetic autonomic nervous system, through catecholamine release into maternal circulation, alters uterine contractile activity (Lederman, 1996) and, by arterial vasoconstriction, may reduce uteroplacental perfusion and restrict fetal growth.

The hypothalamic-pituitary-adrenal (HPA) axis during pregnancy also could affect birth outcomes. Corticotropin-releasing hormone may control the timing of birth and be associated with preterm birth (Sandman, Wadhwa, Chicz-Demet, Dunkel-Shetter, & Porto, 1997). Beta-endorphin (βE), released from the placenta and from the pituitary into maternal circulation in response to HPA activation, could cause disregulation of the developing fetal nervous system (Wadhwa, Dunkel-Shetter, Chicz-DeMet, Porto & Sandman, 1996). Of the three neuroendocrine substances measured (ACTH, βE, and cortisol), ACTH was found to be the most sensitive indicator of maternal psychological stress.

Another pathway, also through the HPA axis, may alter immune system response, rendering the gravida less resistant to infection (Herbert & Cohen, 1993). The fetus also may have altered adaptive responses that could persist into extrauterine life (Coe, Wiener, Rosenberg & Levine, 1985). The addition of biochemical and psychoneuroendocrine measures of anxiety in pregnancy provides construct validity and theoretical explication when they correlate with psychosocial measures of anxiety and with birth outcomes.

Conclusion. Strong evidence exists that maternal anxiety and personality factors, operating through neuroendocrine pathways, effect maternal and fetal/newborn birth outcomes.

REGINA LEDERMAN

See also
STRESS
STRESS MANAGEMENT

PRIMARY AND MENTAL HEALTH SERVICES INTEGRATION

Epidemiological Profile

Just recently, the first US Surgeon General's *Report on Mental Health Research and Services* declared mental health "fundamental to a person's overall health, indispensable to personal well being and instrumental to leading a balanced and productive life" (Satcher, 1999, p. v). Despite the fundamental importance of mental health, a growing public health concern centers on the fact that 20% of Americans are affected by mental disorders per year and yet nearly half of persons with severe mental illness fail to seek treatment for a variety of reasons related to accessibility, affordability, stigmatization, and fragmentation of services. The current mental health care system defined separate from primary care has failed to provide services to the majority of persons, including children, who are challenged with a mental health disorder. In fact, mental disorders are often not detected early and when detected are often not adequately treated. Estimates range from one third to one half of adult primary care patients with mental illnesses are not accurately diagnosed (Katon et al., 1992; Von Korff, Burke, & Teitlebaum, 1987). A similar pattern is found in pediatric populations whereby primary care providers tend to not recognize mental health problems (Richardson, Keller, Selby-Harrington, & Parrish, 1996). In fact, psychosocial problems have been identified as the new morbidity of pediatric populations (American Academy of Pediatrics [AAP], 1993). Even a large proportion of children identified as having mental health disorders do not receive appropriate treatment (Richardson, Keller, Selby-Harrington, & Parrish, 1996). However, quality of life is often significantly improved when a mental health disorder is detected early and treated properly.

The Surgeon General's Mental Health Report (U.S. Department of Health and Human Services [DHHS], 1999) presents an historic opportunity to improve the delivery of mental health services with particular emphasis placed on accessible, affordable, effective, and culturally sensitive treatments. Epidemiological studies have indicated that individuals with psychiatric disorders are often and exclusively seen in primary care settings (Katon & Gonzalez, 1994, Katon et al., 1995; Richardson et al., 1996). The primary care provider is often challenged to not only accurately diagnose mental health conditions but to treat these disorders. In 1989, the National Institute of Mental Health (American Psychiatric Association, *Diagnostic and statistical manual of mental disorders-IV*, 1994) initiated a series of meetings on how to diagnose and treat mental disorders in primary care. The resultant conversations began to bridge the gap between the professional organizations representing primary care and psychiatric care.

Various professional organizations have policy statements that encourage advanced training on mental health disorders within preservice primary care curricula and postservice continuing education programs (AAP, 1993). Nursing as a discipline has had a long tradition emphasizing the importance of integrating biopsychosocial aspects of health within nursing practice. Graduate programs for nurse practitioners have emphasized enriching primary care curricula with psychiatric knowledge and skills (Magyary & Brandt, 1998).

Growing Evidence in Support of Integration

The growing emphasis on the integration of primary and psychiatric care has occurred simultaneously with the scientific emphasis on the integration of the mind-body duality. Recent advancements in science support the conceptualization of wellness and health as a dynamic integration of the mind and body expressed through complex systems using terms such as biobehavioral, biopsychosocial, and neurobehavioral. The design of health service delivery systems needs to acknowledge and enhance the vital interplay between the physical and mental aspects of health. Too often, one system of care treats physical problems and another system treats mental problems without a systematic integration of both aspects of health. And yet a growing body of scientific evidence suggests that physical and mental health may directly or indirectly influence each other. Blount (1998) notes that the majority of patients do not dichotomize their health concerns as either psychological or biophysical, but rather view health as an integrative mind-body undifferentiated entity. Patients are more satisfied with primary care that is based on an integrated concept of health that fits how they present their symptoms, often resulting in better adherence to treatment regimes which leads to better outcomes (Blount, 1998).

Within the past 15 years, with the reorganization of the health care service delivery system, an increased number of studies have been funded to examine the *efficacy and cost effectiveness* of assessment and intervention protocols that interface primary care and psychiatry. Katon et al. (1992) note that primary care patients with mental health disorders are often associated with patterns of high utilization rates of health care services, medically unexplained somatic symptoms, a variety of chronic physical diseases, and significant functional disabilities (Katon et al., 1992).

Recent studies on the integration of primary care and mental health care services provide preliminary supportive evidence that patient care improves, thus resulting in better clinical outcomes as well as financial cost savings. Within pediatric populations, the benefits of primary care-based psychological consultation services that included individualized brief targeted therapy for common school, behavior, and psychosomatic problems resulted in significant improvement in functioning, high satisfaction in services, and a reduction in medical care utilization, especially acute primary care visits (Finney, Riley, & Cataldo, 1991).

Within adult populations, depression is one of the most commonly presented mental health disorders in primary care. The Agency for Health Care Policy and Research (1993) has funded studies to enhance the early detection and treatment of depression within the primary context. One such multifaceted intervention study designed to treat major depression based on a collaborative care model resulted in improved adherence to the treatment regimen, decreased depressive symptoms, and improved satisfaction with care in comparison to the "usual care" control group (Katon et al., 1995).

Likewise, other adult populations with mental conditions appear to benefit from integrating primary and psychiatric care. A primary care model using psychiatric consultation service applied to primary care patients who have a chronic pattern of subthreshold somatization syndrome resulted in significant improvement in physical functioning while simultaneously reducing medical care costs (Smith, Rost, & Kashner, 1995). The results provided promising evidence that even minimal contact through consultation may have therapeutic value for guiding primary care providers in their early detection and treatment of subthreshold mental health conditions as well as decreasing medical costs. However, the minimalist consultation service approach for patients who exhibit symptoms above threshold and thus present with somatization disorders may require a more elaborate intervention involving group treatment and thus a different collaborative psychiatric model.

Even a more elaborate psychiatric consultation service consisting of a single in-depth evaluation session accompanied with written treatment protocols to be implemented by the primary care provider with patients characterized as "psychiatrically impaired high users of health care" did not necessarily improve psychiatric status nor decrease utilization. Different *health care* utilization patterns may require differential models of collaboration ranging from screening to more elaborate services involving short-term collaborative psychiatric care with the primary care provider. Consideration also need to be given to the chronicity and severity of the mental health disorder coupled with the risk/protective profile of family/environmental factors. Perhaps a subgroup of patients require more intensive psychiatric services conducted by psychiatric professionals within the primary care clinic.

Models of Integrated Care

The majority of empirically tested models of integrative care entailed two components (a) advanced training of primary care providers and (b) availability of psychiatric services integrated within primary care services. Primary care providers were involved in a training program that advanced their knowledge and skills to detect and treat mental disorders that commonly present in primary care. The emphasis on managed care and cost containment places the primary care provider at the center of the new health care system with an expansion of responsibilities to include the early detection of mental health disorders, the implementation of brief intervention for common mental health disorders, and the recognition for referral for more complicated mental health. The Primary Care Version of the Diagnostic and Statistical Manual of Mental Disorders (*DSM-IV-PC*, 1995) was developed as a user-friendly approach for diagnosing mental disorders in the primary care setting with an emphasis on clinical, educational, and research utility. However, primary care providers cannot be expected to address the full range of mental health disorders or very complex severe disorders, and yet referral is often not a viable option (Blount, 1998).

Some level of psychiatric care within the primary care clinic was a second commonality across the majority of the studies. The availability of psychiatric services ranged from a simple one-time consultation to a more elaborate in-depth assessment coupled with intervention, particularly for those patients who presented with more than one disorder or required adjustment in their therapeutic regimen. The differential use of on-site psychiatric services needs to be further studied and evaluated for its benefit to patients as well for its cost effectiveness and thus accessibility.

Future Questions for Research

Questions about the breadth and depth of psychiatric services integrated within primary care need to take into account variability attributed to (a) patient variables (type, severity, chronicity, and complexity of the mental disorders, occurrence of comorbid conditions; and the environmental context); (b) provider characteristics (level of training and expertise in mental health); and (c) health care system characteristics (structural and size characteristics including geographic rural versus urban location). Studies have shown that integration of primary and psychiatric care results in improved recognition and treatment of mental disorders in primary care; however the long-term impact on patient outcomes is less clear (Katon & Gonzales, 1994). With the advancement of sophisticated health services research, the type, level, intensity, and specificity of collaborative intervention models are being more carefully defined and measured, thus allowing for the examination of the interplay among the structure, process, and outcome variables as exemplified by Starfield's (1992) Primary Care Evaluation Model (Katon & Gonzales, 1994). Study protocols and designs that are multifaceted and complex would allow for the evaluation of more sophisticated questions on the design and benefits of integrated services.

DIANE MAGYARY

See also
MENTAL DISORDERS PREVENTION
MENTAL HEALTH POLICY

PSYCHODRAMA IN NURSING

Definition of Psychodrama

Psychodrama facilitates insight and cognitive, emotional, and behavioral integration; shifts attitudes; and develops new skills. Before psychotropic drugs were available, it was actually used by Moreno to manipulate psychotic delusions so that the patients' behaviors would be less bothersome to the community. Now psychodrama is used as an adjunctive therapy, helping patients to identify and handle interpersonal conflicts that arise as a result of being mentally ill. It is also useful with healthy individuals who want to increase the quality of their relationships.

Although psychodrama was originally created as a form of group psychotherapy, its techniques can be incorporated into individual treatment by nurses in both inpatient and outpatient settings. Visintainer and Wolfer (1979) illustrate how nurses can help patient's cope by rehearsing behavior. They present what is known in psychodrama as the role-training technique (Hale, 1985, p. 58). The purpose of role training is to provide the kind of insight that occurs through enactment about potential conflicts and alternative ways of interacting. It also serves as a rehearsal for living. Role training has a pre- and posttest built into the process. At the beginning the protagonist enacts how he approaches a situation, and at the end he reenacts the same situation incorporating what he has learned.

Although a variety of mental health professionals become psychodramatists, psychiatric nurses are especially well suited for this advanced practice certification specialty. In contrast to physicians, whose main concern is diagnosing and treating illness, nurses help patients to respond to the effects of illness and treatments. Psychodrama, which enhances empathy and improves relationships, can play a vital part in strengthening support systems necessary in the process of preventing illness and maintaining and promoting health.

Nurses have made significant contributions to psychodrama practice and to bringing psychodramatic methods into nursing education and research. Nurses have also introduced innovations in the use of psychodrama with special populations. Drew (1991) describes how her psychodramatic work using role reversal, self-presentation, psychodramatic encounter and sociometric exercises decreased isolation and interaction and support among chronic mental patients in a day treatment program.

Using process theory (Sabelli, 1989) as a unifying framework, Raaz, Carlson-Sabelli, and Sabelli (1992) have suggested ways to use psychodrama with patients who have dissociative disorders. Carlson-Sabelli (1999) has incorporated psychodramatic techniques with puppet play to create a Therapeutic Puppet Theatre for abused and traumatized children, also a process theory approach. This approach provides a method for assessing the effects of trauma and abuse while at the same time broadening the range of expression of feelings and presenting options for new behavior.

Psychodrama is used in nursing education to diminish anxiety, promote empathy, learn alternative ways of handling situations, and explore issues. The use of psychodrama in nursing education of senior baccalaureate nursing students has been well described by Drew (1990). Psychodrama is not only a powerful means of psychotherapy, it is a powerful way to learn.

Drew (1993) also introduced reenactment interviewing based on the psychodramatic role reversal as a method for phenomenological research. She reports the use of this method (Drew, 1997) to explore the nature of nurses' meaningful experiences with patients and to discover how these nurses recognized and understood the significance of these experiences. She reports that understanding what the nurse finds personally meaningful when caring for patients leads to increased self-awareness. This awareness promotes empathy and engagement and mitigates depersonalization associated with contemporary health care.

Nurses also contributed to development of sociodynamics, a recent offspring of sociometry (Carlson-Sabelli, Sabelli, & Hale, 1994; Sabelli & Carlson-Sabelli, 1995). Sociodynamics expands sociometry by applying catastrophe theory and additional methods of nonlinear dynamics to study processes that are too complex to be studied with metric methods. Sociodynamics enriches sociometry by studying conflicting motivations and emotions and measuring the complex, contradictory nature of the dynamics underlying choice. Sociodynamics also broadens sociometry by studying trajectories of patterns of change in human interactions over time and in open groups. Researchers have empirically demonstrated that preferences are more predictable than choices, suggesting that preference data rather than choice data should be used when measuring interpersonal perceptual accuracy (Carlson-Sabelli, Sabelli, Patel, & Holm, 1992).

Kipper (1986) has made a substantial contribution to the knowledge base about the therapeutic value of psychodramatic interventions. His book *Psychotherapy through clinical role playing* serves as a clinical guide for practitioners who use clinical role playing in treatment, even though they do not consider themselves psychodramatists. Evidence supporting the use of psychodramatic techniques is integrated throughout this scholarly work.

Role-reversal (Moreno, 1959) is considered the cornerstone of psychodrama. In a concept analysis and reinterpretation of the research literature on the psychodramatic role reversal technique, Carlson-Sabelli found that 91% of the research is about sociodramatic role reversal—exchanging roles with fantasy characters or generalized others, rather than real people. Reported here is evidence that the sociodramatic role reversal promotes attitude shift and decreases anger and aggressive attitudes toward specific others with whom one has an unresolved conflict. It brings individuals who hold opposing attitudes closer together if their initial positions are compatible, but it forces them apart if their initial positions are incompatible. Role reversal also has been shown to promote loss of inhibition and increases self disclosure (Kipper & Har-Evan, 1984).

The effectiveness of psychodrama in the treatment of mental illness has not been well researched. There are no studies indicating that psychodrama as a therapeutic modality is effective in increasing the quality of interpersonal interactions of psychiatric patients. These studies are very much needed. Tools necessary to conduct these studies have recently become available.

In designing research it is important to acknowledge that psychodrama does not cure mental illness. If one agrees that psychodrama facilitates participants in identifying and changing patterns of relating, freeing them to encounter others spontaneously, it becomes possible to consider ways to measure these outcomes. One might also want to compare the effects of psychodrama treatment with other adjunctive therapies, purporting to do the same thing with patients who are well stabilized in their individual medication regimes.

In addition, each psychodrama session has a life of its own and has different meaning and impact on each of the patients in the group. It is not enough to describe the intervention as "psychodrama." Rather it is necessary to capture qualitative elements in a psychodrama session. Tracking tools necessary to conduct these studies are available.

Interpersonal profile trajectory plots (Carlson-Sabelli & Sabelli, 1992), coupled with two tools that track process elements of a psychodrama session, the Hollander curve (Hollander, 1969), which depicts the rise and fall of emotion and intensity of catharsis and the Goldman spiral diagram (Goldman & Morrison, 1984), which diagrams the content, sequence, and depth of scenes from periphery to core and back, provide tools to answer questions concerning crucial questions of efficacy such as "Does psychodrama treatment contribute to the development of new patterns of relating in interpersonal relationships?"

Remer and Betts (1997) have introduced interpersonal psychodramatic simulation (IPS) methods of research. These methods also arise from nonlinear dynamics (Remer, 1997) and will become important in future research of human dynamic systems.

LINNEA CARLSON-SABELLI

See also
CREATIVE ARTS
INTERPERSONAL COMMUNICATION

PSYCHOSOCIAL ADJUSTMENT AND THE FAMILY

According to the World Health Organization, the family in most societies is under severe pressure to survive as a unit. In industrialized nations, the destructive forces include economic factors, single parents doing the work of two, physical and emotional illnesses that cripple the well-being of the family. Whereas in third-world countries, the issues may be categorized as sheer survival. In most cultures, the family, as the core social unit, provides for basic physical needs, and in a broader sense, the opportunity for emotional interaction that contributes to individual psychological, social, and cultural development.

In recent decades, the definition and purpose of family have changed substantially. Still, a family may be conceptualized as "a social context of two or more people characterized by mutual attachment, caring, . . . commitment, and responsibility to provide for individual growth, supportive relationships, health of members and of the unit, and maintenance of the organization and system during constant individual, family and societal change" (Craft & Willadsen, 1992).

If the family is considered to be the core social unit, and if the stressors imposed on it are recognized, the need to study and articulate what can be learned about families in health and illness, how they cope—or don't cope—and how to care for them effectively is urgent. Although families are burdened with care of persons afflicted with old age, childhood disabilities, chronic illness, and disease, Gillis (1991) contends that "very little data exist to suggest nursing interventions that affect families. Rather, we have been successful in showing that when we intervene with families we improve outcomes for individuals."

Gillis warns that "while improving individual health may be reason enough to intervene with families as clients, we need more well-conceptualized family nursing intervention studies in which the outcome for the family is adequately measured."

A literature search revealed a plethora of studies in which psychosocial outcomes and predictors were examined, as well as interventions. Key terms, such as adaptation/psychological, social support, stress/psychological, family relations/ spouses/caregivers, chronic disease/chronic illness, led to many citations in Medline, Social Science Citations, CINAHL, PsychInfo, and Dissertation Abstracts. By narrowing the search to nursing, the citations could be organized in categories. The categories with exemplar studies are presented below. Many studies that deserve citation are not included due to space constraints. Key words that are indicative of aspects of adjustment are shown in bold print.

Psychosocial Family Adjustment and Children

Infancy and early childhood constitutes the focus of many studies. Harrison and Magill-Evans (1996) compared mothers and fathers of 54 term infants with 49 preterm infants by observing interaction with the infant in the home during a structured task when the child was 3 and 12 months old. Parents of preterm infants had lower **interaction** scores than parents of term infants. Fathers of both term and preterm infants had lower interaction scores than mothers. The investigators suggest that the results need to be considered in relation to other research findings to prevent premature stereotyping and the vulnerable child syndrome.

Pridham, Schroeder, Brown, Nyamathi, Wenzel, Keenan, Leake, and Gelberg (1999) suggest that "**adaptiveness**" of a mother's caregiving behavior is related to sensitivity to her infant's needs and preferences and to her appropriate, creative, mature **responsiveness** to her infant" (p. 472). The authors compared 44 mothers of full-term infants to 33 mothers of premature infants at four time points, 1, 4, 8, and 12 months postterm. The highest adaptiveness scores were at 4 months and the lowest at 8 months. At 8 months, the mother's education had a significant positive effect on adaptiveness, mother's symptoms of **depression** had a negative effect, and infant weight-for-age had a positive effect.

Children with disabilities, acute illness, and chronic disease have major implications for parents, the family as a unit, and health care providers. When mothers of children with Down's Syndrome believe, for example, that their family's relationship with health care providers is positive and family centered, they feel more satisfied with the care that their child is receiving and they are more likely to seek help from providers (Van Riper, 1999). Higher levels of individual and family **well-being** are reported by mothers who (a) want, and believe they have, positive **family-centered relationships** with providers; and (b) feel more satisfied with care received. Van Riper suggests that the results contribute to a better understanding of the role that health care providers play in individual and family **adaptation** to chronic conditions.

Theoretical frameworks of adaptation are emerging as guides to nursing interventions. For example, a review of literature related to **psychosocial adaptation** in childhood epilepsy led to a model for psychosocial nursing practice (Austin, 1996). Several instruments for assessing need for psychosocial nursing care are recommended. Clawson (1996) also conceptualized family **adaptation** to a child with chronic illness as a continual developmental **process of adjustment** and **change** in a family system. Family responses occur across a continuum from optimal to ineffective adaptation.

The nursing literature reflects an increasing focus on interventions with studies to evaluate effects. For example, Melnyk, Alpert-Gillis, Hensel, Cable-Beiling, and Rubenstein (1997) conducted a pilot test of the effects of an intervention program (COPE = creating opportunities for parent empowerment) on critically ill children in a pediatric intensive care unit and their mothers. The findings suggested positive effects among mothers, that is, they (a) provided more support to their children during intrusive procedures, (b) provided more **emotional support** to their children, (c) reported less negative **mood** state and less parental **stress** related to their children's emotions and behaviors, and (d) reported fewer **posttraumatic stress symptoms** and less parental **role change**.

If childhood death is the outcome, Moriarty, Carroll, and Cotroneo (1996) contend that differences in **distress** within couples who experience sudden death of a child require attention. In their samples of couples, women had significantly greater global distress than men and significantly greater distress in most symptom dimensions that were identified. **Hostility** scores within couples, which were high, were similar. The authors suggest that the findings may be indicative of basic **relationship** problems requiring intervention.

Psychosocial Family Adjustment and Elders

The effect of chronic life-threatening illness on the family is a major problem confronting the present day health care system. Increasingly, family members must assume responsibility for daily management of care, a burden that has a significant effect on family **psychosocial adjustment**. In a qualitative study of six family members, six hospitalized elders, and four nurses by Li, Stewart, Imle, Archbold, and Felver (2000) three domains were identified: family members **providing care** to the patient, **working together** with the health care team, and **taking care** of themselves. The authors hypothesize that all three dimensions of family care actions need to be present for successful family care of elders when hospitalized.

The emphasis on **caregiver burden** is prominent. Conceptualizing caregiver burden as the effect of stressors on family members caring for a physically or mentally ill person, Faison, Faria, and Frank (1999) studied 88 caregivers of elderly chronically ill persons. Increased activities of care performed by the caregiver was positively correlated with caregiver burden. Sons as caregivers reported significantly less burden than did daughters or other relatives. The authors concluded that community health and home health nurses must be able to recognize those factors associated with caregiver burden to effectively render care to clients as individuals and families as units. Consistent with this recommendation, an examination of how patterns in risk for **depression** over 1 year among 188 dementia caregivers suggested that objective (**behavior problems** of the relative) and subjective (**role captivity** and overload) factors constitute primary **stressors** as predictors (Alspaugh, Stephens, Townsend, Zarit, & Greene, 1999).

These findings support a main principle set forth by Gillis (1991), that is, in promoting psychosocial adjustment among families, the individual patient must be treated in the context of the family system. Schumacher (1996), therefore, reconceptualized family caregiving using a grounded theory approach. An investigation of the family caregiver role acquisition among 19 family caregivers and 20 persons with cancer, interviewed across the course of chemotherapy, indicated that **caregiving** could not be understood in isolation from **self-care**. **Patterns** of involvement fluctuated **over time** in both self-care and caregiving. The reconceptualization emphasized the dyadic nature of family-based illness care and change over time.

Needs of caregivers include information on community services, strategies to improve their ability to manage their relatives' care, and perhaps individual counseling to address diverse needs and specific goals (Larsen, 1999). Ultimately, the relative may require placement in a nursing home. Care of a family member with dementia, and perhaps institutionalization, are extremely difficult emotionally. Therefore, studies of the impact on caregivers of persons with Alzheimer's disease are prominent. Winslow (1997) examined whether **formal support** and **coping** would mediate the effects of primary **stressors** and caregiver characteristics on **yielding the role**, **anxiety**, and **physical health**. The data suggested that decreased physical health of the caregiver was best explained by caregiver overload. **Anxiety** was explained by lower levels of care receiver dependency, higher levels of caregiver overload, and higher levels of caregiver anxiety measured 1 year later. Yielding of the caregiver role was explained by the direct effect of higher levels of care receiver problem behaviors as well as more use of formal supports. **Spouse relationship** had a negative effect and **care receiver dependency** had a positive effect on yielding of the role through the mediating influence of formal support, thus reinforcing the important role of health care providers.

It is interesting to note the "cutting edge" research in which older caregivers of spouses with dementia exhibited increased activation of the hypothalamic-pituitary-adrenal axis and a **poor antibody response** to an influenza vaccine (Vedhara et al., 1999), indicating greater vulnerability to infectious disease than the population of a similar age. The authors conclude that the **poor immune response** to influenza virus vaccination in **chronically stressed** caregivers can be attributed to a compromised immune system.

Psychosocial Family Adjustment and Illness

With changes in health care delivery and cost, hospital stays are shorter, and patients are discharged with higher levels of acuity. The impact on family adjustment to breast cancer among partners of patients include, for example, levels of **emotional distress** and **mood disturbance** at 3 days and 18 months postsurgery, which differ significantly from population means (Northouse, 1989a). Higher levels of emotional distress and lower levels of **adjustment** among partners as compared to patients have been noted to continue for as long as 3 years (Baider & Kaplan-DeNour, 1984). As the person most intimately involved in the events related to an illness and treatment, partners attempt to **cope** with **fear** of the illness and **demands** that the illness places on their lives. As demands escalate, increased **depression** among partners poses issues in **marital adjustment** (Lewis, Woods, Hough, & Bensley, 1989).

Although a male partner is often identified in a family as the person most closely associated with the woman facing a diagnosis of breast cancer and treatment, patients who are single, divorced, or widowed must seek **support** from other sources. Conceptualizing **psychosocial adjustment** as the perceived impact of thc diagnosis and treatment of breast cancer on the **vocational**, **domestic**, **social**, **sexual**, and **emotional** aspects of life, Budin (1998) noted that **social support** and **symptom distress** were significant predictors of psychosocial adjustment among 101 unmarried women in the late postoperative recovery phase.

Intervention studies include the work of Samarel, Fawcett, and Tulman (1997), who studied the effect of support groups with coaching on **adaptation** to early stage breast cancer. The intervention consisted of an 8-week cancer support group (CSG) with and without coaching. CSG with coaching resulted in a higher quality of **relationship with the significant other**. However, CSG had no effect on **symptom distress**, **emotional distress**, or **functional status**.

Emerging from these investigations is the critical factor of time and **change** over the course of diagnosis, treatment, and recovery. **Psychosocial adjustment** of partners/spouses of patients with cancer may be characterized by **stages** of **the illness trajectory**, that is, time of diagnosis, period of first remission, first recurrence, and period of metastatic disease (Morse & Fife, 1998). Hoskins et al. (1996) identified four **phases** in the breast cancer experience as diagnostic, postsurgical, adjuvant therapy, and ongoing recovery, concluding that phase-specific health care is essential in promoting **emotional and physical adjustment** in both the patient and the family. Pasacreta and Pickett (1998) also concluded from a review of literature that the majority of cancer patients experience **emotional turmoil** at transition points along the illness trajectory. Patients and families confront **psychosocial issues** that are influenced by **individual**, **sociocultural**, **medical**, and **family** factors.

It may be concluded that the increase in chronic disease with shortened hospitalizations is accompanied by an increase in home care, with added **adjustment problems** for both patients and their families. As noted by Penninx et al. (1998), the effect of **psychosocial coping resources** on **depressive symptoms** among older persons with no chronic disease is more positive as compared to persons with recently symptomatic diabetes mellitus, lung disease, cardiac disease, arthritis, or cancer. **Having a partner**, many **close relationships**, greater **feelings of mastery**, greater **self-efficacy expectations**, and high **self-esteem** have a direct favorable effect on **depressive symptoms**.

It has been noted that common effects of a mental disorder on a caregiver are within the marital **relationship** and **home management** arenas. Laidlaw, Falloon, Barnfathner, and Coverdale (1999) found that 28% of caregivers of persons with an obsessive compulsive disorder were severely **burdened** by their care provider role, and 35% were extremely **distressed** at the prospect of ongoing care provision. According to the authors, caregivers require **support**, and may be considered to be consumers of mental health services themselves. Similarly, the **psychological well-being** of patients with a physical disorder, such as, multiple sclerosis, and their entire family is critically important to **successful rehabilitation** of the patient (Taylor & Taylor, 1998). In both emotional and physical disease, a **sense of control** in the context of chronic illness is impacted by the patient's perceived control over symptoms (PCS) and progression of the disease (PCDP), which in turn affects patient and caregiver outcomes (Wallhagen & Brod, 1997). Control over symptoms is, therefore, significantly associated with **patient well-being**, and **caregiver well-being**.

Family Psychosocial Adjustment and Cultural Diversity

Cultural diversity must also be included in theoretical frameworks for nursing interventions. In a study by Waters (1999), family members' expected **support** from critical care nurses according to **cultural affiliation** of African American, Hispanic, or White as measured by the Professional Support Questionnaire for Critical Care Nurses Working with Family Members (PSQ) indicated that although responses from family members waiting to visit a critically ill relative admitted to the intensive care unit differed significantly on some items, universal values of equitable care, dignity, and respect emerged. The author concluded that nursing interventions that respect cultural uniqueness, as well as universal needs of family members coping with an ill family member, need to be developed.

Conclusions

Intervention studies for families pose a number of theoretical and methodological problems. The issues for families confronted with the crisis of a potentially lethal diagnosis are extremely complex, cross all cultures, and affect the family as a whole system. Usual roles are altered with outcomes of **interpersonal tension** in both patients and partners. Partner levels of interpersonal tension and **somatic symptoms** often are equal to, or greater than, that of the patient, indicating the enormous complexity of the interrelationship of partners' **physical, emotional, and social adjustment** in families.

The distinction between family-as-context and family-as-patient is important. The family-as-context means that nursing interventions are delivered to an individual member within the social context of the family, whereas family-as-client, or patient, means that assessment, planning, intervention, and evaluation occurs for the family unit as a whole. When addressing the latter, questions related to psychosocial adjustment in the family are pertinent. Can a nurse focus on the family while dealing with individuals? How receptive are family members to the care nursing offers the family? What influences this receptivity? What characteristics of the health care system enhance the delivery of family nursing services? What are the significant psychosocial outcomes of family nursing? What are the actual costs of family caregiving? What are the costs of replacement services and lost opportunities due to illness or compromised health in the burdened caretaker?

As indicated in the present brief review of studies, the identification of constructs thought to be indicative of psychosocial adjustment, and their conceptualizations, vary enormously. Predictors of psychosocial adjustment are equally varied and include satisfaction with health care, life stress unrelated to the illness, demographic characteristics, stage of the disease, time since diagnosis, current treatment and side effects, initial emotional status, prior psychiatric morbidity, and social support. A move toward greater consistency in constructs, with valid and reliable instruments for measurement, would enhance the progress in development of interventions. Finally, alternate forms of instruments would permit assessments to capture the important changes that occur over time.

CAROL NOLL HOSKINS

See also
PSYCHOSOCIAL ADJUSTMENT
STRESS
STRESS MANAGEMENT

PSYCHOSOCIAL INTERVENTIONS

The health outcomes of clients may be improved through psychosocial or psychoeducational interventions. Psychosocial interventions include individual and group psychotherapies and educational interventions. An intervention may be defined as a programmatic attempt at altering the course of some life span developmental phenomenon. Interventions may be classified as concrete technologies involving such parameters as the goal: enrichment, prevention, or alleviation; the target behavior: cognition, social interactions, or attitude; the setting: family, classroom, community, or hospital; and the mechanism: training-practice, psychotherapy, or health delivery (Baltes & Danish, 1980).

Nurses are implementing psychosocial and psychoeducational interventions and testing the results of their efforts for many health problems and chronic illnesses. There are a number of integrative literature reviews, including meta-analyses conducted by nurse researchers. Meta-analyses will be reviewed to provide depth and breadth to this summary.

Surgical Patients

Devine and Cook (1986) evaluated 49 studies for the effect of brief psychoeducational interventions on the length of postsurgical hospitalization. The interventions consisted of information, skills training, and psychosocial support and were provided by nurses, physicians, psychologists, pastoral counselors, and social workers. The results showed that these interventions had a positive influence on recovery, pain, psychological well-being, and satisfaction with care among hospitalized adult surgery patients. Not only did these patients have better outcomes; there were positive cost effects across a wide range of patients, treatment providers, and hospital settings. The interventions reduced the hospital stay on average by 1 1/4 days.

Hypertensive Patients

In a meta-analysis of 102 studies, Devine and Reifschneider (1995) evaluated the effects of psychoeducational care on blood pressure, knowledge about hypertension, medication compliance, weight, compliance with health care appointments, and anxiety. A nurse was the primary author in 23% of the studies. Three psychoeducational interventions—education, behavioral monitoring, and relaxation—had small to medium benefits for blood pressure. Usually, the nonrelaxation interventions were directed to promoting adherence and were conducted in outpatient health care facilities. The majority of participants were taking antihypertensive medications, and blood pressure measurement was part of the routine care. In studies with relaxation only and relaxation with biofeedback, the interventions occurred in lab-type settings, and subjects were not taking antihypertensive medications.

Cancer Patients

Devine and Westlake (1995) evaluated psychoeducational intervention studies provided to 5,326 adults with cancer by means of meta-analysis. In this review the results were analyzed to determine how educational and psychosocial care provided to adults with cancer affected seven outcomes: anxiety, depression, mood, nausea, vomiting, pain, and knowledge. A nurse was the primary author in 34% of the studies. The authors found a statistically significant beneficial effect for all seven outcomes. However, it was not possible to determine which type of psychoeducational care—for example, education, muscle relaxation, other relaxation, muscle relaxation with guided imagery, multiple behavioral interventions with relaxation, or education and relaxation—was the most beneficial.

Caregivers

Taft (1995) in a qualitative study interviewed 40 family and professional caregivers with the aim of describing and classifying the specific interventions that could be used as alternatives to physical and chemical restraints in dementia care. She found seven domains of caregiving approaches: (a) social (providing activities, relating, empathic caring, and supportive touching); (b) psychological (being responsive, seeing the world from the recipient's perspective, offering choices, following the recipient's lead, and reframing); (c) functional (assisting with activities of daily living, providing cues, providing supervision, providing rest periods, and assisting with instrumental activities of daily living); (d) behavioral (diversion, noninterference, going along, time-away, delaying, confrontation, and using fibs); (e) environmental (modifying stimuli, providing safety, limiting access, providing personal identification, and using signs); (f) medical (using psychotropic and other medications); and (g) cognitive (helping to remember and reorienting).

Relaxation Training

Hyman, Feldman, Harris, Levin, and Malloy (1989) reviewed 48 experimental studies of nonmechanically assisted, educational relaxation techniques to control a variety of clinical symptoms. Treatment interventions consisted of nonpharmacological methods, such as Benson's relaxation technique, Jacobson's progressive muscle relaxation, rhythmic breathing, Lamaze, autogenic training, hypnosis, transcendental meditation, yoga, Zen, and imagery. Biofeedback was included only when an alternative relaxation technique was used as an additional treatment in the study because biofeedback requires complicated technology not readily available to practicing nurses. Subjects suffered from chronic continuous or acute clinical symptoms, and the average age was 41. In summary, all treatments except Benson's relaxation technique demonstrated positive results for chronic problems such as insomnia, headaches, and hypertension.

Technology Interventions

The use of computers as a psychosocial intervention is a novel idea in nursing. The findings from studies in two populations of caregivers of the elderly with Alzheimer's disease and persons living with AIDS are innovative (Brennan, Moore, & Smyth, 1995; Ripich, Moore, & Brennan, 1992). A project nurse monitored each of the Computer Links and was seen as a group facilitator and a troubleshooter for the participants. The nurse read all public areas daily and maintained the currency of the electronic encyclopedia. In this role the nurse moderator interacted with users via typed messages by reviewing all public messages and also reviewed any personal mail and typed responses to individuals or to the group. There were 102 Alzheimer's disease caregivers, who averaged two encounters per week for sessions lasting an average of 13 minutes. The decision-making confidence of the caregivers was enhanced through this unique psychosocial intervention. There were 31 persons living with AIDS who used the network for catharsis and self-disclosure. They identified group cohesiveness with their new family as very important. Overall, persons living with AIDS with high rates of Computer Link use expressed high levels of satisfaction with the network.

Psychosocial and psychoeducational interventions are a primary method of improving the health of clients and patients entrusted to nurses' care. There is a beginning knowledge base, documented on the outcomes of these interventions to improve the health status of individuals. Nurse scientists and practitioners must continue to develop, test, and document the effects of these interventions and their impact on phenomena of concern to nursing.

GRAHAM J. MCDOUGALL

See also

COGNITIVE INTERVENTIONS

QUALITY OF LIFE

Quality of life research is an extensive field, with scholars who have thought carefully about the parameters, indicators, diversity, and variability of the dimensions of quality of life (Benner, 1985; Spilker, Simpson, & Tilson, 1991). However, there is no universally accepted definition of quality of life. A consensus among researchers seems to be that its components should include a person's satisfaction with his or health and function, economic status, family life, and spiritual, occupational, and psychosocial well-being. The scope of the research typically includes a general assessment of perceived well-being and subsets of health-related components of quality of life. General overall assessment of quality of life typically gauges the health and functional abilities of the person; the health-related aspects are often measured as symptom experiences, disease management, economic effect of disease and treatment, and level of wellness.

Definitions of quality of life vary greatly. Early studies measured patient functional capacity, illness status, and longevity. Currently, components measured include impact of an illness and its treatment, socioeconomic status, and cultural or personal characteristics influencing a person's ability to have a fulfilling life. Many researchers now use a health-related framework that defines quality of life as measures of rehabilitation following disease or disability. Rehabilitation indexes often use measures of a person's ability to carry out routines of daily living and roles of life (e.g., homemaker, employee, student).

Numerous measures that represent quality of life have been developed, and many of the early definitions were unidimensional. Early definitions of quality of life were often measures or ratings of physical function made by the physician. Both the unidimensional and the outside rater approaches to measurement of quality of life have been criticized as too simplistic as well as inaccurate. Nurse researchers indicate that qualitative methods are preferable to questionnaires. However, the ability to follow changes over time by using quantitative methods is important for researchers (Jalowiec, 1992). Utilizing quantitative methods is also appropriate with large sample sizes. Discussions about the validity of using subjective versus objective measures of quality of life have ended in the notion that both are available but must be discussed in relation to the purpose of the research study.

In the 1980s the Adjusted Quality of Life Years Utility Index was developed (Torrance, 1987). This formula-oriented definition of quality of life included the cost of medical treatments over the expected number of years survival and patients' preferences for living with the treatment. This approach and definition added the economic factor and the individual's opinions to quality of life measures. The World Health Organization's 1995 position paper on quality of life assessment broadens the view of quality of life beyond health without illness.

The current regulations by the Food and Drug Administration requiring quality of life to be a component of drug studies have resulted in numerous specific and narrow measures of medication efficacy, commonly using single-item indicators and linear analog scales. Many instruments have been developed for specific populations of patients, resulting in illness-, functions-, and symptom-oriented measures that reflect treatment outcomes (Smith, 1993).

Nurse researchers and others have expanded the definitions of quality of life to include a person's satisfaction with health and function, economic status, family life, occupation, and psychosocial well-being (Padilla et al., 1983). In 1989 the Institute of Medicine staff published a monograph on the quality of life measures they recommended for use. Padilla's quality of life instrument for cancer patients was the only nurse-authored questionnaire in the monograph. Medical studies and clinical trials have often employed health-rating scales. Judgment analysis also has been used in assessing quality of life (McGee, O'Boyle, Hickey, O'Malley, & Joyce, 1991).

In a unique instrument, Ferrans and Powers (1992) measured not only a person's satisfaction with health, family, economic status, and psychospiritual well-being but also measured the importance of each of those areas to the person. This comparison between importance and satisfaction ratings by the person better reflects quality of life unique to each individual's life goals. Self-comparison of importance versus satisfaction also allows for following changes in a patient's quality of life over time. One conclusion common to all researchers, in the past and currently, is that quality of life for individuals with incomes below the poverty line will be low, regardless of health and family status or self-perceived well-being.

The paradigm has shifted to a multifactoral basis of measurement: multiple variables which obtain a variety of subjective perceptions of each patient that go beyond the physical aspects of life. There are differences in a single-person quality of life measure, which measures personal function, and a community-oriented concept, which reflects the person's ability to have an effect on the greater society. Nurses have also expanded the notion of quality of life beyond the individual and his or her disease state. Research with family caregivers and discussion of family and community quality of life are being formulated for further study by the authors.

CAROL E. SMITH
CAROL GASKAMP

See also
PSYCHOSOCIAL ADJUSTMENT

RELAXATION TECHNIQUES

A relaxation technique is any intervention that produces the relaxation response. This response is characterized by decreases in blood pressure, pulse, respiratory rate, muscle tension, anxiety, and increases in skin temperature. Recent developments in the field of psychoneuroimmunology and society's renewed attention to holistic approaches to health care are expanding the parameters being examined as outcomes of relaxation techniques. Indices such as T lymphocyte and natural killer cell (NK) counts are being used to measure outcomes of relaxation interventions. In the past, nurses tended to measure only psychological outcomes, such as anxiety, as outcomes of relaxation training interventions. However, an increasing number of stress management studies conducted by nurse researchers are measuring both psychological and physiological parameters (Hyman, Feldman, Harris, Levin, & Malloy, 1989; Snyder, 1997).

Since the pioneering work of Edmund Jacobson on progressive muscle relaxation in the 1930s, numerous interventions that produce the relaxation response have been identified. Commonly used relaxation techniques include autogenic therapy, biofeedback, humor, imagery, music, massage, progressive muscle relaxation, sensation information, and therapeutic touch.

Nurses, along with researchers in the biobehavioral sciences, have conducted research about the efficacy of many of these techniques. Although an increasing number of studies using relaxation interventions are being conducted by nurses, few programs of research have evolved. Sensation information (Johnson, Rice, & Endress, 1978) and therapeutic touch (Quinn, 1984) are examples of interventions for which programs of research have evolved. Explorations by nurse researchers on the efficacy of imagery, massage, and music in reducing stress are increasing (Snyder, 1997). Eight studies on imagery were published in nursing journals during the 1991–95 time span, as well as seven studies using massage and four studies using music.

Despite the increase in the number of published reports, many studies continue to be characterized by small sample sizes and lack of methodological sophistication. Thus, a sound scientific basis to guide practitioners in selecting specific relaxation techniques for use with a client is lacking. Attention also must be given to other variables that may have an impact on study results. For example, in several studies on massage the results differed for male and female subjects (Snyder, 1997).

Another factor that impedes the development of a scientific basis for relaxation techniques is the widespread use of the term *relaxation training* without authors specifying the technique being tested. Because numerous techniques can be used to produce relaxation, it is important that descriptions of the techniques be provided to inform other researchers and practitioners of the outcomes from specific relaxation techniques. When multiple interventions are included, study designs should provide for the examination of each intervention.

Complementary therapies, which encompass many of the relaxation interventions, are being more widely accepted and used. Findings from well-constructed studies are needed to guide the use of such interventions. Nurse researchers can play a key role in furthering the scientific basis for relaxation interventions.

MARIAH SNYDER

See also
MUSIC THERAPY
STRESS MANAGEMENT

RESOURCEFULNESS

Resourcefulness involves the ability to maintain independence in daily tasks despite potentially adverse situations (i.e., learned resourcefulness) (Rosenbaum, 1990) and to seek help from others when unable to function independently (i.e., help-seeking behavior) (Nadler, 1990). Researchers report that elders who are socially resourceful and seek help from others have better psychological and physical health (Rapp, Shumaker, Schmidt, Naughton, & Anderson, 1998). However, older adults tend to be self-reliant and engage in self-care activities rather than seeking out formal or informal help, and hence they may not use their help-seeking skills to their best advantage. Elders with both high learned resourcefulness and help-seeking have been found to be less anxious or depressed and have better daily functioning than those high on learned resourcefulness alone or help-seeking behavior alone (Zauszniewski, 1996). Hence, both learned resourcefulness and help-seeking behavior are important for physical and psychological health and should be viewed as complementary, rather than as substitutes for one another (Nadler, 1990; Zauszniewski, 1996).

Resourcefulness is believed to be socially learned (Rosenbaum, 1990) and, therefore, can be taught. In a pilot study, the skills constituting learned resourcefulness were taught to healthy community-dwelling elders who improved in their performance in daily activities (Zauszniewski, 1997a). Currently, a 4-year clinical trial is examining the effectiveness of teaching learned resourcefulness (self-help) skills and help-seeking behaviors in elders with chronic conditions. The separate and combined effects of teaching self-help and help-seeking skills are being investigated in relation to the physical functioning and psychological well-being of elders.

Conceptualization

The cognitive-behavioral skills constituting learned resourcefulness are self-help strategies that are acquired through interaction with others and are used to control the potentially disturbing effects that certain internal processes, including cognitions, emotions, and sensations, may otherwise have on the performance of daily activities (Rosenbaum, 1990). Through formal or informal instruction, individuals acquire throughout life this basic repertoire of skills that enables them to cope independently (without the help of others) with stressful situations (Rosenbaum, 1990). Thus, learned resourcefulness refers specifically to internal resources rather than seeking external resources such as help from others.

The dimensions of learned resourcefulness include redressive self-control (e.g., use of positive self-instructions for thought, mood, and pain control), reformative self-control (e.g., problem-solving strategies and postponement of the need for instant gratification), and belief in coping effectiveness (perceived self-efficacy). While redressive self-control is directed at resuming normal functioning that has been disrupted, reformative self-control is directed at disrupting the customary way of functioning and adopting a new behavior (Rosenbaum, 1990). The perceived self-efficacy dimension refers to one's self-evaluation of the ability to attain the desired (health) goal.

Learned resourcefulness has been studied in adults with arthritis (Braden, McGlone, & Pennington, 1993), diabetes (White, Tata, & Burns, 1996), hypertension (Picot, Zauszniewski, & Delgado, 1997), cardiac problems (Doerfler, Pbert, & DeCosimo, 1997), cancer (Braden, Mishel, & Longman, 1998), and chronic pain (LeFort, Gray-Donald, Rowat, & Jeans, 1998). Using resourcefulness skills has been found to enhance health-promoting behaviors, including smoking cessation and curbing alcohol intake (Carey, Carey, Carnike, & Meisler, 1988) and changing eating habits (Kennett & Nisbet, 1998). Highly resourceful persons also have greater daily functioning, better daily task performance and social role functioning (Zauszniewski, 1994, 1995), and less anxiety and depression (Zauszniewski, 1997a). Although learned resourcefulness has been related to numerous positive health outcomes in adults, there is limited systematic investigation of the impact of learned resourcefulness in children and adolescence.

However, seeking help from others is another important strategy that can be used to overcome difficulties associated with illness and to promote physical and psychological health (Rapp et al., 1998). Help-seeking behavior refers to accessing resources external to the individual, rather than mobilizing internal resources (i.e., learned resourcefulness). Help-seeking behavior includes utilization of formal health services and informal help from family members. Among elderly persons the use of formal and informal support was found to reduce both physical and psychological symptoms (Blaum, Liang, & Liu, 1994).

Both learned resourcefulness and help-seeking behaviors are important for health promotion and therefore viewed as components of resourcefulness (Nadler, 1990; Zauszniewski, 1996). The findings from the clinical trial in progress will determine the separate and combined effects of teaching learned resourcefulness and help-seeking on physical and psychological health outcomes. While the combined effects of the two interventions are expected to be significantly greater than their individual (separate) effects, the results from the separate analyses of the two interventions (learned resourcefulness training and help-seeking behavior training) will indicate whether the combined effects are additive or interactive.

Operationalization

Learned resourcefulness has been consistently measured using the Self-Control Schedule (SCS) (Rosenbaum, 1980). The SCS consists of 36 Likert-type items using a 6-point scale. Subjects indicate the degree to which each item describes their behavior, ranging from extremely descriptive to extremely nondescriptive, and a higher composite score indicates greater resourcefulness. Internal consistency estimates ranged from .78 to .85 in adults, including samples of elders (Rosenbaum, 1990; Zauszniewski, 1997a). As theoretically expected, the SCS has moderate relationships with locus of control, religious orientation, anxiety (Rosenbaum, 1990), depressive cognitions, and psychosocial attributes (Zauszniewski, 1997b) to support its construct validity. Although there are few studies of children's resourcefulness, a measure for children that contains 32 items exists with an acceptable internal consistency coefficient of .78 and construct validity demonstrated through significant correlations with measures of social adjustment and depression (Rimon, 1980).

Though the SCS is a psychometrically sound measure of learned resourcefulness, it does not reflect the broader conceptualization of resourcefulness in which both self-help (learned resourcefulness) and help-seeking skills are essential. Therefore, to obtain an estimate for help-seeking behavior, Zauszniewski (1998) developed 12 additional items. The 12 additional items follow the same format as the SCS and ask respondents whether seeking help from others is descriptive of them in specific contexts. These items are embedded within the SCS measure and the psychometric properties of the revised measure, called the Resourcefulness Scale (Zauszniewski, 1998) are currently being tested in elders.

Intervention

Since resourcefulness skills are learned, principles of cognitive behavioral theory provide the framework for crafting interventions to teach the self-help (learned resourcefulness) and help-seeking behaviors. The interventions are short-term, structured, time-limited, and consist of six weekly 2-hour sessions with 10 to 12 individuals per group. Instructional techniques include coaching; modeling; rehearsal; performance feedback; shaping; and the use of praise, approval, and support. Nursing strategies such as assessment, education, motivation, guidance, and support enhance the instructional methods. The small group sessions incorporate group discussion, verbal instruction, handouts, and assignments between sessions. While learned resourcefulness skills and help-seeking behaviors may be taught in separate interventions, they may also be integrated into a single intervention program.

Learned resourcefulness training (LRT) teaches specific skills that include coping strategies, problem-solving, positive self-talk, priority setting, and decision-making. Help-seeking behavior training (HSBT) incorporates all means of seeking help from family, friends, clergy, health care professionals, counselors, and so on and focuses on encouraging, motivating, and inspiring both curative and preventive help-seeking to promote physical and psychological health. An intervention combining LRT and HSBT for elders focuses on current health-related issues that involve changes in health status or the aging process and the self-help (learned resourcefulness) and help-seeking skills that are appropriate to these issues.

For elders, the structured protocol uses their perception of their functional health status as a forum for identifying and discussing past successful coping skills that may be used to solve present problems. The problem-solving process is taught and applied to the use of both learned resourcefulness and help-seeking strategies. Teaching elders to seek help from others involves teaching them to differentiate normal, healthy aging from symptoms that are serious and warrant prompt attention. Upon making this distinction, elders are taught the priority-setting and decision-making skills that are a part of resourcefulness, and how these can be applied to particular situations. Specific guidelines are given to the elders for using resourcefulness skills and seeking out help from others who are available to them for preventive or curative (immediate) services.

Conclusion

It is reasonable to expect that highly resourceful individuals are the most healthy in physical functioning and psychological well-being. However, since it was first identified 20 years ago (Rosenbaum, 1990), resourcefulness has evolved from its original restricted focus on the use of internal resources and self-help skills to a broader conceptualization that encompasses help-seeking behaviors that involve the use of external resources (Nadler, 1990; Zauszniewski, 1996). After two decades, the context of resourcefulness research has progressed from healthy college students to adults with various psychological and physical conditions and to community-dwelling and chronically ill elders. In addition, research methods in studies of resourcefulness have evolved from standard psychometric studies to designs that characterize individuals with high or low resourcefulness to the investigation of predictive models to the testing of interventions that teach resourcefulness to elders. However, in general, studies of resourcefulness in children and adolescents are few, and many opportunities in this area exist.

JACLENE A. ZAUSZNIEWSKI

See also
NURSE-PATIENT INTERACTION
NURSE-PATIENT RELATIONSHIP

SELF-EFFICACY

Bandura's (1997) general self-efficacy construct provides a useful explanation for how people exercise influence over their own motivation and behavior. Perceived self-efficacy refers to beliefs in one's capabilities to organize and execute the courses of action required to produce given attainments. This influence may entail regulating one's motivation, thought processes, affective states, and actions; or it may involve changing environmental conditions, depending on what one seeks to manage. Self-efficacy judgments determine the behavior to be chosen and affect the amount of effort one devotes to a task, as well as the duration of one's persistence when difficulties are encountered. Bandura postulated four principal sources of self-efficacy information: (a) enactive mastery experiences that serve as indicators of capability; (b) vicarious experiences that alter efficacy beliefs through transmission of competencies and comparison with the attainments of others; (c) verbal persuasion (and allied types of social influences) that one possesses certain capabilities, and (d) physiological and affective states from which people partly judge their capability, strength, and vulnerability to dysfunction.

According to Bandura (1997), efficacy beliefs vary across activity domains, levels of demands within the domains, and different environmental circumstances of performance. Therefore, self-efficacy in psychosocial functioning is best determined by measures tailored to particular domains of functioning rather than by a global test. Self-efficacy scales must reflect these dimensions in their measurement and should include level, generality, and strength. Levels of task demands represent varying degrees of challenge or impediment to successful performance. These levels predict routine activities to be carried out regularly. Self-efficacy strength is a measure of an individual's ability to execute the requisite activity at different levels of task demands. The strength domains are presented as "can do" rather than "will do" because *can* is a measure of capability, whereas *will* is a statement of intention. Nursing knowledge of various developmental phenomena and life course events in health and illness has increased, using the construct of self-efficacy as an outcome or an intervention strategy incorporated into a nursing model.

Pender and Pender (1987) developed the health promotion model to explain the occurrence of behaviors directed toward increasing the level of wellness, rather than behaviors targeted specifically to decreasing the probability of illness. The health promotion model is a synthesis of findings from studies on factors related to health-promoting behaviors, and the model attempts to explain why individuals engage in health actions. Pender's model is appropriate for continued investigation because, being derived from social learning theory, it stresses the importance of cognitive mediating processes in behavior regulation.

Determinants of the health promotion model are cognitive-perceptual factors, modifying factors, and variables affecting the likelihood of action. The modifying factors indirectly influencing patterns of health behavior are demographic characteristics, biological characteristics, interpersonal influences, situational factors, and behavioral factors. The cognitive-perceptual factors are the primary motivational mechanisms for the acquisition and maintenance of health-promoting behaviors and include perceived self-efficacy. Nursing investigations of developmental phenomena and life course events have included self-efficacy as a predictor as well as an outcome of a tailored intervention.

Natural Disaster

Murphy (1987) investigated the influence of global self-efficacy and social support on the mental health of individuals who experienced a natural disaster, volcanic eruption. One to 3 years postdisaster, the victims continued to experience physical and mental distress. Self-efficacy was positively related to mental health; social support was not. The findings showed that the individuals relied more on themselves and believed in their own abilities to cope with their losses. Even though social support was not a predictor of mental distress, the findings suggested that if there was someone to turn to, the identified stressor was more manageable.

Cardiac Recovery

Self-efficacy was found to be a strong predictor of recovery from cardiac illness. It has been studied as a variable to predict exercise performance and as a theoretical framework for designing nursing interventions to increase exercise. Gortner (Gortner et al., 1988) was the first nurse researcher to design a self-efficacy-driven exercise intervention; it was tested in 67 patients recovering from cardiac surgery. The experimental intervention contained a counseling aspect focusing on emotional reactions. At 3 months postsurgery participants in the intervention group had higher self-efficacy than did participants in the control group. Gortner and Jenkins (1990) later tested education and telephone monitoring in 149 cardiac surgery patients during their recovery phase. Patients in the experimental group at 8 weeks had greater walking, lifting, and general activity. Self-efficacy expectations were a significant predictor for self-reported activity up to 24 weeks following surgery. These studies provide evidence of support for continued development of nursing interventions based on self-efficacy theory in patients recovering from cardiac surgery.

Family Roles

The parent role creates new stressors for individuals, and this phenomenon of parenting efficacy has long-term effects on both the parents and the child. The results of investigations by Gross and her colleagues (Gross, Fogg, & Tucker, 1995) showed that low perceived efficacy fosters depression in mothers of toddlers and may determine whether the mother goes on to develop chronic depression. The investigators created a program to build parenting confidence in ability to handle toddlers' behavioral problems using mastery modeling and self-efficacy theory. The mothers who participated in the program increased their sense of parenting efficacy and experienced lower familial stress and child behavior problems. The mothers who did not participate became more critical and had more negative interactions with their children.

Memory Aging

General or specific incidents of forgetting are often used by older adults to interpret the effectiveness of their memory ability and awareness. Self-efficacy in psychosocial functioning is best determined by measures tailored to particular domains of functioning, rather than by a global test. Memory self-efficacy is defined as beliefs about one's own capability to use memory effectively in various situations. Knowledge about memory is distinct from memory self-efficacy. Thus, it is possible that an older individual may have extensive and accurate knowledge about how memory functions but also may believe that his or her ability to remember in a given context is poor. More older adults than younger adults have poorer memory self-efficacy, and low memory self-efficacy has a number of adverse consequences. McDougall (1994) determined that healthy elders attending adult educational programs, without major chronic illness or depression, had decreased memory self-efficacy. This perception led them to believe that they had limited memory capacity, that they could do little to affect their memory, that anxiety and stress easily influenced their memory, and that it would inevitably decline with age.

If the individual perceives memory to be a decreasing function with age, then he or she is quick to interpret faulty performance as an indicator of declining memory capacity. Those who have low self-efficacy may give up trying because of doubts about achieving a desired level of performance. Conversely, the individual who views memory ability as a skill to be developed and practiced may achieve higher memory capacity. Nurses are able to assist older adults to view their cognitive abilities realistically and not promote negative views and stereotypes about cognitive aging. These studies offer examples in which nurse scientists investigated life-span phenomena incorporating self-efficacy theory as a component in the quest to develop nursing knowledge.

GRAHAM J. MCDOUGALL

See also
COGNITIVE INTERVENTIONS
PSYCHOSOCIAL INTERVENTIONS

SMOKING CESSATION

It is estimated that 25% of the adult population in the United States are current smokers (Centers for Disease Control, 1994). According to the National Youth Tobacco Survey, 34.8% of all U.S. high school students use some form of tobacco, with 9.2% of middle-school students and 28.4% of high school students categorized as current cigarette smokers (Centers for Disease Control, 2000). Acquisition of a regular smoking pattern usually requires 2 to 3 years of experimentation. Onset of tobacco use generally occurs between years 11 to 18, with experimentation increasing dramatically by age 15 (United States Department of Health and Human Services, 1994). Among adults, male smoking prevalence is slightly higher, although females are expected to surpass men early in the twenty-first century (Pierce, Fiore, Novotny, Hatziandreu, & Davis, 1989). Prevalence is disproportionately higher among: (1) those with a high school education or less aged 20 and older (34%); (2) blue-collar workers (36%); (3) military personnel (42%); and (4) minorities (33–55%) (United States Department of Health and Human Services, 1991).

Psychiatric comorbidity is more common among smokers as compared to the general population. Regular smoking has been reported to occur more frequently among individuals who had experienced a major depressive disorder than among individuals who had never experienced major depression or among individuals with no psychiatric diagnosis (Glassman et al., 1990). Further, smokers with major depression were observed to be less successful in achieving long-term abstinence from smoking. It has also been estimated that 15 to 20% of heavy smokers have current alcohol dependence or abuse; approximately 80% of alcohol/drug abusers in treatment are classified as smokers (Hughes, 1995). Finally, a very high percentage of patients with schizophrenia smoke and many express little interest in cessation (Ziedonis, Kosten, Glazer, & Frances, 1994).

Over 400,000 deaths annually in the United States have been attributed to smoking (Centers for Disease Control, 1993). Economically, the costs of smoking and tobacco are significant, with $50 billion spent annually in the United States on health-related expenditures (Centers for Disease Control, 1994). Another $47 billion is allocated annually to indirect costs, such as lost productivity (Herdman, Hewitt, & Laschober, 1993). The health benefits of smoking cessation are well described in persons of all ages. Over time, the survival rates of former smokers approach those of persons who never smoked (Doll, Peto, & Wheatley, 1994).

While psychiatric comorbidity has been shown to increase the risk of relapse after smoking cessation, evidence suggests that smoking cessation treatment is efficacious among smokers with psychiatric diagnoses. In general, smoking cessation interventions delivered by nurses have been determined to be effective (Houston-Miller, Smith, DeBusk, Sobel, & Taylor, 1997) although nurse-managed studies with smokers who have been diagnosed with a psychiatric disorder have yet to be described. Presented below is a brief review of major studies that have examined cessation in smokers with a psychiatric comorbidity.

Smoking Cessation Treatment: Research Findings

According to the Smoking Cessation Clinical Guideline published by the Agency for Health Care Policy and Research (AHCPR), clinician support, problem-solving skill training, and nicotine replacement therapy (NRT) are recommended as the three major elements of treatment (Fiore et al., 1994). Nicotine products, including the transdermal patch, gum, spray, and inhaler have been evaluated as efficacious and are available for use in therapy (Fiore et al., 1994). The effectiveness of combination NRT products has also been examined and determined to be effective (Fagerstrom, 1994; Kornitzer, Boutsen, Dramaix, Thijs, & Gustavsson, 1995). In addition, a nonnicotine agent, the antidepressant bupropion hydrochloride, has been recommended recently for treatment of smoking cessation (Hurt et al., 1997).

With regard to smokers with psychiatric comorbidity, the number of investigations examining the effectiveness of these various pharmacotherapies is limited. In a double-blind crossover design, Hartmann and colleagues (1991) observed that transdermally administrated nicotine reduced the number of cigarettes smoked each day in 13 psychiatric patients who were not actively attempting cessation. The majority of the patients (77%) were diagnosed with schizophrenia or schizoaffective disorder and had been smoking more than one pack of cigarettes each day for 19 years on average. This finding suggested that NRT may represent a potential adjuvant form of therapy among psychiatric patients who smoke. More recently, Ziedonis and George (1997) reported that among 24 patients with schizophrenia who were treated with nicotine replacement, motivational enhancement therapy, and relapse prevention behavioral therapy, 50% of patients completed the program. Forty percent of all patients decreased their smoking consumption, and 13% were biochemically confirmed as abstinent at 6 months posttreatment. These preliminary results also suggest that the AHCPR recommendation of nicotine replacement in combination with behavioral counseling can be effectively implemented in smokers with psychiatric disease.

Level of functioning and severity of illness may be important determinants of smoking status and eventual success in quitting among those with a psychiatric illness. In a descriptive study of 300 chronic psychiatric patients, Hall and others (1997) reported that former smokers were more likely to live independently and were less likely to have a drug or alcohol problem. Former smokers also had significantly lower scores on the Brief Psychiatric Rating Scale, indicating that better functioning patients may be more likely to quit the behavior.

Treatment for nicotine dependence has not been shown to exacerbate the use of other addictive substances. In a prospective, nonrandomized controlled trial with a 1-year outcome (n = 101), Hurt and colleagues (1994) demonstrated that cessation rates were 11.8% and 0% in the intervention and control groups, respectively. Intervention group participants received inpatient behavioral counseling that included a structured relapse prevention program. Most importantly, treatment for nicotine dependence did not interfere with abstinence from alcohol or other drugs, as evidenced by 31.4% and 34% relapse rates for the intervention and control groups, respectively. While there is concern that abstinent smokers with other drug dependencies will increase their other drug use, this preliminary evidence suggested that this is not the case. Similarly, the institution of smoke-free units in psychiatric settings has not been associated with an increase in aggressive or disruptive behavior, discharges against medical advice, use of medications or restraints, or admission refusals (Resnick, 1993).

To date, the majority of studies examining smoking cessation among patients with psychiatric comorbidity have been pilot, or preliminary, in nature. These studies should be replicated, using well-controlled randomized clinical trial designs. In addition, future research should investigate whether treatment tailored specifically to the psychiatric smoker represents a more effective approach to long-term abstinence. Research studies that determine the effectiveness of nurse-managed approaches with psychiatric smokers are also lacking and should be conducted.

MARY ELLEN WEWERS

See also
ALCOHOLISM
DRUG ABUSE
DUAL DIAGNOSIS

STRESS

The term *stress* first appeared in the *Cumulative Index to Nursing and Allied Health Literature (CINAHL)* in 1956. Nursing's interest in stress as a focus of research has mushroomed since 1970. Although the word *stress* is familiar to many and has become part of our everyday vocabulary, the term conveys divergent meanings, and multiple theories have been proposed to explain it. Most of the theories attempting to describe and explain stress as a human phenomenon can be categorized under one of three very different orientations to the concept: response-based, stimulus-based, and transaction-based. The response-based orientation was developed by Hans Selye. Selye (1976) defined stress as a nonspecific response of the body to any demand. That is, regardless of the cause, situational context, or psychological interpretation of the demand, the stress response is characterized by the same chain of events or same pattern of physiological correlates.

Defined as a response, stress indicators become the dependent variables in research studies. Nurse researchers who have used the response-based orientation measure catecholoamines, cortisol, urinary Na/K ratio, vital signs, brain waves, electrodermal skin responses, and cardiovascular complaints as indicators of stress. The demand component of Selye's definition is treated as an independent variable, whereas hospitalization, surgery, or critical care unit transfer were commonly the assumed stressor in much of the nursing research using this orientation. The response-based model of stress is not consistent with the nursing philosophical presuppositions that each individual is unique and that individuals respond holistically and often differently to similar situations (Lyon & Werner, 1987).

The stimulus-based theoretical explanation treats stress as a stimulus that causes disrupted responses. As a stimulus, stress is viewed as an external force similar to the engineering use of the term to represent dynamics of strain in metals or an external force directed at a physical object. Defined in this way stress becomes the independent variable in research studies. The most frequently cited example of a stimulus-based theory is the life event theory proposed by Holmes and Rahe (1967). Stress is operationalized as a stable additive phenomenon that is measurable by researcher-selected life events or life changes that typically have preassigned normative weights. The tools most commonly used to measure stress from a stimulus-based orientation are the Social Readjustment Rating Scale (SRRS) and the Schedule of Recent Experiences (SRE). Nurse researchers who have used the stimulus-based orientation have used the SRRS or SRE or developed new tools such as the Hospital Stress Rating Scale (HSRS) (Volicer & Bohannon, 1975). The primary theoretical proposition of the stimulus-based orientation is that too many life events or changes increase vulnerability to illness. Results of studies using the life event perspective have failed to explain illness, accounting for only 2% to 4% of the incidence of illness.

The third way to conceptualize stress is a transaction between person and environment. In this context stress refers to uncomfortable tension-related emotions that arise when demanding situations tax available resources; and some kind of harm, loss, or negative consequence is anticipated. (Lazarus & Folkman, 1984). In the transactional orientation, stress represents a composite of experiences, including threatening appraisals, stress emotions (anxiety, fear, anger, guilt, depression), and coping responses. As such, the term *stress* has heuristic value but is a difficult construct to study. Use of a transactional theoretical orientation requires that the researcher clearly delineate which aspects of the person-environment transaction are to be studied. Commonly, the independent variables in experimental and quasi-experimental studies based on the transactional orientation are personal resources such as self-esteem, perceived control, uncertainty, social support, and hardiness. Appraisal of threat versus appraisal of challenge is commonly studied as a mediating factor between resource strength and coping responses. Dependent variables often include somatic outcomes such as pain, emotional disturbances such as anxiety and depression, and well-being. The transactional model was deemed by Lyon and Werner (1987) to be compatible with nursing's philosophical suppositions.

Lyon and Werner (1987) published a critical review of 82 studies conducted by nurses from 1974 to 1984. The studies reviewed fell evenly across the three different theoretical orientations, and approximately 25% of the studies were atheoretical in nature. In 1993, Barnfather and Lyon edited a monograph of the proceedings of a synthesis conference on stress and coping held in conjunction with the Midwest Nursing Research Society. This critical review of the research covered 296 studies published from 1980 to 1990. Both the 1987 and the 1993 critical reviews noted a disturbing absence of programs of research, making it difficult to identify what we have learned from the discipline's research efforts. Lyon (1993) noted in a preliminary synthesis of findings from the critical review that the transactional orientation has dominated nursing research studies since the late 1980s.

The significance of nursing research in the area of stress grows even more important in the era of managed care and capitated pay for health care services. It is widely recognized that as many as 65% of visits to physician offices are for illnesses that have no discernible medical cause, and many of those illness are thought to be stress-related. Furthermore, productivity in the workplace is thought to be greatly affected by the deleterious effects of stress. Future directions for nursing research in the area of stress will focus on (1) effects of psychological stress on the somatic sense of self, functional ability, the experience of illness, and aberrant behaviors such as abuse and use of alcohol and drugs; (2) the identification of patterns of variables that predict vulnerability or at-risk status for stress-related illness experiences and aberrant behaviors; (3) intervention studies designed to alter factors that make a person vulnerable to stress-related illnesses; and (4) intervention studies to evaluate the effects of various stress management strategies including cognitive restructuring on stress-related illnesses and aberrant behaviors.

BRENDA L. LYON

See also
STRESS
STRESS MANAGEMENT

STRESS MANAGEMENT

Stress management involves strategies to both decrease stress and prevent stress. Actions taken to decrease stress or alleviate it once experienced are commonly referred to as coping strategies or behaviors. Some of the coping strategies frequently used by nurses include taking action, drawing on past experiences, using problem-solving techniques, using humor, talking over problems with co-workers, accepting the situation, taking breaks (escaping from the situation), using diversions, using relaxation, and exercise (Lewis & Robinson, 1986; Petermann, Springer, & Farnsworth, 1995). Actions taken to prevent stress involve balancing demands and resources, focusing on the positive in difficult situations, maintaining perceived choice and sense of personal control, building social support, and viewing difficult situations as challenges that can bring gain or benefit through learning (Dionne-Proulz & Pepin, 1993; Lyon, 1996).

In addition to the research conducted on stress management strategies used by nurses, nurse researchers also have studied the effects of stress management interventions with various patient and client population groups. Snyder (1993) critically reviewed all 54 stress-related intervention studies appearing in the nursing literature from 1980 through 1990. The types of stress management interventions used included relaxation strategies (e.g., progressive muscle relaxation, imagery, meditation, breathing techniques, massage, music), educational strategies, and use of social support groups. A major flaw of most of the intervention studies was an inadequate description of the intervention used, and there was a lack of attempts to explain the theoretical link between the intervention and outcome measures. Manipulation checks as a way to assure that subjects mastered the intervention and to verify that subjects actually used the intervention also were lacking in the intervention studies. Studies using sensation information (e.g., Johnson, Rice, Fuller, & Endress, 1978) and studies using progressive relaxation techniques (e.g., Pender, 1985) have demonstrated positive effects on health-related outcomes such as less anxiety and an increased sense of well-being.

Future directions for nursing research should focus on the effectiveness of stress management interventions for both nurses and patients or clients. For meaningful results, however, it will be imperative that the researcher clearly define and delineate interventions and offer testable theoretical formulations that explain how the intervention affects outcome variables. It is also essential that the researcher incorporate manipulation checks into the methodology to verify that subjects have implemented a strategy correctly and that the intervention actually altered the target variable as proposed in the theoretical formulation.

BRENDA L. LYON

See also
MUSIC THERAPY
RELAXATION TECHNIQUES
STRESS

VIOLENCE AS A NURSING AREA OF INQUIRY

Violence is well recognized as an important health problem in the United States, and nursing research, practice, policy, and advocacy have all been instrumental in addressing the problem. The United States is one of the most violent countries in the industrialized world. Each year homicide and suicide claim more than 50,000 lives, and 2.2 million people are injured by violent assaults. If the trend continues, death rates from firearms will surpass motor vehicle crashes by the year 2003 (U.S. Public Health Service, 1995). Since the 1985 Surgeon General's Conference on Violence, a public health approach has been recognized as an important framework for research and interventions to reduce violence and ameliorate its effects.

The term *violence* originates from the Latin *violare*, to violate. The victims of violence are violated, physically, emotionally, spiritually, and socially. Nurses encounter victims and perpetrators of violence in every health care setting, with a variety of injuries and other health problems. The holistic approach of nursing addresses all aspects of human responses to violence. Nursing scholarship has also recognized the complex interaction of community factors (structural inequalities and erosion, residential mobility, poverty, lack of career opportunities, housing, cultural norms and biases, and population density) and individual and family risk factors for violence that require preventive measures.

Violence against Women

The largest body of nursing research is focused on violence against women. Ann Burgess's ground-breaking studies of rape in the early 1970s initiated a program of nursing research to address the cognitive processing of trauma and later focused on the concerns of rape victims about HIV infection (Campbell, Anderson, Fulmer, et al., 1993). Nurse researchers have studied children who have been sexually abused and have done work on identifying response patterns in children and adolescents exploited in sex rings and pornography as well as the development of a model of children's responses to sexual abuse that explains their acute and chronic symptoms.

Other nurse researchers have focused on incest survivors, exploring both the long-term difficulties they experience and the positive aspects of adaptation, healing, and empowerment. Work with rape victims has included examination of self-esteem and primary prevention techniques.

Battered Women. Nursing studies related to domestic violence have resulted in a diverse but impressive body of nursing knowledge. A recently published review (Campbell & Parker, in press) of 20 years of nursing research on domestic violence documented a significant prevalence of abused women in a variety of health care settings with significant physical (chronic pain, headaches, and backaches; risk of sexually transmitted disease; and sleep disturbances) and mental health problems (depression, low self-esteem, substance abuse, and anxiety). Battered women's perceptions of less than adequate care given by health professionals has been supported by studies of the attitudes of physicians and nurses that identified the paternalistic and blaming attitudes of many of these professionals. Related to these issues, an experimental nursing intervention study tested a training program for emergency room nurses that resulted in a significant increase in appropriate identification and documentation of battered women in the nurses who received the training.

Judy McFarlane and Barbara Parker (Campbell & Parker, in press) have documented a higher prevalence of abuse during pregnancy (16% to 17%) than was shown in other research studies. This higher prevalence may be related to the use of nurse-conducted personal interviews. Findings of various studies have suggested that universal screening of all women (including adolescents) for intimate partner abuse at *each* health system encounter should become routine nursing practice. Nursing research has also supported the link between abuse during pregnancy and low-birthweight infants, substance abuse, smoking, and depression.

There was also substantiation in nursing research of the significant strengths of battered women, indication of normal processes of grieving and recovering, and the fact that leaving battering relationships is a process that occurs over time, the majority of women leaving or making the violence end. Landenburger (Campbell & Humphreys, 1993) used grounded theory to develop a theory of entrapment and recovery from an abusive relationship that was later used as a basis for clinical nursing intervention.

Understanding dating violence among adolescents is recognized as significant not only because of the injuries and suffering experienced at the time but also because of its relationship to adult domestic violence. The prevalence of dating violence varied between 9% and 61% in various studies. These differences may be related to differences in definition. One nursing study of adolescent dating violence in North Carolina revealed that many adolescents denied abusive relationships but reported numerous abusive events. Twenty-four percent of these adolescents reported extreme violence, including episodes of rape or use of weapons. In one midwestern city a nursing study found the prevalence of dating violence among nursing students to be similar to the prevalence among American women overall, thus the need for nursing faculty to be alert for signs of abuse.

The contribution of nursing research to the field of domestic violence is noteworthy because of its activist and feminist (i.e., woman-centered) assumptions and stance. Nursing scholars have developed close collaboration with shelters for abused women, paid particular attention to the safety and empowerment of women and their children, and documented strengths as well as problems. Nursing research has proceeded from the assumption that the locus of responsibility for battering lies not only with individual perpetrators but also with our societal structures and attitudes that facilitate or fail to prevent the battering of female partners. There has also been a beginning sensitivity and inquiry about ethnic and cultural differences in women's responses to battering from nursing investigators such as Doris Campbell, Sara Torres, Rachel Rodriguez, and Diane Bohn (Campbell & Parker, in press).

Children of Battered Women. In the United States at least 3.3 million children ages 3 to 17 witness domestic violence each year. There is a strong correlation (40% to 77% concordance) between domestic violence and violence against children. Nurse researchers have studied some of the effects on children witnessing or experiencing family violence. These effects include more physical health problems, higher levels of internalizing behaviors (depression, social withdrawal), low self-esteem and self-efficacy, lower social competence, higher levels of externalizing behaviors (aggression, hyperactivity, conduct problems), anxiety reactions, posttraumatic stress symptoms, and school problems. Children who were abused also showed a high incidence of subsequent violent behavior and arrests. The qualitative studies of Humphreys and Henderson (Campbell & Parker, in press) have provided new insights into the experience of children living with domestic violence and into their concerns, for example, worries about their mother's actual (battering) or potential (smoking, pregnancy) health problems.

Child Abuse

According to 1990 data, over 2.7 million children in the United States were victims of child maltreatment in that year, and this number has remained high (U.S. Public Health Service, 1995). Nurses have contributed to the view that child abuse is the result of a complex interaction of individual, family, environmental, and societal factors (Campbell & Humphreys, 1993) and to the recognition that disability and twinship place children at risk for abuse. Factors that influenced clinicians' identification and management of child abuse and family violence were found to be education and attitudes towards the abuser. Nurse researchers in the United States and the United Kingdom have demonstrated the effectiveness of home visits in screening, intervening, and preventing child abuse.

Adolescent Violence

Youths are increasingly involved as perpetrators and victims of violence. Homicide is a leading cause of death among 15–19-year-olds nationally. Risk behavior surveys indicated that a large percentage of students in grades 9 through 12 reported carrying a weapon in the 30 days preceding the surveys. These indicators, along with the increase in juvenile arrests, raise concerns about our youth and their access to firearms. In recognition of these trends, the midcourse review of Healthy People 2000 includes a new objective addressing physical fighting by adolescents (U.S. Public Health Service, 1995).

More research on youth violence by nurses and social scientists is needed. The research in this area by nurses has been rather limited. Cull (Campbell, Harris, & Lee, 1995) examined the influence of being a victim of violence on self-care practices of adolescents, and Lee used epidemiological methods to examine the effects of gun violence on youths and adults. More studies are needed to examine the etiology and prevention of youth violent behavior and the effects on our children of witnessing violence. Nurses play a significant role in schools and in the community and have the opportunity to evaluate interventions in these settings.

Elder Abuse

Elder maltreatment is an important topic that has received very little attention. It is estimated that 700,000 to 1 million older Americans experience mistreatment each year. Nursing research on this topic has focused on an understanding of predictive factors, instrument development, and clinical decision making. This research, led by Fulmer and Phillips (Campbell, Anderson, Fulmer, et al., 1993), has influenced policy on such issues and leads the way to an important avenue of nursing research.

Summary, Critique, and Future Directions

Nursing research has made substantial contributions to the health problem of violence. There have been methodological shortcomings in terms of relatively small sample sizes and unsophisticated designs. There is also a scattering of studies in many different directions, impeding accumulation of nursing knowledge in specific areas. However, many study findings have been corroborated by findings from other disciplines.

Attention to culture and ethnicity, use of qualitative and quantitative data, a holistic perspective, strong clinical grounding, and the advocacy positions of prior nursing research should be continued to advance the body of nursing knowledge about the causes and interventions related to violence. More longitudinal, comparison group, and large sample studies are needed, especially those that develop and test midrange nursing theory. Further documentation and investigation of health consequences and costs of violence must build on existing nursing research. The effects of violence should be incorporated in other programs of nursing research in maternal-child health, substance abuse, HIV/AIDS, gerontology, international health, and community health. Studies that test nursing interventions with victims of violence, their families, and groups at risk are needed to demonstrate the value of nursing care in making the health care system a primary, secondary, and tertiary prevention site.

JACQUELYN C. CAMPBELL
JOAN KUB
LINDA LEWANDOWSKI

See also

ELDER ABUSE
WORKPLACE VIOLENCE
YOUNG WOMEN AND DEPRESSION

WORKPLACE MISTREATMENT

Research findings from studies of perceived workplace mistreatment indicate that its occurrence has measurable negative consequences on individuals and work performance in organizations. This paper summarizes what is generally known about such conduct and behaviors in the learning and work environment of colleges and universities. It also illustrates the uses and benefits associated with an assessment checklist that was developed by the author in the course of research and service delivery regarding workplace conflict at a major research university. While this dysfunctional behavior was studied outside a conventional treatment setting, the research drew extensively on perspectives in psychosocial/mental health nursing and knowledge from cognate fields. Moreover, the client education and preventive approach that has been used over time parallels interventions generally used in nursing research and service delivery.

This author defines workplace mistreatment as behaviors or situations that are unwelcome, unwanted, unreasonable, inappropriate, or excessive and that also violate the human rights of those who experience such mistreatment. Examples include yelling, swearing, namecalling, or physical actions such as pushing or hitting someone. Such conduct creates a sense of hostility, intimidation, or fear on the part of those who are the recipients of such actions. This dysfunctional behavior has negative consequences for the individuals as well as the institutions where it occurs.

Studies documenting the occurrence of mistreatment in the educational setting have been reported by several researchers. In medicine, Silver and Glicken (1990) surveyed all students in one medical school and a sample of medical school administrators nationally. The students reported yelling or shouting by residents and faculty. Physical abuse was rare. However, the deans and other administrators denied the existence of verbal or any other abuse in the faculty/resident-student relationship in their institutions. Sheehan, Sheehan, White, and others (1990) collected survey information from third-year medical students in one medical school. The mistreatment led to cynicism among over three fourths of the third-year students. Their findings were similar to those reported in the study by Silver and Glicken (1990). The American Medical Association's Council on Ethical and Judicial Affairs (1994) has stated that perceptions of abuse and misconduct may be our only guides for identifying behaviors that lead to trainee and supervisory conflict. Larson and Martinson (1990) found that nurses generally expected verbal abuse by physicians, with operating room nurses reporting a high degree of vulnerability to such mistreatment. They indicated that help was needed to understand and cope with abusive communication. By working together with hospital executives and staff members, they were able to develop a policy and program for reducing and preventing verbal abuse.

In the general university setting several different approaches and findings have been reported. Student athletes were surveyed in a study sponsored by the

American Institute for Research (1988). This is one of the largest studies in this subject area. In a random sample of 3000 varsity athletes, 1240, or 41.3%, responded. Mental abuse from coaches was considered pervasive and frequently reported among football and basketball players. The abuse extended to being asked to ignore injuries and to place their athletic participation above academic performance. Based on a random sample of 11% of the faculty and staff at a major research university (with a 51% response rate), Price Spratlen (1994, 1995) reported that 23% of respondents had experienced some form of mistreatment. Applying strict criteria, this level reflected a rather stringent standard that had to be met before mistreatment was considered valid. A later records review of 40% of the faculty and staff who had used the services of the ombudsman's office reported a 27% incidence of workplace mistreatment. Coworkers were equally as likely as administrators to engage in such misconduct. In another culture (a university in Finland), Bjogvist, Osterman, and Hjelt-Back (1994) found expressions of aggression and workplace harassment. Females reported being harassed significantly more than men. Individuals in higher status positions and roles were more likely to harass someone than a person in a lower status position.

Common threads of evidence in all the literature substantiate that perceived mistreatment results in negative psychosocial outcomes. Some of the most common are fear, anxiety, depression, and increased physical symptoms on the part of recipients. Lower productivity, morale, high absenteeism, and job turnover have also been documented. With respect to nursing research in the area of psychosocial and mental health, the studies that are reported here have provided a foundation on which to further expand our knowledge of perceived mistreatment and how to prevent its occurrence.

LOIS PRICE SPRATLEN

See also

VIOLENCE

WORKPLACE VIOLENCE

WORKPLACE VIOLENCE

Background on Fatal and Non-fatal Assaults

Workplace violence is defined as "violent acts, including physical assaults and threats of assaults, directed toward persons at work or on duty" (National Institute for Occupational Safety and Health (NIOSH), 1996). Homicide is the leading cause of occupational injury death among women. In 1990, homicide bypassed machine-related injury to become the second leading cause of occupational injury death among all workers. Over 1000 workers are murdered on the job each year. Workers employed in retail trade are at highest risk of homicide with a rate of 1.60 per 100,000 workers, representing 38% of all homicides. Nearly 80% of workplace homicides involve the use of a firearm (NIOSH, 1996). Nonfatal workplace assaults are much more common, and although they share many of the same risk factors as workplace homicides (e.g., contact with the public, working with unstable or volatile persons, working alone or in small numbers, working in high-crime areas, working late at night or during early morning hours, working in community-based settings), health care rather than retail workers represent the majority of victims. According to the Department of Justice's National Crime Victimization Survey (NCVS), more than two million incidents of workplace violence occurred in the workplace each year from 1992 to 1996 (Warchol, 1998). Twelve percent of all victims reported physical injuries; 6% of workplace crimes resulted in injury that required medical treatment. Only 44% of the incidents of workplace violence were reported to the police.

Health Care Workers and Workplace Violence

Among the victims of workplace violence included in the NCVS, professionals in the mental health field had an incidence rate of 79.5 per 1000 workers compared with an overall rate of 14.8 per 1000 workers. Overall, nurses had an incidence rate of 24.8 per 1000 workers, the highest incidence rate in the "medical" category (Warchol, 1998).

The Bureau of Labor Statistics (BLS) figures indicate that the health care sector leads all other industry sectors in nonfatal workplace assaults. In 1993, 38% of all nonfatal assaults against workers that resulted in lost workdays occurred in the health care sector; 27% were in nursing homes and 11% in hospitals. Workers in "nursing and personal care facilities" have a rate of 38 per 10,000 nonfatal assaults compared with a rate of 3 per 10,000 in the private sector. In 45% of reported cases of nonfatal workplace assault, the perpetrator of the assault is a health care patient (BLS, 1995).

Mental Health and Workplace Violence

The problem of violence in mental health care facilities has an extensive history, with the first documented case of a patient fatally assaulting a psychiatrist in 1849 (Bernstein, 1981). Until the 1990s, most studies that examined the risk of violence to psychiatrists and other therapists focused on the victim's role, the assaultive patient's characteristics, and contextual factors surrounding the assault. Only recently have environmental risk factors been a focus of research and nurses and aides the subject of study.

A recent study of the problem within mental health compared the number of formal incident reports and the workers' compensation claims from a Washington state psychiatric hospital with the number of reported incidents of assault reported on a survey that measured attitudes and experiences related to assaults. Seventy-three percent of staff surveyed reported at least a minor injury related to an assault by a patient in the past year. Only 43% (85/197) of those reporting moderate, severe, or disabling injuries related to assault filed for workers compensation. The survey found an assault incidence rate of 437 per 100 employees per year, a rate that underestimated incident reports of assault by a factor of more than 5 (Bensley et al., 1997).

The Occupational Safety and Health Administration (OSHA) defines an occupational injury as one that results in death or in "lost workdays, loss of consciousness, restriction of work or motion, termination of employment, transfer to another job, or medical treatment (other than first aid)." This definition was used by Carmel and Hunter (1989) to conduct a 1-year study of injuries in a 973-bed maximum-security forensic hospital in California. They found that nursing staff sustained 16.0 injuries per 100 staff compared with a rate of 8.3 per 100 full-time workers in all industries combined, and 14.2 per 100 full-time workers in the construction industry (Bureau of Labor Statistics, 1991). Carmel and Hunter's data suggest that at this maximum security hospital, the rate of injuries from assaults alone put workers at a higher risk than workers in the most hazardous industry in the country, the construction industry (Lipscomb & Love, 1992).

Speculation about the cause of the violence in hospitals include the use of violence in the general society as a means of solving problems, the use of mind-altering drugs and alcohol abuse, and the ready availability of weapons. All of these may contribute to violence in health care settings. The high rate of violence in psychiatric settings has been attributed to (1) deinstitutionalization of the chronically mentally ill, (2) the right of involuntary patients to refuse psychotropic medications, (3) the change in the involuntary commitment criterion from "in need of treatment" to "dangerousness," and (4) shorter hospital stays and frequent readmissions of violent patients and the blurred boundary between mental illness and criminality (Lipscomb & Love, 1992).

Environmental Risk Factors

A number of environmental risk factors have been associated with patient assaults, including staffing, security, time of day, and containment activities (Carmel &

Hunter, 1989; Fineberg, James, & Shah, 1988; Jones, 1985). Inadequate training, policies, and procedures have also been identified as contributing to assaults (Bernstein, 1981; Hodgkinson, Hillis, & Russell, 1984). Three studies have shown that training in the management of assaultive behavior can reduce injury from assault (Carmel & Hunter, 1990; Infantino & Musingo, 1985). By contrast, Lee et al. (1999) found that among 105 nurses who had filed a worker's compensation claim for work-related assault injuries, the presence of security personnel reduced the rate of assault, while the perception that administrators considered assault to be part of the job, having received assault prevention training, a high patient to personal ratio, working primarily with mental health patients, and working with patients who had a long hospital stay strongly increased the risk of assault.

Patient Characteristics as Risk Factors in the Mental Health Setting

Much effort has been directed toward predicting violent behavior by psychiatric patients despite evidence that efforts at predicting "dangerousness" have been less than successful (Bernstein, 1981; Werner, Yesavage, Becker, Brunsting, & Isaacs, 1983). The one patient characteristic that has been singled out as a strong risk factor for violence is a history of violent behavior. Drummond et al. (1989) reported that they reduced assaults against staff by 91% by flagging charts of patients with a history of assaultive or disruptive behavior. A number of studies have documented that a small percentage of patients are responsible for the majority of assaults (Hillbrand, Foster, & Spitz, 1996; Jones, 1985) supporting the view that patients with a history of violent behavior place health care workers at greatest risk of future assaults and making evident the need for history taking and communication regarding a history of violence. In addition, the environment must be made safe for all health care workers through the use of currently available engineering and administrative controls such as security, alarm systems, adequate staffing, and training.

Violence Prevention and Training

Many psychiatric settings now require that all patient care providers receive annual training in the management of aggressive patients. However, few studies have examined the effectiveness of traditional aggression/violence management training. Those that have (Carmel & Hunter, 1990; Hurlebaus & Link, 1997; Lehmann, Padilla, Clark, & Loucks, 1983) generally found improvement in nurses' knowledge, confidence, and safety after taking an aggressive behavior management program.

In 1996, the Occupational Safety & Health Administration published "Guidelines for Preventing Workplace Violence for Health Care and Social Service Workers." They describe the key elements of any proactive health and safety program, including management commitment and employee involvement; a written violence prevention program; a worksite analysis; hazard prevention and control; medical management and postincident response; training and education; and record-keeping and evaluation of the program. The effectiveness of these guidelines in preventing violence within the mental health setting is currently being evaluated by the author. Research is also needed to evaluate intervention directly at primary, secondary, and tertiary prevention of violence across health care settings.

JANE LIPSCOMB

See also
VIOLENCE
WORKPLACE MISTREATMENT

YOUNG WOMEN AND DEPRESSION

Major depressive disorder (MDD) is common among premenopausal women. The National Co-Morbidity Study showed a 12-month MDD prevalence in women of 12.9% and a lifetime prevalence of 21.3% (Kessler, McGonagle, Zhao, et al., 1994). Depressive disorder begins early in adolescence for many women, and its incidence peaks before menopause. Women most commonly experience the chronic recurrent form of the disorder and often have comorbid seasonal affective disorder, premenstrual syndrome (PMS), and anxiety disorder. Recurrent MDD is characterized by its spontaneous onset, severity, and longevity and is accompanied by significant impairment of familial, social, and occupational functioning. For women managing demanding familial and occupational careers, MDD is a powerful barrier to personal success and well-being.

Despite its impact, MDD often is not detected or appropriately treated in women. One reason is women's tendency to seek health care in primary care settings, where physicians do not often recognize or treat MDD. This is lamentable because effective treatment modalities have been developed and evaluated through empiricism, and guidelines exist for practice in primary care settings. Neither these treatment modalities nor the derived guidelines, however, are gender-specific. Depression treatment for women often does not address their specific relational needs and is not culturally sensitive, nor does it consider specific barriers like poverty, child care needs, or transportation (Hauenstein, 1996).

Because of this, women frequently stop treatment before securing symptom remission.

Descriptive studies of women with MDD have linked the disorder to biological phenomena and interpersonal distress (Weissman & Olfson, 1995). Researchers using data from female twins have identified at least four interacting risk factor domains: early traumatic experiences, genetic factors, temperament, and interpersonal relationships (Kendler, Kessler, Neale, Heath, & Eaves, 1993). Recently, Hauenstein (1996) has developed a theory-based, biopsychosocial causal model of depression for rural disadvantaged women to guide nursing intervention.

The Nursing Practice Paradigm for Depressed Women depicts two major pathways leading to depression. One portrays depression as occurring relatively spontaneously in vulnerable women. Excessive stress reactivity, early trauma, and the cyclical mood disturbance attendant on PMS are widely regarded as altering specific neurotransmitter and hormonal physiological systems. These alterations lead to MDD without an apparent external precipitating event.

Uncompensated environmental or personal stress triggers these same physiological mechanisms in the second pathway. Emphasized here is the role of physical, cognitive, emotional, and social resources in reducing the deleterious effects of external and internal stressors. This perspective permits nursing intervention to be directed to both reducing stressor effects and augmenting personal resources. Empiricism supporting the model is described elsewhere (Hauenstein, 1996, 1997).

The model depicts four goals of nursing intervention: depression prevention, reduction in stress responsiveness, prevention of stress dysregulation, and promotion of recovery from MDD. Outcomes from several major research clinical trials of MDD treatment demonstrate that both somatic and psychosocial intervention are key to enacting these goals of treatment.

Nonpharmacological, somatic interventions for depressed women are supported by the nursing practice paradigm and are an important area for nursing research. Predominant among these are stress-reduction modalities, sleep-restoration techniques, dietary manipulation, and exercise. Stress-reduction techniques, including deep-breathing exercises, meditation, and progressive muscle relaxation, have shown promising effects in reducing excessive stress responses that initiate central neurotransmitter and peripheral cortisol changes antecedent to MDD.

Regular aerobic exercise improves neurotransmitter and hormonal responses to stress, thereby creating a more dynamic and effective stress response system. Diet regulation also is necessary, to manage cyclical weight gain associated with carbohydrate craving that is seen in 75% of women with affective disturbance. Sleep-restoration techniques and diet address circadian and appetite disturbances prominent in depression. One nursing researcher is pioneering research in sleep deprivation and phase variation interventions that promote circadian rhythm restoration in women (McEnany, 1990). Still, significant nursing research demonstrating improvement in physiological and psychological functioning with the use of nonpharmacological somatic therapies is sorely needed.

Psychosocial therapies are requisite to achieving the goals of the nursing practice paradigm and are critical in effectively treating women's depression. There is vigorous debate about what strategies are most effective in reducing depressive symptoms and improving functioning. Research has shown that cognitive-behavioral therapy is most effective in those with prominent cognitive dysfunction, and interpersonal therapy works best for those with predominately social dysfunction. Because women's relationships are critically important to them and pessimism and poor self-esteem are common, it often is impossible to determine where the greater source of dysfunction lies. Nursing has much to contribute in identifying factors that lead to an effective match between treatment modalities and specific characteristics of young women.

The nursing practice paradigm does not provide guidance about the needed intensity of treatment for depressed women. Most clinical trials have shown that brief treatment of 3–6 months is adequate to secure symptom remission. There are several issues germane to women's depression, however, that are not addressed in these studies. Women with comorbid personality disorder often require sustained intervention beyond that supported by outcomes of these trials. Needed treatment intensity also may vary among groups of women. Women with a history of current or past trauma may require frequent, sustained psychosocial treatment during different phases of treatment while the biological, psychological, and social concomitants of trauma are addressed. Women with recurrent MDD may require much different intensity and duration of treatment than do women who are early in their trajectory for recurrent illness or experiencing a first episode.

Somatic and psychosocial treatment for premenopausal rural women with MDD based on the nursing practice paradigm is currently under investigation (Hauenstein, 1997). Each aspect of the model is tested, with the basic premise of reducing risks for depression while augmenting client resources. Somatic therapies implemented include stress reduction modalities, sleep restoration, dietary regulation, exercise, and augmentation of social support. Antidepressant medication is provided according to specific criteria. Psychosocial treatment is provided as well, aimed at increasing personal resiliency, problem solving, and use of social support. Cognitive-behavioral therapy and psychoeducation predominate among treatment strategies used.

Treatment is implemented according to a structured protocol in 12 sessions delivered in 3 months, with a protracted period of maintenance and follow-up for 12 months. Treatment is administered by clinical nurse specialists in collaboration with each woman's primary care provider and is offered in the client's home to overcome specific barriers to treatment.

Early outcomes indicate that women show symptomatic improvement with the described nursing intervention. Functional role limitations also are reduced with intervention. Treatment gains appear to be maintained for at least 6 months. Preliminary data indicate, however, that rural, low-income women may not tolerate the intensity of treatment involved in the 12-week sequence. About half of women entering treatment fail to complete the 12 sessions.

Early findings from this study illustrate the numerous challenging problems for nurses in providing depression treatment for women. Novel nursing approaches that illuminate unique etiological factors in specific populations of women are needed as well as innovative programs that match therapies to discrete populations. Intervention intensity and longevity also are fruitful areas for nursing research. Because nurses are often positioned to care for depressed women, nursing research and practice can contribute to reducing this health care need.

EMILY J. HAUENSTEIN

See also
CHRONIC MENTAL ILLNESS
RELAXATION TECHNIQUES

Part II

PATHOLOGIC CONDITIONS AND NURSING INTERVENTION

INTRODUCTION

The second section of the *Psychiatric Mental Health Nursing Research Digest* will review the nursing research on pathologic conditions and related nursing interventions. Pathologic conditions refer to psychiatric disorders that often cause significant functional impairment and may result in frequent hospitalizations. Because these conditions are generally chronic in nature, other individuals, especially family members may be actively involved in the care and treatment of those diagnosed with a psychiatric disorder. Therefore, the development of research-based nursing interventions that effectively address the needs of both the client and the family should be a major aim with this population.

Pathologic conditions may cause disturbances in thought, mood, and behavior and typically include schizophrenia, major depression, and bipolar disorder. The majority of entries in this section focus on these three disorders. The schizophrenia research on self-monitoring, symptom management, and coping strategies is well summarized in the entry by O'Connor, while studies of prodromal symptoms, illness course, family burden, and comorbidity are highlighted by Farrell. Martinez and Adamson examine one of the nursing interventions frequently used in the hospital setting, seclusion and restraint. The current research on depression in families is surveyed by Badger, and Wykle and Zauszniewski review geriatric depression, the most common psychiatric disorder in older persons. In addition, McCrone and Lenz describe the association between anxiety and depression and increased mortality rate following coronary artery bypass graft surgery. Finally, McDougall explores the research on gender differences, treatment issues, and caregiver burden related to bipolar disorder.

Schizophrenia, depression, and bipolar disorder are generally considered to be enduring and potentially disabling. Kane, therefore, outlines the current studies on health promotional behaviors, supportive interventions, and quality of life with chronic psychiatric illness. In a related entry, Lyon, Kane, and Parker examine the research on health concerns of women with severe and persistent mental illness. Findings suggest that women diagnosed with chronic psychiatric disorders are more likely to suffer from coexistent medical conditions and higher mortality rates.

Another group of entries includes the nursing literature on substance abuse. Sullivan stresses the importance of educating nurses to perform careful screening and intervention since chemically dependent individuals are frequently encountered in the hospital and community setting. Furthermore, substance abuse is often diagnosed in conjunction with psychiatric illness, according to Phoenix. In fact, recent findings indicate that dual diagnosis is prevalent in nearly half of those diagnosed with schizophrenia and in a majority of those diagnosed with bipolar disorder or antisocial personality disorder. Other topics of nursing research in the area of substance abuse include intervention strategies, nurses' attitudes, and drug addiction among nurses. Naegle's entry, which appears near the end of this section, synthesizes the current literature on substance abuse and addiction in registered nurses.

Mental health research with children is the focus of three of the entries in this section. According to Elder, child abuse and neglect may be related to substance abuse, anxiety, depression, and crime. Research from medical, psychosocial, and cultural perspectives is surveyed with a strong emphasis on the need for further inquiry. Murray describes the studies on sibling psychosocial adaptation to the childhood cancer experience. He looks at predictors of adjustment, coping strategies, and nursing interventions. Mohr reviews Webster-Stratton's extensive research on the prevention and treatment of conduct disorder in children.

Several entries on cognitive disorders are also included here. For example, McDougall outlines the research on psychosocial interventions for cognitively impaired older adults. In addition, Vermeersch and Foreman describe the studies that examine commonly used screening instruments in the assessment of delirium and report inadequacies in intervention research and in nursing education related to this disorder.

Correctional mental health research is the subject of an entry by Allen, Lovell, and Rhodes. Because of the increasing numbers of incarcerated mentally ill who are receiving inadequate treatment, the authors emphasize the need to designate this area as an important one for future research. Nursing inquiry with this vulnerable, underserved population may facilitate the reforms necessary for improved psychiatric intervention and rehabilitation.

Two entries in this section examine the nursing research with another vulnerable and underserved population, the homeless. It has been estimated that nearly one quarter of the homeless community suffer from some form of mental illness. McNamee and Lindsey report that most nursing studies on homeless health are descriptive in nature and seldom address health promotion and disease prevention. Kempe highlights the research on mood disorders in the homeless and asserts that while there has been an increase in research on the needs and problems of this community, nursing intervention studies are limited in number.

Other critical and timely topics included are eating disorders and the psychological sequelae of HIV. Although the incidence of eating disorders is increasing, according to Stein and White, few nursing studies had been undertaken in this area until recently. Much of the research is etiology based and looks at behavior, cognition, biology, and social factors. Kirksey, Hudson, Bunch, and Holzemer outline three major studies on symptom management and quality of life for persons living with HIV.

Research on suicide is the subject of two entries at the close of this section. According to Demi, nursing studies on suicide are few and typically explore suicidal messages, thoughts, behaviors, and attitudes. Moreover, much of the research focuses on the suicide survivors, namely, family members and therapists. In a related entry, Strickland reviews the current literature on intervention strategies and risk factors for suicide in Alaska Native and American Indian youth.

Finally, Murphy surveys the studies on responses to traumatic events. Individual responses may be emotional, cognitive, biological, or behavioral. Recent findings suggest that posttraumatic stress disorder is most effectively treated using multiple methods.

In conclusion, the nursing research on pathologic conditions in mental health must focus on the development of effective intervention strategies that will improve the quality of life for both the client and the family. Individuals diagnosed with a psychiatric illness, a substance abuse disorder, or a cognitive disorder often require a great deal of family and community support. Furthermore, the constraints imposed by the present system of managed care and the limited community resources available frequently create a need for families to assume a much greater role in the care and treatment of a family member diagnosed with a psychiatric illness. It is, therefore, essential to provide both client and family with the knowledge and assistance they will need for continued illness management and prevention of reoccurrence.

PATRICIA A. WILKE

ACUTE CONFUSION/DELIRIUM

Delirium or acute confusion is a disturbance of attention and cognition reflecting an acute brain failure (American Psychiatric Association, APA, 1994). It is a common and devastating symptom of underlying pathophysiology that adversely affects the patient, the family, and the caregivers (Inouye, Rusing, Foreman, Palmer, & Pompei, 1998; O'Keefe, 1999). Delirium creates behaviors that are unsafe and difficult to understand or manage. Hospitalized patients with delirium experience greater functional decline, morbidity, and mortality than nondelirious patients. They are more likely to experience residual cognitive impairment months after hospitalization and are at greater risk for dementia. Delirious patients consume more nursing resources due to their unsafe behaviors and increased dependency (Brannstrom, Gustafsson, Norberg, & Winblad, 1989; Ludwick, 1999; Sullivan-Marx, 1994; Williams, Ward, & Campbell, 1986). With the expected rise in the proportion of older persons and their increased use of health care services, the delirious older adult is rapidly becoming a major concern for nurses in all settings.

Despite the difficulties delirium creates for patients and caregivers, it has received little attention from researchers until the last 10 years. The major studies supporting nursing assessment, diagnosis, prevention, and treatment of delirium with recommendations for future nursing practice and research are presented here.

Assessment and Diagnosis

The assessment of delirium in practice and research is fraught with difficulties. These difficulties stem from the unstable nature of the phenomenon, differential diagnosis, lack of standardized tools, and failure of health practitioners to recognize or identify delirium (Foreman, Wakefield, Culp, & Milisen, 2000).

The DSM-IV criteria highlight the unstable nature of delirium; that is, it must develop acutely and vary diurnally (APA, 1994). The instability of both the presence and severity of the phenomenon make identification difficult for practitioners as well as researchers who must "capture" the phenomenon when it occurs (Bucht, Gustafson, & Sandberg, 1999). This instability also may explain to some extent the range of prevalence rates, which vary from 14 to 80% depending on the setting and population studied.

The practice guidelines recently developed by The American Psychiatric Association (APA, 1999) attempt to facilitate the differential diagnosis of delirium from dementia and depression. Although the guidelines are based on available research, the diagnostic criteria lack specific behavioral patterns and are not well grounded in research. In fact, very little is known concerning the natural history of delirium, the behavioral patterns, and how these patterns vary with etiology or treatment (Liptzin, 1999). Despite these flaws, the *Diagnostic and statistical manual of mental disorders-IV* criteria (American Psychiatric Association, 1994) are an attempt to standardize the diagnostic process and facilitate the differential diagnosis.

Several screening tools have been developed as well as tools to measure the severity of delirium. The most common tool to assess delirium is the Mini Mental Status Exam (MMSE) developed by Folstein et al. (1975) to measure cognitive functioning. Although this tool is used widely in both practice and research, it fails to distinguish delirium from dementia and more recently has been criticized because it fails to assess right brain functioning (Trzepacz, 1999).

Some screening tools for delirium or acute confusion are being used in research though not in practice. The primary advantage of these scales is their clinical utility (Rapp et al., 2000). The primary disadvantage is their lack of standardization. Several tools are available to measure the severity of delirium. Most are based on the criteria set out by the APA (1994). These tools require more training to use and may tend to miss the quieter forms of delirium that have more serious consequences for the patient (Foreman et al., 2000).

Physicians and nurses both underrecognize and underreport delirium (Johnson, Kerse, Gottleib, Wanich, Sullivan, & Chen, 1992). Physicians and other medical subspecialists record nonspecific terms versus a diagnosis of delirium. Of the criteria for delirium, both nurses and physicians tend to record disorientation most often and attention deficit (the key feature of delirium) the least often (Johnson et al., 1992).

Interventions

Intervention research has been sparse, as the etiology of delirium and its pathogenesis has not been well established. What intervention strategies have been developed flow from two models of delirium: vulnerability model (Inouye et al., 1999; Neelon & Champagne, 1992) and the cholinergic model (Trzepacz, 1999).

In the vulnerability model of delirium, two main factors lead to the development of delirium: predisposing or risk factors and precipitating factors or acute insults. Preexisting conditions that predispose an individual to delirium include existing cognitive impairment, severe physical illness, multisensory impairment, and evidence of dehydration. Precipitating factors are those involving the acute physical illness, its treatment, and the treatment environment that work cumulatively and simultaneously to supercede the individual's compensatory systems, culminating in delirium. Examples of some precipitating factors include: physical restraints and other immobilizing devices, malnutrition, polypharmacy, and any iatrogenic event, such as the use of bladder catheters (Inouye et al., 1999; Neelon & Champagne, 1992).

Treatment of existing delirium is focused on identifying the preexisting, predisposing, and precipitating factors then eliminating or lessening their impact. Neelon and Champagne (1992) organized the interventions into a hierarchy with vital functions first, followed by internal regulation, interpersonal interaction, and external stability. In other words, the nurse would administer oxygen before trying to reorient the patient. Neelon and Champagne's hierarchy emphasizes the necessity of attending to vital physiologic functions before attending to the interpersonal and environmental interventions.

Inouye and colleagues (1999) used the vulnerability model to identify those at greatest risk and provide preventive interventions. Specific protocols were developed for six identified risk factors: cognitive impairment, sleep deprivation, immobility, visual and hearing impairments, and dehydration. Results from their study are promising in terms of targeted outcomes and cost: the number and duration of episodes of delirium were reduced in hospitalized older patients. However, there was no significant effect on the severity of delirium or on reoccurrence rates. Once delirium occurred, the intervention was less effective and efficient.

Trzepacz's cholinergic model is based on studies of the neuropathogenesis of delirium (Trzepacz, 1999). Various researchers have described the changes in neural metabolism and neurotransmitter production and transmission during episodes of delirium in selected patient groups. One of the most promising observations is the decline in acetylcholine during a delirious episode. Such changes in neurotransmitters are the basis for the use of antipsychotics and benzodiazepines in treating the hyperactive forms of delirium. This model also can account for the positive impact of specific preventive strategies, such as oxygen. Treatment of less agitated forms of delirium is not as clear as the neuropathologic changes are not as well known. Likewise, there is growing evidence that the neuropathology of delirium may vary with the specific etiologic event, such as hypoxia versus drug intoxication.

In a review of prevention and treatment studies, Cole (1999) drew several conclusions. First, interventions were generally more effective in surgical patients, especially elderly persons. Second, the more the intervention targeted a specific risk factor (e.g., hypoxia), the more effective it was. Third, interventions carried out by nurses alone were as effective as those involving physicians.

Conclusions and Recommendations

The APA (1999) and the University of Iowa Gerontological Nursing Interventions Research Center (Rapp et al., 1998) have developed protocols for the detection and diagnosis of delirium. Both protocols are based on the available research and make a strong case for the use of routine screening using an instrument designed specifically for delirium, especially with elderly persons. These tools vary in their clinical utility and should be carefully evaluated before use in practice. As with any instrument, these tools help in the detection of delirium but are not sufficient for the diagnosis.

Protocols for the prevention and treatment of delirium are still under development. Some recommendations are available through the APA and Iowa group, but again, little research is available to support the wholehearted implementation of either protocol. In particular, little is known about which patient groups are best treated with physiologic interventions, medications, or environmental/behavioral interventions. Neelon and Champagne's hierarchy holds the most promise for nursing practice, but the intervention protocols need further development and testing with a wide variety of patient populations.

Nursing research needs to focus on the following areas: The natural history of delirium in various patient populations (including children, young adults, and the middle aged) using in-depth case study. Studies that correlate physiologic parameters with specific behaviors are critical to further our understanding of the phenomenon and the pathophysiology. Screening tools need to be compared across patient populations for their psychometric properties and clinical utility. Prevention and intervention protocols need to be further developed and tested across settings and populations. The actual costs associated with delirium need to be further explicated, especially in out-patient and home-care settings.

Nursing educational programs need to include delirium as thoroughly as heart failure, attending especially to the vulnerability and effects on the older adult. Routine screening for delirium using a specific tool should be included in all physical assessment classes and interventions for prevention and treatment added to basic medical-surgical courses. Of particular importance is conveying the attitude that delirium is an indication of acute brain failure regardless of the person's age and should be treated quickly and aggressively by the entire health care team.

MARQUIS D. FOREMAN
PATRICIA E. H. VERMEERSCH

See also
COGNITIVE DISORDERS

ALCOHOLISM

The DSM-IV diagnostic category of alcohol dependence is commonly called alcoholism. Alcohol dependence is a disease characterized by abnormal alcohol-seeking behavior that leads to impaired control over drinking (National Association on Alcohol Abuse and Alcoholism [NIAAA], 1993). A diagnosis of alcohol abuse refers to a pattern of use that results in detrimental effects on health or social life that may eventually lead to alcohol dependence.

Alcohol dependence (alcoholism) is a primary, chronic disease with genetic, psychosocial, and environmental factors that influence its development and manifestations. Alcoholism results after prolonged, continuous, or periodic use of alcohol. Alcoholism is noted when control over drinking is impaired, when preoccupation with alcohol occurs, and when use continues despite adverse consequences. The disease often is progressive and fatal. Distortions in thinking, most notably denial, result (Sullivan, 1995).

Alcohol is a depressant drug and is the most commonly used and abused substance of addiction. It is widely available, can be legally acquired by persons over 21 (in most states), and is relatively inexpensive.

Prolonged use of alcohol results in numerous physiological and psychological effects. Alcohol is metabolized by the liver; women may metabolize alcohol less efficiently than men. Liver damage often occurs as a result of prolonged use. Alcohol-induced cardiovascular injury, immune system impairment, and neurological disorders also can occur. Alcohol withdrawal syndrome is usually mild and self-limiting but in about 5% of cases can result in delirium tremens, which can be potentially fatal.

In contrast with other health problems, there is no definitive physical finding or laboratory test for alcoholism. Tests for liver function reveal end-stage organ damage; they do not detect the primary disorder.

Alcohol use has occurred throughout recorded history. Alcoholism has often been considered a moral failing caused by the availability of alcohol. The temperance movement and Prohibition were attempts to control alcoholism. The establishment of Alcoholics Anonymous in the early 1930s and the acceptance of alcoholism as a medical condition in the mid-1950s were more therapeutic efforts to address alcoholism.

Reflecting absence of societal interest and the health care community's lack of understanding, research and clinical reports about alcoholism have been sparse in the nursing literature and in nursing science. Prior to 1989, studies of alcohol abuse or alcoholism were often descriptive, addressed nurses' attitudes toward clients with alcohol problems, or studied nurses who were recovering from alcoholism (Naegle, 1995). Nurse researchers who have contributed to the early literature on alcoholism include Haack, Hughes, Naegle, and Sullivan, among others.

In fact, information about alcoholism has been scant in nursing curricula. Thus, nursing students and presumably future clinicians and scientists were not aware of the extent of alcoholism as a health problem, and few studies of this serious illness were pursued. Nurses, however, care for clients with alcoholism regularly. It has been estimated that 30% of hospitalized patients have disorders secondary to alcohol abuse, such as trauma, falls, cirrhosis, pancreatitis, or cardiovascular disease (NIAAA, 1993). Further, 15% to 20% of clients seen in primary care settings are estimated to have alcohol disorders (Fleming & Barry, 1992).

Recent initiatives by the federal government have attempted to ameliorate the lack of content and expertise in nursing education. Beginning in 1989, the National Institute on Alcohol Abuse and Alcoholism (NIAAA), the National Institute on Drug Abuse (NIDA), and the Office of Substance Abuse Prevention (now the Center for Substance Abuse Prevention) established initiatives to improve substance abuse education in schools of nursing through model curriculum projects and faculty development programs. Three curriculum models are now available, and more than 60 faculty fellows from 13 schools of nursing have been prepared through the federal faculty development grants; some have now received funding for alcohol research from NIAAA. Reports of this work, however, are in progress and not yet available in the literature. However, empirically based studies examining clinical interventions are beginning to appear in the literature (Mudd, Boyd, Brower, Young, & Blow, 1994; Wing & Thompson, 1995).

The potential for improved access to information about alcoholism exists through the curriculum models and the expertise of faculty, some of whom will continue alcohol research efforts and will encourage alcohol research among their students. It must be noted, however, that most schools of nursing do not have faculty trained in these projects and must rely on individual initiative to develop or enhance alcohol-related content.

Alcohol remains the most widely used and abused drug in America. Nurses will continue to encounter the consequences of alcohol abuse and dependence among their clients. It is essential that nurses be cognizant of the dire results of excessive alcohol consumption and be participants in the efforts to rehabilitate alcoholic clients. Although past research has focused on such issues as alcohol abuse content in nursing education or nurses with alcohol problems—both important topics—nonetheless, future research must target intervention strategies to improve the care of clients with alcohol disorders. The health of millions of clients with alcohol problems depends on it.

ELEANOR J. SULLIVAN

See also
DRUG ABUSE
VIOLENCE AS A NURSING AREA OF INQUIRY

BIPOLAR DISORDERS

Emil Kraepelin (1856–1926) created the diagnosis of manic-depressive insanity in 1896, and it continues to influence present day psychiatry. His intellectual curiosity was in the nosological dichotomy between schizophrenia (dementia praecox) and bipolar disorder (manic-depressive insanity). A recent metaanalysis of a sample of Kraepelin's primary data suggests that his original classification is supported by clinical evidence (Jablensky, 1999). This chapter reviews selected nursing and multidisciplinary research studies published on bipolar disorders and retrievable from PubMed. With the exception of two references, the review covers the period 1995 to 2000. The emphasis is on gender differences, late life, treatment, and illness burden for the patient and family members. This paper does not review studies of genetic markers, substance abuse comorbidity, schizophrenia, and psychosocial interventions in which the principal investigator was not a nurse.

There is a continuing debate regarding the clinical manifestations of mania in pure and mixed episodes. When they compared signs and symptoms of 316 patients with mania and those mixed bipolar disorder, Cassidy, Murry, Forest, and Carroll (1998) found substantial rates of dysphoria, lability, anxiety, and irritability. Surveys provide important data regarding treatment and relapse. Shepherd and Hill (1996) found that 89% of the national respondents from a manic depression fellowship in England reported at least one hospital admission. In a survey of forty-two nurse practitioners, 76% prescribed psychotropic medications for their clients even though depression and anxiety disorders were the most frequent conditions, with bipolar disorder and schizophrenia seen less often (Flenniken, 1997). Akiskal and Pinto (1999) support a broadening of the bipolar spectrum and a partial return to Kraepelin's broad concept of manic-depressive illness by focusing on the clinical subtypes I through IV. They believe this approach will augment the utilization of mood stabilizers.

Weissman and colleagues' (1996) study ($N = 38{,}000$) conducted on major depression and bipolar disorders included the United States, Canada, Puerto Rico, France, West Germany, Italy, Lebanon, Taiwan, Korea, and New Zealand. The researchers found that the lifetime rates were consistent across countries, from .3 per 100 in Taiwan to 1.5 per 100 in New Zeland. In addition, the sex ratios were nearly equal, however, the age at first onset is earlier (average, 6 years) than the onset of major depression (range, 24.8–34.8 years). In Denmark from 1971 to 1993, Kessing (1998) analyzed the discharge diagnoses of 20,350 first-time admitted patients with affective, depressive, or manic-cycle disorders and found that the risk of recurrence was progressive regardless of age, gender, and type of disorder.

Gender Differences

Women have a higher incidence of rapid cycling bipolar disorder (RCBD), defined as the presence of at least four affective episodes per year (Kilzieh & Aksikal, 1999). Leibenluft (1996) found that bipolar women have more depressive episodes and fewer manic episodes than bipolar men do. Women also report greater overall impairment, later onset mania, and often experience mixed episodes (Robb, Young, Cooke, & Joffe, 1998). Tondo and Baldessarini (1998a) metaanalyzed 10 studies with a total of 2057 patients with bipolar disorders and found that among women and men with RCBD, the percentage of women was higher than men (72% vs. 28%). The risk of rapid cycling was inconsistently greater among women than men (30% vs. 17%). Leibenluft, Ashman, Feldman-Naim, and Yonkers (1999) found that even though women were overrepresented in samples of patients, they concluded there was no association between menstrual cycle and mood in women with RCBD. Pregnancy poses special risks to the fetus, even though the rate of bipolar disorder recurrence during the first 40 weeks after lithium was discontinued was the same for pregnant and nonpregnant women (Viguera et al., 2000).

Treatment Concerns

Treating RCBD with standard therapies is difficult since lithium is insufficient to prevent the frequency of the episodes in up to 82% of cases (Kruger, Braunig, &

Young, 1996). Various mood stabilizers such as carbamazepine and valproate, neuroleptics, antidepressants, calcium channel blockers, l-thyroxine, benzodiazepines, and electroconvulsive therapy (ECT) are being used. Several authors concluded that antidepressant treatment might actually worsen RCBD. In a longitudinal analysis of 51 patients with treatment-refractory bipolar disorder, antidepressant-induced cycle acceleration occurred in 25% of the sample and was associated with being female and younger (Altshuler et al., 1995). Neuroleptic treatment in bipolar disorders poses the risk of developing tardive dyskinesia, akathisia, and acute dystonia. Brotman, Fergus, Post, and Leverich (2000) reviewed treatment-refractory bipolar disorder in the records of 133 patients treated at the National Institutes of Mental Health (NIMH) and found only 12 of the group previously treated with neuroleptics required these drugs at discharge. They concluded that neuroleptic treatment should be minimal. After a retrospective review of 178 NIMH patients' records treated between 1974 and 1996, Frye et al. (2000) found a 78% improvement rate was achieved. However, over time, each 5-year cohort of patients required increasing numbers of medications to achieve the same degree of improvement at hospital discharge.

Simon and Unutzer (1999) found insured patients with bipolar disorder costs were significantly higher than age- and sex-matched general medical outpatients, patients treated for depression, or diabetes. In the bipolar disorder group, mental health and substance abuse services accounted for 45% of the total costs. Unutzer, Simon, Pabiniak, Bond, and Katon (2000) found that in pharmacy records of bipolar disorder patients ($N = 1246$), 83% of the subjects filled a mood stabilizer prescription during the 1-year study period; however, 75% of the subjects had at least one interruption in medication use. In addition, 50% of the subjects had one 7-month period without a recorded blood level or monitoring of their medications for adverse effects. Lithium treatment reduces morbidity with greater benefits in bipolar type I and II patients (Baldessarini & Tondo, 2000; Tondo, Baldessarini, Hennen, & Floris, 1998b). After a long period of declining use, the number of Medicare beneficiaries treated with ECT between 1987 and 1992 has steadily increased from 12,000 to 15,560 (Rosenbach, Hermann, & Dorwart, 1997). In the outpatient setting, over the same time, ECT expenditures have increased from 7% to 16%, with a patient receiving an average of eight treatments. Those patients living in the Northeast compared to those patients living in the West received more ECT treatments (8.3 vs. 6.7).

Burden of Care

Family members are stressed by a relative with chronic mental illness. Honig, Hofman, Rozendaal, and Dingemans (1997) found that when compared to the control group, relatives in a treatment group showed a significant change from high to low levels of expressed emotion. In a study of 266 caregivers of patients with bipolar illness, 93% of the caregivers reported moderate or greater distress in burden (Perlick et al., 1999). In addition, the caregivers' illness beliefs were strongly predictive of the burden experienced.

Nursing research has focused on qualitative investigations of the caregiving experience of caring for a relative with bipolar disorder, as well as caring for the individual with the illness. Clement (1996) found that women married to men with bipolar disorder have more problems with separation-individuation than women married to men without this mental illness. Jeon and Madjar (1998) found 14 caregivers lived each day without long-term plans, looked at the world through the ill family member, and observed how the outside world responded to the illness. Rose (1998) found that 15 caregivers focused on the essence of the ill person, found a place for self, and helped the relative move forward. Hume, Barker, Robertson, and Swan (1988) hypothesized that life events had a greater influence on relapses in patients with bipolar disorder than was previously believed; whereas Barker (1994) hypothesized that locus of control and cognitive vulnerability may be important cognitive factors that predict the clinical picture of the illness. Pollack's (1996) research program focused on both quantitative and qualitative methods to learn more about bipolar patients' informational needs, coping abilities, and self-management strategies. Patients need information on managing the disorder, relating to others, managing daily life, relating with self, and living in society. Bonin (1999) developed a predictive model of lithium compliance based on Pender's Health Promotion Model and found that being female, being older, living with a partner, and evaluating perceived treatment benefits and obstacles were predictive of lithium compliance.

Late-Onset Bipolar Disorder

In the older adult population, a diagnosis of bipolar disorder is uncommon (VanGerpen, Johnson, & Winstead, 1999). Webster and Grossberg (1998) found 10% of 1700 geriatric patients admitted to an acute inpatient psychogeriatric unit had late-life psychosis. Whereas Blixen, McDougall, and Suen (1997) found that 17% of the older adult patients on a psychogeriatric unit had bipolar disorder (7%) and psychosis (10%). The clinical manifestations often consist of delusions and hallucinations, and clinical manifestations are of greater severity, lower comorbidity, and a higher incidence of bipolar I disorder rather than unipolar disorder (Benazzi, 1999). Shulman and Herrmann (1999) found the prognosis to be poor with high morbidity and mortality rates. Treatment in elderly psychiatric patients often includes clozapine, which was found to be safe in a low mean dose of 134 mg daily (Barak, Wittenberg, Naor, Kutzuk, & Weizman, 1999).

In summary, descriptive research continues to be the primary emphasis in studies of bipolar disorder. Ongoing work with assessment and diagnosis of the illness is a major thrust of multidisciplinary efforts with a particular emphasis on drug trials. Continued research on late-life mania is needed. Nurses have primarily focused on caregivers without developing research-based strategies to assist the patients who have to live with bipolar disorder. Given the availability and number of internet-based support groups, there were no studies identified in which these psychosocial interventions have been tested for their efficacy. Future knowledge development is directed toward psychosocial and self-help interventions with the internet and its ability to offer support to the individuals who must adapt and cope with living with chronic mental illness.

GRAHAM J. MCDOUGALL

CHILD ABUSE AND NEGLECT

Child abuse and neglect, also known as "maltreatment," represent a component of violence in society that poses major threats to the integrity of families (Gelles & Cornell, 1990; Strauss, Gelles, & Steinmetz, 1980). Many of society's problems such as substance abuse, anxiety, and depression (Downs & Harrison, 1998), as well as sexual dysfunction and crime (Creighton & Noyes, 1989; Geffner, 1992; Hobbs, Hanks, & Wynne, 1999) are thought to be closely associated with child abuse and neglect. Therefore child abuse and neglect must be viewed as priorities and addressed vigorously by nurses and other health practitioners. The priority was suggested at the 1992 Second Invitational Conference on Research Priorities in Nursing Science by the National Center for Nursing Research (Staff, 1993, p. 4) and remains an identified research focal area by the current National Institute of Nursing Research and the National Academy of Sciences (1998).

The author's recent review of the literature shows that to advance knowledge in the area of child abuse and neglect, there must be (a) clear definitions of clinically relevant terminology spanning multiple disciplines; (b) theoretical models and frameworks for organizing and testing knowledge; and (c) sound research initiatives leading to the systematic investigation of diagnostic and intervention methods focusing on early recognition and family-centered treatment of children.

Defining Child Abuse and Neglect

"Child abuse" is legally defined as "Any form of cruelty to a child's physical, moral or mental well-being" (Nolan & Nolan-Haley, 1990, p. 239). Examples of child abuse include overt physical abuse defined as "inflicted acts causing physical injury" (Dubowitz & DePanfilis, 2000, p. 15) such as hitting, grabbing, burning, and shaking, as well as emotional abuse, which may be more subtle and difficult to detect. In addition, children who witness family violence and abuse are themselves victimized (Hobbs, Hanks, & Wynne, 1999; Stuart & Laraia, 1998). "Child abuse" is also used to describe the form of sexual attack that may or may not amount to rape (Nolan & Nolan-Haley, 1990). In the Child Abuse Prevention and Treatment Act of 1974 the definition of child abuse was expanded to include not only cruelty but also negligent treatment or maltreatment of a child under the age of 18 by a person who is responsible for the child's welfare (American Association for Protecting Children, 1986). "Child neglect" is defined as "omissions in care resulting in significant harm or the risk of significant harm to children" (Dubowitz & DePanfilis, 2000, p. 10). Legal definitions do not specify what qualifies as "significant harm" or "risk of harm." Consequently, health care professionals and local child welfare agencies are left to interpret the definition in the context of specific cases. As one might imagine, this ambiguity can be problematic to clinicians and researchers. Helfer and Kempe (1987) offer some clarity by discussing child maltreatment in a family context and defining it as any interaction or lack of interaction between family members that results in nonaccidental harm to the individual's physical or developmental states.

Need for Clinically Applicable Theoretical Models

To advance science in a particular area, it is important to employ an organizing framework with clearly defined theoretical concepts. Unfortunately, research in child abuse and neglect has been hindered by unclear concepts and theoretical frameworks specific to certain disciplines. Professionals involved in the care of maltreated children and their families often view their clients through their own professional lenses rather than seeking to formulate more globally understood and accepted perspectives. These specialized and fragmented perceptions lead to what has been described as a "jigsaw puzzle approach to child maltreatment." Efforts must be directed toward combining individual "pieces" to form a more functional "overall picture" (Hobbs, Hanks, & Wynne, 1999, p. 3). Critical to a comprehensive approach is an understanding of the medical and the psychosocial perspectives as well as the cultural context.

Medical Model. The medical model of child maltreatment focuses on the nonaccidental aspect of injuries. Traditionally, emphasis has been on assessing child physical and sexual abuse with more recent attention on sequelae related to emotional abuse and neglect. For the most part, diagnosis and treatment remain child centered. However, recently more attention has focused on family pathology, particularly related to conditions such as Munchausen Syndrome By Proxy, which is difficult to diagnose without assessment of the perpetrating parent (Monteleone, 1998).

Psychosocial Models. Numerous psychosocial theoretical perspectives have been proposed as explanations for child abuse and neglect. Yet there is no universally accepted model. Focus is often on disturbances in the parent-child relationship related to negative parental childhood experiences, marital or child-rearing stress, and impoverished living conditions with related environmental stressors. Bowlby's (1969) attachment theory has been a core concept in many research studies. Garbarino (1977) and Belsky (1980) propose that an anxious or insecure attachment is a critical concept in child maltreatment within complex familial ecology. Theoretical frameworks for studying child neglect, such as the newly developed Parental Environmental Cluster Model (Burke, Chandy, Dannerbeck, Watt, 1998), are needed to facilitate intervention development and testing in all areas of child maltreatment.

Cultural Context. Others contend that child abuse should be viewed from a broader social perspective (Paulk, 1999; Williams & Vine, 1999). Stress incurred through poverty, unemployment, racism, and inequality among individuals are all theorized to have an impact on the prevalence of child maltreatment in modern society (Hobbs, Hanks, & Wynne, 1999). Building on this theoretical base, McKinney and Frank (1998) suggest using King's theory of dynamic interacting systems (King, 1981) to examine the effect of personal, family, and community stressors on abuse victims. Cowen (1999) discusses how treatment for neglectful families should include nurses as child advocates and a multidisciplinary team approach to improve family functioning and promote safe and nurturing home environments.

Building Knowledge Through Research

As discussed, knowledge regarding child maltreatment is fragmented. There is an urgent need to develop appropriate theoretical frameworks that are multidisciplinary and facilitate systematic research. Critical to this endeavor is a discussion of limitations related to previous research and current directions in the area of child abuse and neglect.

Over the past decade substantial progress has been made in understanding the symptomatology associated with child maltreatment. However, prevention and intervention research studies are rare and often have methodological limitations (Kaplan, Pelcovitz, & Labruna, 1999). Particularly troubling are marked discrepancies in the findings from retrospective and prospective studies. Downs and Harrison (1998) note methodological limitations resulting from differences between data from official records and self-report measures. Furthermore, research has failed to identify any factors that are present in all abusing families and absent in all nonabusing families.

Current knowledge gaps reflect inherent difficulties in child maltreatment research. For example, child abuse and neglect are sensitive topics, therefore subject recruitment and retention as well as data collection can be particularly challenging. In addition, the complexity of child maltreatment mandates a variety of research methods. While it is critical to identify high-risk families and intervene early, it is also important to understand the phenomenon of maltreatment. Both quantitative and qualitative approaches are indicated. Well-designed and executed empirical research can provide essential data for evaluating current and future diagnostic and treatment methods while sound qualitative research is needed to further define and develop theoretical models.

Current findings indicate that future research should focus on the identification and treatment of high-risk children within the context of their families and society. Some factors thought to contribute to child maltreatment include unrealistic parental beliefs and limited parenting skills, inappropriate foster care placements, familial stress related to unemployment and single-parent households, inexperienced adolescent mothers, cognitively impaired parents, parental substance abuse and other mental illnesses, child developmental disorders, and chronic illness within families (e.g., AIDS). Also worthy of further investigation is the repetition of abuse that may result from inadequate parenting and parent role-modeling over several generations (Jackson & Saunders, 1993; Patterson, 1998).

Summary

Clearly there is a need to further understand all aspects of the child maltreatment phenomenon, characterize complex maladaptive family systems, develop suitable multidisciplinary theoretical models and frameworks, and empirically evaluate interventions aimed at modifying unhealthy parent-child interactions. As front-line interveners, nurses are not only legally and ethically responsible to report suspected abuse but are well-positioned to build research programs addressing each of these knowledge gaps.

JENNIFER HARRISON ELDER

See also

CHILD AND ADOLESCENT MENTAL HEALTH INTERVENTIONS
CULTURAL ASPECTS

CHILDHOOD CANCER EXPERIENCE AND SIBLING PSYCHOSOCIAL ADAPTATION

Cancer is the principal antecedent of disease-related death among children in the United States. Over 7500 new cases of childhood cancer were diagnosed during

1996. Furthermore, the occurrence of cancer among children is escalating. Treatment of many childhood cancers has improved greatly, with over 60% of children diagnosed expected to survive (National Childhood Cancer Foundation, 1997). Many childhood cancers are now perceived as chronic diseases involving repeated hospital stays and long-term, intensive treatments (Cohen, 1985). The overwhelming demands of this disease, including the prognosis, are unpredictable elements that cause enormous stress for all family members (Cohen, 1985; Murray, 1999a). The family must learn to integrate the child's illness and treatment into their everyday lives as they endeavor to regain a sense of normalcy (Murray, 1998).

The demands of childhood cancer on ill children and their parents have been studied for over 40 years now. Despite progress in this area of research, very little importance has been placed on examining the effects of the cancer experience on healthy siblings. With pediatric health care providers today, there is a growing cognizance that the psychosocial needs of healthy siblings are less adequately met than those of other family members (Murray, 1999a). A review of the literature by Murray (1999a) reveals that siblings are particularly susceptible to adjustment difficulties (depression, anger, anxiety, feelings of guilt, and social isolation), and they experience similar stress to that of the ill child. The need to prevent adjustment difficulties has been emphasized by clinicians and researchers throughout the research literature (Murray, 1999a).

Clinical investigations conducted over the past several decades have explicated psychosocial adjustment difficulties siblings' face when they have a sibling with childhood cancer. Research on siblings has made some advancement over the past few years. Research has broadened from a retrospective approach distinguishing psychosocial problems following the ill child's death (Binger et al., 1969; Cain, Fast, & Erickson, 1964) to an exploratory approach identifying stressors during the illness experience (Cairns, Clark, Smith, & Lansky, 1979).

Although researchers have identified many negative effects of the cancer experience on siblings, using qualitative research methodology they have identified positive effects as well. Iles (1979) and Kramer (1981) found both positive and negative effects of having a sibling with cancer. Positive consequences included increased sensitivity and empathy for the patient and others, enhanced personal maturation, and an increased appreciation for life. Negative consequences included emotional stress, sense of emotional deprivation, decrease in parental tolerance, increase in parental expectations, anger, and guilt. Further descriptive exploratory research by Havermans and Eiser (1994) also found that siblings became more empathetic toward others and valued life more.

Additional exploratory and descriptive research has been conducted that identifies some siblings adjust to the stressors of the childhood cancer experience with minimal disruption (Koch-Hattem, 1986). Van Dongen-Melman, De Groot, Hahlen, and Verhulst (1995) investigated the after effects of the childhood cancer experience on well siblings. The researchers found no differences between siblings of children that survived childhood cancer and controls on emotional and behavioral problems.

Studies on variables found to predict sibling adjustment to the cancer experience have also been conducted. Using a longitudinal exploratory approach, Spinetta (1981) found several age-related differences with adaptation. Siblings between the ages of 4 and 6 had significantly lower self-concept scores and a more negative attitude toward self than the child with cancer. Siblings between the ages of 6 and 12 years had more maladaptive levels of anxiety, depression, and maladaptive responses (e.g., acting out behaviors). Cohen (1985) identified predictors of sibling adjustment to include parent depression, marital adjustment, annual family income, neighborhood/community social support, parent-sibling communication about the illness, and time since diagnosis. Wang and Martinson (1996) found inadequate knowledge, reduced family communication, and insufficient support to be adjustment predictors. Another study in 1996 conducted by Sloper and While found adjustment difficulties were related to the degree of disruption of family life caused by the illness and resources available to the family to cope with the effects of such disruption.

To identify and describe coping strategies used by siblings to contend with the stressors imposed as a result of the cancer experience, the following studies were conducted. Walker (1988) conducted a qualitative study and found coping strategies used by siblings included wishful thinking, talking to others, attention-seeking behaviors, and solitary play. Heffernan and Zanelli (1997) described playing with friends to be an effective coping strategy for siblings.

More recent research endeavors have been targeted at recognizing what behaviors or interventions health care providers understand to be most significant in promoting the siblings' coping efforts with the effects of childhood cancer and its treatment (Walker et al., 1992). In a Delphi study by Walker et al. (1992), common sibling facilitative behaviors included making siblings feel special, encouraging consistent discipline for all children, and encouraging visits to the hospital/clinic. In 1995, Murray conducted a descriptive study investigating interventions used by pediatric oncology nurses to provide support to siblings of children with cancer. Results indicated that the two most frequently used nursing interventions to provide support to siblings were (a) encouraging parents to spend time with their healthy children; and (b) providing honest responses to questions asked by siblings.

To obtain an understanding of a sibling's experience with the childhood cancer experience, a phenomenological study was conducted by Murray (1998). Themes that emerged through the data included: emotional intensity, increased empathy for others, personal growth, need for support, and desire to help others.

Previous research has identified that pediatric oncology nurses report barriers to providing support to siblings, Murray (1999b) found pediatric oncology nurses frequently reported staffing shortages, lack of access to siblings, institutional constraints, role boundary issues, and lack of support for sibling support groups as common barriers to meeting the needs of siblings. The findings of this investigation suggest that additional research is needed to determine the best way to provide interventions for siblings given the barriers reported.

Studying the meaning of the childhood cancer experience for healthy siblings and identifying interventions aimed at promoting adaptation is in the early stages (Murray, 1999a; Wang & Martinson, 1996). Additional quantitative and qualitative studies are needed to fully address the childhood cancer experience for healthy siblings.

Advances in pediatric oncology have significantly improved the rate of survival in children with childhood cancers. As greater advances are made with these diseases, understanding the impact not only on the patient, but also on other members of the family is critical. Siblings of childhood cancer patients are considered to be vulnerable to adjustment difficulties. The need to identify, and implement in clinical practice, nursing interventions to provide psychosocial support to healthy siblings is essential.

LT. COLONEL JOHN S. MURRAY

The views expressed in this article are those of the author and do not reflect the official policy or position of the United States Air Force, Department of Defense, or the US Government.

See also

CHILD AND ADOLESCENT MENTAL HEALTH INTERVENTIONS
STRESS

CHILDHOOD PSYCHOPATHOLOGY

Although we do not know the extent or prevalence of mental illness in children, psychopathology in children appears to be a relatively common occurrence. Overall estimates of developmental, emotional, and behavioral disorders in children have ranged from 14% to 22% of all children with more severe forms of diagnosable mental disturbances estimated to occur in approximately 8% to 10% of all children (United States Department of Health and Human Services, 1999). This translates to as many as 10 million children in the United States who suffer from psychiatric problems that are sufficiently severe to compromise their ability to function optimally. Moreover, these estimates do not include a substantial number of children who manifest subclinical or undiagnosed disturbances that may place them at high risk for the later development of more severe clinical problems.

Despite these facts, nursing research in the area of child psychopathology is scant, reflecting what Hyman (June 21, 1999) refers to as a "an alarming lack of skillful researchers in the area of childhood mental health." Textbooks contain many references to articles written by nurses, but when one looks closely at these references they are primarily expository in nature. Thus, finding references that represent what nurses have contributed to this field presents a singular challenge. By far the most prolific nurse researcher in the area of childhood psychopathology is Carolyn Webster-Stratton, who has studied conduct disordered children and their families for over two decades. This brief article discusses conduct disorder and reviews Webster Stratton's contribution to the prevention and treatment of this condition as well as their implications for nursing.

Conduct Disorder

Webster-Stratton's research involves children with Conduct disorder. Conduct disorder is a disruptive behavior disorder (APA, 1994) that is comprised of aggressive and antisocial behaviors involving the infliction of pain or the denial or the rights of others (e.g., initiating fights, breaking into others' homes, firesetting). Some of the causal influences in the development of early onset conduct disorder are: male gender, genetic risk, neuropsychological deficits, low verbal IQ, family discord, discordant parent-child interactions or abuse history, attachment disruption, low socioeconomic status, and neighborhood influences (Craig & Pepler, 1998). Children with conduct disorder invariably have poor prognoses.

Review of Literature

Because they are the most powerful and proximal influence on their children, Webster-Stratton's program of research has focused specifically on the role of their parents. One early research study was concerned with the interactions of clinic-referred parents and their conduct disordered children with those of non-clinic "normal" parents who had children without conduct problems. Examining the interactions for negative and positive affective components, results indicated that clinic parents exhibited considerably more negative verbal interactions with and more negative nonverbal affect toward their children that the nonclinic sample. Moreover, the children in the clinic sample exhibited fewer positive behaviors with their mothers than children in the nonclinic sample (Webster-Stratton & Fjone, 1989).

Further studying parents and their interactions with young children Whipple and Webster-Stratton (1991) examined the role of parental stress in physically abusive and nonabusive families with conduct disorder. Parental stress was found to play a critical role in abusive families who were found more likely to be living in poverty, had less education, more frequently reported a history of child abuse, and were more likely to abuse drugs or alcohol. The mothers in abusive families were more often depressed and reported more stress due to life events and more marital dissatisfaction and social isolation than the nonabusive group. Furthermore, the fathers in the abusive group spanked their children more, and the mothers exhibited a high frequency of negative and critical statements to their children. Children from abusive households had significantly more behavior problems.

With respect to interventions with parents, she and her colleagues examined the effects of a videotaped modeling group discussion program. This program consists of 10 videotapes of modeled parenting skills that are shown by a therapist to groups of 8 to 12 parents. Following this BASIC program parents are offered an ADVANCE program that involves components of personal control, communication skills, problem solving skills, and strengthening social support and self care. The ADVANCE component was added to target other parental risk factors, such as marital distress and anger management. A series of five randomized studies was conducted to evaluate the effectiveness of the BASIC program in terms of improving the quality of parental attitudes and parent-child interactions, reducing parents' reliance on violent disciplinary practices, and reducing the number of child conduct problems. Comparison groups consisted of nonintervention as well as other intervention groups of parents. The results of these studies revealed that the program was highly effective in improving child and parental behaviors. The mothers were found to be less critical and more positive of their children, and children were more independent and less negative with their mothers. Moreover, it was effective in terms of achieving sustained improvement in children's conduct disorders in over 60% of the BASIC intervention group families (Webster-Stratton, 1981, 1982a, 1982b, 1984, 1990; Webster-Stratton, Kolpacoff, & Hollinsworth, 1988).

When the ADVANCE treatment was added and evaluated with 78 parents who were randomly assigned to the BASIC or BASIC and ADVANCE programs, both groups improved at short-term follow-up. But the ADVANCE group produced additional improvements in terms of parents' communication and problem-solving skills.

Most recently the effectiveness of the BASIC and an additional training component (PARTNERS 2), which included a teacher training component, was evaluated with 394 Head Start mothers, teachers, and family service workers. Head Start centers were randomly assigned to the intervention condition (BASIC plus PARTNERS 2) or to a control condition that involved the regular Head Start program. Mothers in the intervention group were observed by teachers to make fewer negative remarks, use less physical discipline, and were more positive and consistent in their discipline styles than the control group. Intervention children exhibited significantly fewer conduct problems and more positive affect than control children (Webster-Stratton, 1998).

Implications

The brief summary of a sample of Webster-Stratton's research illustrates study of only one childhood disorder. But it shows great promise for future prevention interventions that would target families that are at high risk for having conduct disordered children. By assessing families for risk factor profiles, the videotaped programs could represent a potential early intervention that could assist in breaking the cycle of an exceedingly devastating condition.

Future Directions

Webster-Stratton's program of research into conduct disordered children serves as a paradigm for psychiatric nursing research. Not only does her research inform assessment strategies, but the intervention that she and her colleagues have developed shows promise as an overall program of treatment. Moreover, it is cost effective—a not insignificant consideration in this managed care environment.

Further research efforts with conduct disordered children, as well as children with other conditions and their families should include:

- Research strategies that are not only focused on the effectiveness of interventions, but that attempt to understand mechanisms that moderate or mediate long-term adaptation.
- Efforts to identify "resilient" children and their families to design intervention and prevention strategies on what can be learned from this population.
- Teasing out the differences between families who are "ready to change" and become engaged in a treatment program and those who are not. Developing different intervention strategies for the families who are more resistant.
- Coordinated efforts employing a similar framework for research that would take into account both development and context. This would require working in multidisciplinary teams.

Conclusion

Our nursing research showings in the area of childhood psychopathology are meager and our practices suffer accordingly in the absence of an empirically grounded knowledge base. We only have to look at the history of exposés involving the practices in many of our child psychiatric units and residential treatment facilities to see the results of this neglect.

The field of child psychopathology is overshadowed by the persistent, unmet mental health needs of children in the United States. The present system within which children are treated is inadequate at early identification, early intervention, and outreach to vulnerable low-income, minority populations who are disproportionately at risk (Knitzer & Aber, 1995). Disparity exists between the number of children who are in need of mental health services and those who receive any services at all. The traditional treatment delivery system is inadequate to meet the developmental and mental health needs of our most vulnerable groups of children in high-risk environments (United States Department of Health and Human Services, 1999). These children are inadequately served, and those who receive services often receive culturally inappropriate and contextually irrelevant care (Crittenden, 1992).

Given these facts, it is time for nurses to meet this public health challenge. Webster-Stratton's work represents an exciting starting point, as well as an example that we would do well to emulate.

WANDA K. MOHR

See also
CHILD AND ADOLESCENT MENTAL HEALTH INTERVENTIONS
CHILD FAILURE TO THRIVE

CHRONIC MENTAL ILLNESS

Chronic mental illness is more recently referred to as serious and persistent mental illness (SMI), in deference to the victims of psychiatric disorder and to reflect more accurately the intensity and course of various disease processes. SMI is considered to be a psychiatric condition that persists over time, with a variety of clinical courses and with varying intensity of disability. It presents diagnostic and treatment challenges to clinicians that are beginning to be addressed more directly in the empirical nursing literature. Stress diathesis models of causation and course, pharmacological and other biochemical models of intervention, and psychosocial models of course and intervention are all subsumed within a biopsychosocial framework. Selected empirical studies of SMI are presented chronologically.

Review of Major Studies

Slavinsky and Krauss (1982) compared a nursing social support intervention to a medication management intervention over 2 years in a sample of 47 persons with SMI. Contrary to the hypothesis, the medication group improved in socialization and satisfaction with care, indicating that psychiatric nurses should develop more complex treatment models combining low-stimulation, low-threat atmospheres with a social support emphasis to encourage gradual assimilation into the community rather than attachment to the treatment environment.

Harding and colleagues (Harding, Brooks, Ashikaga, Strauss, & Breier, 1987) interviewed 82 persons with SMI 20–25 years after their discharge into a rehabilitation project from the Vermont State Hospital. Over one-half of the sample had achieved considerable improvement or recovery. Previous longitudinal studies of shorter duration had found little or no change in function at follow-up. Subsequently, Harding and colleagues (DeSisto, Harding, McCormick, Ashikaga, & Brooks, 1987) completed a follow-up study with persons from a Maine state psychiatric facility with no psychiatric rehabilitation discharge program. Findings showed better function for the Vermont group at follow-up.

Hamera and colleagues (Hamera, Peterson, Handley, Plumlee, & Frank-Ragan, 1991; Hamera, Peterson, Young, & Schaumloffel, 1992) examined the process of self-regulation and symptom monitoring in persons with SMI, using the Self-Regulation Interview for Schizophrenia. Target symptoms indicative of the relapse prodrome were identified in a community-living sample of persons with schizophrenia. The majority of subjects' target symptoms were anxiety-related, occurred weekly or more often, and always occurred with decompensation. Though occurring less frequently, psychotic and depressive markers were rated significantly more troublesome than anxiety-based indicators. Subjects reported taking three or more actions to regulate the symptom. The most frequent action was to add new activities or focus on existing ones. A 1-year follow-up of 28 original subjects found that half of the subjects reported using the same indicator or an indicator from the same category.

The data provided support for a symptom self-regulation model. Subjects easily identified indicators of illness that were disturbing and represented the need for action when they were present. Baker's (1995) qualitative study of the ability of persons with schizophrenia to detect early signs lends support to the model of Hamera et al. Baker's interviews indicate that the level of disturbance caused by prodromal symptoms motivate individuals to take action to relieve the distress. The study further explicates the developmental process of individuals with schizophrenia becoming aware of the need to monitor their distress and take action when needed.

Fetter and Lowery (1992) applied attributional models to perspectives on psychiatric rehospitalization by 120 patients and 162 inpatient staff. Findings suggested that patients tended to give internal attributions for the illness relating to their readmission, believing that the cause was not under their control. Staff also were likely to ascribe internal attributions for the readmission but were more likely to see the cause as lack of patient effort, which is considered to be controllable by the patient. These important differences in attribution suggest implications for preventing rehospitalization and for nursing staff education.

The general psychiatric literature documents unexpected high morbidity and mortality rates in psychiatric populations, compared to populations with primarily medical diagnoses. An investigation of 25 persons with SMI recently discharged to the community (Murphy, Gass-Sternas, & Knight, 1995) documents the health risks and health promotion activities of this population. In semistructured interviews, subjects reported high tobacco use, low levels of physical exercise, poor oral health, high-risk sexual behavior, and limited medical and dental care. Health promotion activities included adequate sleep and limited use of alcohol and drugs. The subjects reported a strong interest in participating in health promotion programs. This study suggests that a focus on adequate mental and dental care and the development of health promotion programs for persons with SMI could have a positive impact on the physical and mental health of this population.

In a study of community mental health service delivery (Francis, Merwin, & Fox, 1995), personal characteristics and use of community services were evaluated as predictors of use of inpatient care by 446 clients of this community mental health service. Findings indicated that inpatient hospitalization was predicted by use of community service. Clients who received assistance in obtaining outpatient medical services were less likely to be hospitalized, and those receiving legal and housing assistance were more likely to be hospitalized. These findings suggest that lack of adequate housing and appropriately supervised living settings may be related to inappropriate use of inpatient care as a substitute for community residential placement. This study highlights the need to increase efforts to support nontraditional assistive services to psychiatric clients.

In a retrospective descriptive interview study of 43 persons with SMI in a variety of inpatient and outpatient settings, Chavetz (1996) examined individual life histories to determine the processes, conditions, and events that subjects considered influential in their clinical outcomes. The complex and rich descriptive nature of this qualitative study precludes a full explication here; however, the interviews suggest some general conclusions. The clients perceived the management of their psychiatric illness as a partial result of individual learning and personal decision making. They reported that medication played a pivotal role in illness management, and they acknowledged psychosocial factors such as acceptance of diagnoses, negotiation of treatment, obtaining environmental supports, and relationship development as important in coping with and managing the challenges of the illness.

Further, personal choices seem to involve trade-offs between support and protection; thus, these individuals may accept restricted lives in exchange for clinical stability. Though such restrictions may reflect a real resource deficit, they emphasize how these individuals have relinquished goals and aspirations over time to protect against personal vulnerability and avoid challenging situations. This study characterizes the complex nature of the disabilities associated with severe mental disorder and associated deficits in social and vocational resources, which must be addressed in the development of community nursing intervention programs.

In a similar vein, Perese (1997) investigated the effect of unmet needs of persons with SMI on their quality of life, emergency room usage, and rehospitalization events. In semistructured interviews with 73 persons with SMI and some family members, unmet needs were most frequently cited as lack of friends, social and vocational roles, group affiliations, and self-identity. Poor perceived quality of life was statistically associated with stigma, poor self-identity, and lack of employment. Rehospitalization and emergency room use were related to unmet needs for safety, money, and employment. As with other studies reported here, these findings suggest the need for the development of innovative and meaningful human services that address the complex nature of SMI and its sequelae, including physical, cognitive, interpersonal, resource, and vocational deficits.

Summary and Implications for Future Research

The studies reported here are atypical of the general base of nursing literature regarding SMI in that the samples are large, the methodology is quantitative, and the questions address the illness, its consequences to the individual, and implications for treatment development. The need for substantive nursing research is crucial and includes further investigation of (a) causal attributes and processes, (b) course and outcome, (c) clinical indicators of morbidity and mortality, and (d) symptom regulation and management. There remains a critical demand for empirical investigations to determine those interventions that specifically enhance symptom management, daily coping, adaptation, general health status, and quality of life.

CATHERINE F. KANE

See also
COMMUNITY MENTAL HEALTH
MENTAL HEALTH IN PUBLIC SECTOR PRIMARY CARE
MENTAL HEALTH SERVICES RESEARCH
SCHIZOPHRENIA NURSING RESEARCH

COGNITIVE IMPAIRMENT IN OLDER ADULTS: PSYCHOSOCIAL INTERVENTIONS

Cognitive function includes any and all of the mental operations of attention, concentration, judgment, intelligence or learning ability, memory, orientation, perception, problem solving, and reaction time (McDougall, 1991, 1995; McDowell & Newell, 1996). Additional behavioral manifestations of cognition such as psychomotor ability and social intactness are often included in the definition. Executive function is the individual's ability to engage in goal-directed behaviors such as planning, sequencing, and monitoring of behavior (Dugbartey, Rosenbaum, Sanchez, & Townes, 1999; Goldberg & Bilder, 1986). A disturbance in executive function was added to the Diagnostic and Statistical Manual (DSM)-IV's definition of dementia in 1994. A disturbance of the central nervous system, executive failure includes two constellations: (1) inactivity and affect flatness and (2) behavioral and affective disinhibition.

Cognitive impairment is any disorder affecting any aspect of cognitive function. Since cognitive impairment is a broad construct, a number of descriptors may be used when searching the literature. Examples include age-associated memory impairment (AAMI), Alzheimer's disease (AD), acute confusional states, Alzheimer's disease and related dementias (ADRD), cognition, cognitive decline, confusion, delirium, dementia, mental status, multiinfarct dementia, organic brain syndrome, primary degenerative dementia, pseudodementia, and senile dementia of the Alzheimer type (SDAT). Tests of cognitive function include intelligence tests, clinical neuropsychological tests, and laboratory tests. This chapter reviews aspects of cognitive function and four psychosocial interventions that have been tested with older adults with the aim of improving age-related disturbances in cognitive function. The review is not comprehensive; reports from Cochrane data bases are used to illustrate the systematic reviews that have been conducted on psychosocial interventions.

McGlynn (1990) identified attention and motivation, language and speech, memory, motor disturbance, and social behavior as appropriate rehabilitation outcomes applicable to cognitive and behavioral disturbances. Other authors recommend borrowing theories from the behavioral sciences to examine outcomes of psychiatric treatment. For example, attribution theory predicts that participants will attribute their failures to a lack of effort (an internal unstable and controllable attribute) rather than to lack of motivation, learned helplessness, or decreased confidence in their self-efficacy (Fosterling, 1991). Because deficits in cognitive functions are manifested in numerous disorders, including schizophrenia, alcoholism, and in age-related disorders, psychiatric rehabilitation has evolved from basic training in social and vocational skills to advanced rehabilitation strategies for remission of cognitive deficits (Stuve, Erickson, & Spaulding, 1991). Franzen and Haut (1991) reviewed 87 studies of psychological treatment for memory impairment and found that the treatments used either pure memory or analog tasks or daily activities as proximal outcomes. The types of activities used included direct retraining (improvement through practice), substitution (alternative functional systems), and facilitative activity (behavioral prosthetics).

Knowledge gained from the cognitive sciences has increased our understanding of the basic mechanisms related to cognitive function. Attention is the first cognitive indicator of neocortical dysfunction in early AD, and Parasuraman and Haxby (1993) found in 33 studies of selective, divided, and sustained attention that the cognitive deficits observed in early stages of AD overlapped considerably with the attention concerns of healthy older adults. Burt, Zembar, and Niederehe (1995), who reviewed 99 studies of recall and 48 studies of recognition memory, found an association between depression and memory impairment. Executive functions tested with the Trail Making Test were associated with slower performance of instrumental activities of daily living among community-residing older persons (Carlson et al., 1999; Mahurin, DeBettignies, & Pirozzolo, 1991). Using the Trail Making Test, Lyness, Eaton, and Schneider (1994) found that depressed older subjects did not perform as well as controls on visuomotor scanning tasks. More recently, Royall (1999) found that frontal deficits, manifested as executive dysfunction, rather than mood disturbance, explained the disability of depressed patients.

Rosswurm (1991) developed an attention-focusing program in three skilled nursing facilities for residents with AD or multiinfarct dementia and found significant improvements in perceptual processing of information and in the social interactions of persons in the attention-focusing group. McDougall (2000) examined the effectiveness of an eight-session self-efficacy-based intervention nursing home residents. Forty-five residents from a county nursing home in northeast Ohio participated. Forty-three percent of the sample was depressed, and 46% were cognitively impaired. There were 30 subjects in the experimental and 15 in the comparison group. At pretest, the experimental group had lower scores on the Mini Mental State Exam (MMSE), health, and prospective memory (belonging and message). Class attendance was low (M = 4.48); the dropout rate was 58%. Posttest data were available for only 13 subjects in the experimental group. Immediate story recall significantly ($p < .01$) increased ($M_1 = .67$; $M_2 = 1.33$). The experimental group made significant gains ($p < .0001$) on memory self-efficacy ($M_1 = 35.84$; $M_2 = 41.87$). The scores on the memory items of date and delayed route decreased at posttest. Mortimer (1997), reviewing nine studies of AD, discovered that a large proportion of the older, nondemented individuals who had sufficient numbers of plaques and tangles to meet neuropathological criteria for AD did not manifest any of the symptoms. He hypothesized that greater brain reserve may be due to (1) the number of neurons or density of their interconnections in youth, (2) a collection of cognitive strategies, and (3) the amount of functional brain tissue remaining at any age. The findings of numerous studies indicate that aspects of brain function may be impaired in older adults and indicators or proximal outcomes of cognitive assessment may facilitate remediation strategies if possible.

The Cochrane Database of Systematic Reviews

The Cochrane Database of Systematic reviews chooses topics of interest for integrative literature reviews, and recently, the Cochrane Dementia and Cognitive Impairment Group reviewed the existing literature on four psychosocial treatments for dementia: music therapy (Koger & Brotons, 1999), reality orientation (Spector, Orrell, Davies, & Woods, 1999), reminiscence therapy (Spector et al., 1999), and validation therapy (Neal & Briggs, 1999). This section provides an overview of the findings.

Music Therapy. Nurses are interested in using music therapy as an alternative to medications and restraints or a complementary treatment for people with dementias. Koger and Brotons (1999) analyzed 36 clinical trials using music therapy, the treatment group was composed of at least three adults over 60 years of age with a diagnosis of ADRD. The music intervention was delivered by a trained professional and included a minimum of three sessions. Diverse music techniques such as singing or playing of instruments by patients, listening to live or taped music, dancing or moving to music, and participating in individual or group musical activities were included in the analyses. The outcomes examined included a global impression of change, participation in group social behavior and musical activities, socioemotional skills, cognition, behavior change, verbal expressions, institutionalization, length of stay, and death. The effect of music therapy produced significant improvements. Future emphasis will be on analyses of the protocols to determine the underlying mechanisms (Koger, Chapin, & Brotons, 1999).

Reality Orientation. In this review of eight clinical trials, each trial included at least four elderly persons per group with a DSM or International Classification of Diseases (ICD) diagnosis of dementia; all subjects were greater than 55 years of age who participated in the reality orientation (RO). The RO intervention was defined as attendance at least 10 regular meetings for 3 weeks. The classes varied from 30 to 60 minutes and included the presentation, repetition, and use of orientation information (time, place, and person-related). At least 60% of the subjects in each trial completed the study. The outcomes included aspects of cognitive function such as cognition, short-term memory, orientation, and information and tests of behavior. Spector et al. (1999) found that participation in a classroom-based RO program had short-term cognitive and behavioral benefits for participants. However, to have long-term benefits, an ongoing 24-hour program with a detailed schedule of reinforcement including boards and signs and follow-up may be necessary. Future studies might include quality of life and everyday memory skills outcomes, and the programs may need to be tailored to the individual.

Reminiscence Therapy. This review included one clinical trial with adults 55 years of age and older diagnosed with dementia, cognitive impairment, or a comparable DSM or ICD diagnosis. At least 60% of the subjects attended a minimum of eight sessions during a 4-week to 48-week period and completed the study. The reminiscence intervention consisted of small groups consisting of at least four people, who were involved in the process of reminiscing, which might include photographs, music, and videos from the past. The outcomes included well-recognized cognitive and behavioral tests. Cognitive outcomes included cognition, short-term memory, orientation, and information. Behavioral outcomes included activities of daily living and other tests not related to cognition or emotion. The findings were inconclusive. However, a trend toward improved behavior was observed, and clearly more studies are needed (Spector et al., 1999).

Validation Therapy. Two validation therapy clinical trials consisted of adult participants greater than 65 years of age with a diagnosis of ADRD. Validation therapy was defined as any activity that referred to and drew on the framework of Naomi Feil. The intervention or technique defined by Feil included 14 techniques and approaches: centering, using nonthreatening words, rephrasing, using polarity, imagining, reminiscing, maintaining eye contact, using ambiguity, loving voice tone, matching motions and emotions, linking behavior, using preferred sense, touching, and using music. The length of the intervention was a minimum of 6 months with the group meeting once per week. The findings were statistically nonsignificant, and therefore no conclusions could be drawn. Although observational studies have reported positive outcomes and the literature suggests potential benefits, future research is necessary (Neal & Briggs, 1999).

In summary, many interventions have been tested with cognitively impaired elderly persons. However, whether individuals suffering from a cognitive impairment can benefit from a psychosocial intervention is not clear at this time. Psychosocial intervention studies are difficult to implement and difficult to maintain and complete. The participants are often frail and unable to maintain their participation with the demands of a regularly scheduled psychosocial intervention.

GRAHAM J. MCDOUGALL

See also

MUSIC THERAPY

PSYCHOSOCIAL INTERVENTIONS

CORONARY ARTERY BYPASS GRAFT (CABG) SURGERY: PSYCHOLOGICAL SEQUELAE

Coronary artery bypass graft surgery (CABG) has become an increasingly common treatment for coronary artery disease; more than 407,000 operations are performed in the United States every year (American Heart Association, 1994). Although CABG surgery is usually successful in relieving angina, a significant number of patients report feelings of anxiety and depression both pre- and postoperatively (Duits et al., 1998). Psychological problems experienced before and during the recovery period are as important as physical limitations and comorbidities in determining outcomes such as length of hospital stay, ability to function, and quality of life (Pirraglia et al., 1999; Heijmeriks et al., 1999). Psychologically distressed patients have significantly higher rates of cardiovascular rehospitalization and recurrent "hard events" (cardiac death, myocardial infarction, or cardiac arrest and resuscitation) as well as significantly higher rehospitalization costs (Carney et al., 1988; Allison et al., 1995).

Nurses caring for patients pre- and postoperatively are in a unique position to study the incidence and course of psychological sequelae in patients undergoing CABG surgery. Simple self-report instruments can be administered to identify those at risk for negative psychological outcomes. Intervention strategies could then be developed and tested to determine their efficacy in preventing negative outcomes.

The effects of psychological factors on cardiac disease and recovery from CABG surgery have been documented in numerous studies. Although much of the research focuses on incidence of anxiety and depression through cross sectional analysis, researchers have more recently examined patterns of psychological distress longitudinally (see Table 1). Although women are less represented in the published research, they appear to exhibit a different incidence and course of physiological and psychological sequelae of cardiac disease and surgery.

Major Studies

Depression. A convincing body of research links depression, cardiovascular disease, and mortality. In patients with preexisting cardiovascular disease, significantly higher rates of cardiac events were found in patients with depression. Carney et al. (1988) identified a major depressive disorder (MDD) as the best predictor of any cardiac event (myocardial infarction, death, CABG surgery, or angioplasty) independent of the extent of coronary disease, smoking status, and left ventricular ejection fraction. The incidence of any cardiac event in patients with MDD (77.7%) was more than twice that of patients without MDD (34.9%, relative risk 2.2, and $p < .02$). Although the basis of the relationship between

TABLE 1 Summary of Selected Studies on the Psychological Sequelae of CABG Surgery

Researchers & Study	Sample	Methodology	Outcome
Mumford et al., 1982 Analysis of Intervention Research	34 controlled studies MI or cardiac surgery	Meta analysis	Nonspecific, psychological care was cost effective
Rankin, 1990 Male and female differences in recovery from cardiac surgery	117 patients and families undergoing cardiac surgery	Longitudinal (Preop, 1 month, 3 months)	Females poorer physiological status, longer ICU stays, more deaths, less mood disturbances
Burker et al., 1995 Depression male and female patients undergoing cardiac surgery	141 patients	Longitudinal (Preop, postop 1 day prior to discharge)	47% depressed preop, 61% depressed postop Factors associated: Female gender, high state anxiety, low social support
Ai et al., 1997 How gender affects psychological adjustment one year after CABG surgery	151 patients 112 males 39 females	Longitudinal	Women more likely than men to experience postoperative depression attributable to poor health
Czajkowski et al., 1997 Preoperativecharacteristics of men and women undergoing CABG	759 patients 269 women 490 men	Cross sectional	Women older, more likely to have preoperative medical conditions, less likely to be married, more anxious and depressed
Duits et al., 1997 Prediction of quality of life after CABG	17 prospective studies	Meta analysis	Preoperative anxiety and depression predicted postoperative psychological maladjustment

TABLE 1 *(continued)*

Researchers & Study	Sample	Methodology	Outcome
Timberlake et al., 1997 Incidence and patterns of depression following CABG	121 patients 109 males 12 females	Longitudinal	Preoperativedepression best predictor postop depression. Trait anxiety discriminated depressed and non, pre- and postop
Glassman & Shapiro, 1998 Depression and CAD	10 studies	Meta analysis	
Vingerhoets, 1998 Perioperative anxiety and depression in open-heart surgery	80 patients 67 men 13 women	Longitudinal	Preoperative emotional arousal predicted emotional distress after surgery
Duits et al., 1998 Course of anxiety and depression in patients undergoing CABG	217 patients 176 men 41 women	Longitudinal	Overall decrease in anxiety and depression in postop period. Women more anxiety and depression pre and postop with stronger decrease in early postop period.
Duits et al., 1999 Structural modeling analysis of anxiety and depression in patients undergoing CABG	217 patients 176 men 41 women	Longitudinal	Relationships between anxiety and depression over time weak, at same time points strong
Pirraglia et al., 1999 Depressive symptomatology in CABG surgery patients	237 patients 192 male 45 female	Longitudinal	Low social support, life stressor, moderate to severe dyspnea, little or no help, less educa-

(continued)

TABLE 1 ***(continued)***

Researchers & Study	Sample	Methodology	Outcome
			tion associated with preop depression; longer ICU stays and little help predicted postop depression
Sabourin & Funk, 1999 Readmission of patients after CABG surgery	124 patients 98 male 26 female	Cross sectional	Female gender and obesity predicted hospital readmission

depression and cardiac morbidity and morality remains speculative, it is possible that changes in the autonomic nervous system and platelets found in depressed individuals account for a substantial portion of the association (Glassman & Shapiro, 1998).

Longitudinal studies of recovery from cardiac surgery clearly demonstrate that the process of recovery is neither simple nor experienced consistently in all patients. In a metaanalysis of studies (1986–1996) predicting psychosocial outcome following CABG surgery, Duits et al. (1997) found that preoperative anxiety and depression predicted postoperative psychological maladjustment, while social support, preoperative feelings of control, denial, and optimism contributed to psychological adjustment. The authors conclude that appropriate identification of predictive factors might promote the development of individually designed interventions for patients at risk for postoperative psychological problems.

The course of pre- and postoperative depression has been examined in several recent studies. Researchers investigating the relationship of preoperative characteristics, life stressors, social support, cardiac and neurological outcomes, and other complications with depressive symptomatology found that 43% of the patients experienced depressive symptoms preoperatively, while 23% experienced them postoperatively (6 months). Low social support ($p < .01$), presence of at least one life stressor within a year of surgery ($p < .01$), moderate to severe dyspnea ($p < .01$), little or no available help ($p < .01$), and less education ($p = .05$) were associated with higher preoperative depression. When controlling for preoperative depression, longer intensive care unit stays ($p < .001$) and little or no available help ($p < .001$) predicted higher postoperative depression (Pirraglia et al., 1999).

To examine the incidence and patterns of depression, patients undergoing routine, elective CABG surgery were assessed preoperatively and 8 days, 8 weeks, and 12 months postoperatively (Timberlake et al., 1997). While preoperative depression score was the best predictor of postoperative depression at all times, trait anxiety maximally separated those who were depressed pre- and postoperatively from those only depressed shortly after surgery.

Anxiety. Increased preoperative anxiety in patients undergoing CABG surgery has been documented in several studies (Jelicic & Bonke, 1991). Vingerhoets (1998) found patients with high, moderate, or low anticipatory anxiety maintained these levels of anxiety in the postoperative period (7 days and 6 months), supporting the idea of a linear relationship between pre- and postoperative arousal. Although one third of the patients had clinically relevant anxiety scores preoperatively, by the seventh postoperative day state anxiety scores had dropped significantly and declined slightly more by 6 months. While patients in the high range had a significant drop in anxiety following surgery, their scores remained in the high range. Trait anxiety assessed preoperatively contributed significantly to the patient's postoperative state anxiety levels.

In a longitudinal study (2 weeks pre- to 6 months postoperatively) describing the course of anxiety and depression, Duits et al. (1998) found that anxiety strongly decreased over time, with a slight decrease occurring at the day prior to surgery and a strong decrease 7 days postoperatively, which stabilized at 6 months. A structural model analysis of the data was undertaken to clarify psychological processes (Duits et al., 1999). The results indicated that the personality dimension, neuroticism, was related to pre- and postoperative anxiety and depression. Although relationships between anxiety and depression over time were relatively weak, relationships of anxiety and depression at the same points in time were relatively strong. Preoperative depression led to preoperative anxiety, while postoperative anxiety led to postoperative depression. With respect to this relationship, both depression and anxiety shared a substantial component of negative affect, which may have been responsible for the strong association.

Gender Issues. Although research indicates that the number of women undergoing CABG surgery each year is increasing (Penckofer & Holm, 1990), the outcome of the surgery may not be as beneficial for women as it is for men. Rankin (1989) found that women had significantly more shortness of breath, poorer cardiac functional status, and longer intensive care unit stays than did men. In a large study comparing preoperative characteristics of men and women, Czajkowski et al. (1997) found women to be older (65 ± 9 vs. 62 ± 10 years, $p < .001$), more likely to have a preoperative medical condition, less able to perform activities of daily living, more anxious ($p = .01$), and more depressed ($p < .001$).

In several studies examining depression in male and female patients undergoing cardiac surgery, factors associated with preoperative depression were female gender, trait and state anxiety, and less social support (Burker et al., 1995; Timberlake et al., 1997). Although Duits et al. (1998) found mean levels of anxiety and depression decreased over a 6-month period, men and women appeared to follow different courses. Women reported more anxiety and depression both pre- and postoperatively, but demonstrated a relatively strong decrease in both depression and anxiety in the early postoperative period. In evaluating factors that predicted readmission of patients after CABG surgery, female gender had the highest predictive value (Sabourin & Funk, 1999).

Future Directions

A strong relationship between pre- and postoperative anxiety (trait and state) and depression has been documented, with higher depression scores linked to increased cardiac morbidity, readmission costs, and mortality. Early identification of patients reporting high levels of anxiety and depression preoperatively could lead to the development of individualized treatment interventions whose efficacy could then be tested. In an analysis of the literature, Mumford and associates (1982) found that even modest and nontailored psychological interventions were successful in decreasing length of hospital stays for patients recovering from cardiac surgery or myocardial infarction. Clearly, women are at greater risk than men for negative physiological and psychological outcomes. Future psychiatric mental health researchers need to target this vulnerable population for early identification and intervention.

SUSAN MCCRONE
ELIZABETH LENZ

See also
DEPRESSION IN FAMILIES
STRESS
STRESS MANAGEMENT

CORRECTIONAL MENTAL HEALTH: A RESEARCH AGENDA

Whether nurses are concerned about public health and the well being of marginalized and poor populations, community health perspectives on mental illness and substance abuse, or the management of persons with severe mental illness, the criminal justice system warrants more of our attention. Too few nurses are cognizant of the major reinstitutionalization of America's mentally ill that is occurring in jails and prisons. Nurses need to significantly increase their research into this phenomenon. Currently, about the only research-based claim that nurses in correctional mental health can make is that the numbers of persons with mental illness in prisons and jails is increasing. It seems likely that the United States institutionalizes a larger portion of its mentally ill than ever before and almost certain that the United States incarcerates more mentally ill than any other country in the world. And there's a fair amount of evidence that the treatment persons with mental illness receive in prison is substandard (Jemelka, Trupin, & Chiles, 1989; Kupers, 1999; Lamb & Weinberger, 1998). The scope of the problem is immense: This chapter outlines recommendations for research at the systems, institutional, and individual level. The recommendations are based on gaps in the literature and almost a decade of directing a funded Correctional Mental Health Collaboration between the University of Washington and Washington State's Department of Corrections. This work has included policy design; design, implementation, and evaluation of prison mental health services; and research on imprisoned populations (Allen, Lovell, & Rhodes, 2000; Lovell & Rhodes, 1997).

Systems Research

Because the vast majority of prisoners are held in state prisons and local jails, each state constitutes its own system. Although affected to some extent by federal policy (such as the "war on drugs," which was really a war on low-end drug users in minority populations) and certainly national trends (e.g., determinate sentence reform), generalization across different states is very difficult (Forer, 1994). Not only do state and local laws (and their implementation) vary widely, central dimensions of the correctional mental health "system" reveal dramatic differences. One central difference, for example, is whether mental health treatment in prisons is provided by the correctional system or the mental health system. Each model has its problems, but each also has systemic possibilities for reform. When mental health is provided by corrections, it may be easier to integrate clinical considerations into administrative decision making than when the mental health staff report to noncorrectional personnel. On the other hand, the treatment imperative is in constant risk of being undermined by punishment and custodial commitments. Clinicians who are employed by a mental health system may be better able to retain a treatment priority and facilitate linkage between prisons and community mental health as mentally ill inmates (MIOs). But the ability to influence internal prison practices that have adverse effects on MIOs is weakened.

Who Is Out There?

The first systemic question concerns populations: Where in the correctional system are people with mental illness and what sorts of problems do they have

(Lovell & Jemelka, 1998)? While these questions are basic to formulating any intervention, they are extremely difficult to answer. Even the definition of "mental illness" is more complicated: While the courts have limited the legal obligation to treat to those prisoners who have Axis I diagnoses (e.g., schizophrenia, major depression, bipolar disorders), the separation of these disorders from "personality" disorders is both artificial and a site of considerable internecine conflict. "Madness" is a highly contested condition in corrections—staff use clinical taxonomies to move or resist movement of inmates back and forth between custody and treatment (Rhodes, 1998). And one can argue that various forms of insanity not adequately captured by Axis I cause a great deal of misery to prisoners and staff alike (Haney, 1993). Once one makes necessary (political and ethical) definitional decisions, there are immense problems around availability and interpretation of data. Medical and correctional records are notoriously inadequate and almost certainly underestimate the prevalence of disorders such as major depression that are either adaptive or not disruptive to prison operations. Randomized clinical interviews are certainly the most valid measure but extremely difficult to implement and heavily influenced by prison environmental conditions. In some systems, it may be possible to track previously diagnosed and treated individuals by linking community mental health and correctional records, but based on our experience, this is extremely difficult and underestimates undiagnosed individuals.

How Did They Get There?

For those of us concerned about the incarceration of mentally disabled populations, prevalence only defines the scope of the problem. A central public health concern is how the mentally ill became incarcerated and what can be done to reduce the rate (Steadman & Cocozza, 1993; U.S. Health and Human Services, 1995). Important research issues range from public policy to individual decision making. At the policy level, the drive to reduce judicial sentencing discretion has created legal disincentives to plead "not guilty by reason of insanity" (NGI) (Forer, 1994; Callahan, Steadman, McGreavy, & Robbins, 1991). Conviction leads to a finite time in a state institution (prison) while NGI can lead to indefinite confinement (in a hospital) and contingent release. The vast majority of incarcerated mentally ill persons have one or more chemical dependency—the availability of treatment (and whether mental illness is an exclusion from substance abuse treatment and vice versa) and supportive housing and community treatment are likely contributors to imprisonment and recidivism (Fuller Torrey et al., 1992).

Institutional Research

Clearly there is no simple distinction between "systems" and "institutions," but we are using the difference to focus on the careers of individual MIOs—what happens to them once they are institutionalized? One civil rights issue demanding more attention is length and conditions of sentences served by MIOs. Since their mental illness may interfere with understanding and following prison regulations and their vulnerability may lead to exploitation by inmates and staff, MIOs serve longer sentences under more restrictive conditions than prisoners convicted of identical crimes and receiving identical sentences (Lovell & Jemelka, 1996). Major human rights organizations (ACLU, Amnesty International, Human Rights Watch, American Friends) have objected to our increasing practice of solitary confinement, in violation of several treaties the United States has signed. And MIOs appear in these units—which aggravate their conditions—in very high rates (Human Rights Watch, 1997). Research indicates that mental health treatment—both appropriate medication and psychosocial interventions—can reduce violations of prison rules by MIOs and increase their ability to stay in less restrictive conditions (Lovell, Allen, & Jemelka, 2000). Much more needs to be understood about how the (dis)articulation of prison mental health treatment and community mental health influences the transitions of MIOs released into the community and their recidivism.

Individual Level Research

The role of nurses in the delivery of mental health care to prisoners and the responses of prisoners to various treatment modalities is a major area needing additional research (O'Connor, Lovell, & Brown, 2000). Prisoners reflect America's underclass: They are undereducated, poor, from traumatized families and communities, and disproportionately people of color. They are the same people who circulate through our homeless shelters. In addition to the addiction issues raised above—which are most acute on admissions and nearing release—these inmates suffer a disproportionate number of physical health problems that result from trauma and poverty. Poor diet, physical injuries, fetal alcohol syndrome, brain injuries, and cardiac disease appear to be prevalent. And all these conditions interact with mental illnesses. Nurses who are prepared at an advanced level in both mental health and initial primary care screening and referral skills are perfectly positioned to have a positive influence on this highly vulnerable population (Thomas, Brandt, & O'Connor, 1999). Unfortunately, most mental health care in prisons is delivered by professions such as social workers and psychologists who lack the preparation to manage the biophysiological interventions, complications, and interacting conditions. Although nursing has under attended to its participation in racism, it has begun to commit to more culturally diverse approaches to intervention (Boutain & Olivares, 1999). This is another pivotal arena for practice and research on outcomes.

Conclusion

Nurses who are committed to people with serious mental illness cannot ignore the plight of the vast numbers of such individuals in America's prisons and jails. They work in correctional systems and have a professional preparation to meet the many challenges of correctional mental health. But if their practice is to be based on sound theoretical and empirical grounds, they must increase research in this area.

DAVID G. ALLEN
DAVID LOVELL
LORNA A. RHODES

See also
CHRONIC MENTAL ILLNESS
MENTAL HEALTH POLICY
MENTAL HEALTH SYSTEMS RESEARCH

DEPRESSION AMONG OLDER ADULTS

The most common mental health disorder in late life is depression. It is often manifested as a recurrent illness or as a comorbid condition occurring with chronic health disease. Among older adults living in the community, 3% have a major depression and 10% to 14% have depressive symptoms. Depression has a wide severity and morbidity range and is conceptualized as an abnormal mood state, a pattern of symptoms, or a clinical syndrome ranging from sadness to major depression.

As a mood state, depression is a universal human condition. In general, persons of all ages who experience a lowering of mood or transient feelings of sadness claim to be depressed. Clinically, the concept of depression is used to indicate a collection of symptoms, such as sadness, reduced ability to experience pleasure, pessimism, inhibition, retardation of action, and a variety of physical complaints. Symptoms of depression have been classified into types: physical, emotional, cognitive, and motivational (Beck, 1978).

Emotional symptoms of depression include sadness, dejection, anxiety, irritability, distress, disappointment, frustration, extreme negativity, overt hostility, intense anger, and inability to derive pleasure from previously satisfying activities. Cognitive symptoms include pessimism, negative self-evaluation, expectation of failure, self-blame, learned helplessness, disturbance in thought processes, inability to concentrate, and impaired decision making. The inability to complete even simple tasks, lack of initiative to perform daily activities, procrastination, avoidance of responsibility, and psychomotor retardation or agitation are referred to as motivational disturbances. Physical symptoms of depression are loss of appetite, sleep disturbances, loss of libido, and diffuse aches and pains. Psychosomatic complaints are more dominant in older individuals than in younger persons. Older persons also have a tendency to mask sad moods. Finally, interpersonal aspects of depression are likely to include withdrawal from social activities, increased dependency, acquiescence, dysfunctional communication patterns, and proneness to interpersonal tension and conflict.

Generally, a nursing diagnosis of a major depression is made if five of the following symptoms have been present for at least 2 weeks: changes in appetite, weight loss or gain, agitation, fatigue and loss of energy, feelings of hopelessness and guilt, and suicidal ideation. Be aware that cognitive impairment symptoms may be marked in the older person with depressive illness and may be mistaken for dementia. Differentiation between dementia and depression is a critical part of the nurses' assessment.

As a clinical syndrome, depression is usually qualified by an adjective to specify a particular type or form. Clinically, forms of depression include reactive, agitated, and psychotic. In addition, depression has been classified as endogenous (due to internal processes) or exogenous (due to external factors), terms that refer specifically to etiology. Moreover, depression is called primary when not preceded by any physical or psychiatric condition and secondary when preceded by another physical or psychiatric disorder. Finally, depression has been classified as acute (less than 2 years duration) or chronic (more than 2 years).

As a clinical entity, depression comprises attributes and characteristic signs and symptoms, including a definitive type of onset, course, duration, and outcome. The *Diagnostic and Statistical Manual of Mental Disorders* (DSM IV; American Psychiatric Association, 1994) classifies clinical depression into major, minor, and dysthymic subtypes. Major depression refers to a clinical depression that meets specific diagnostic criteria as to duration, impairment of functioning, and presence of a cluster of physiological and psychological symptoms. Minor depression includes fewer depressive symptoms than does major depression. Dysthymia consists of fewer symptoms than are expressed in major depression but more than in minor depression, and it is more chronic.

Many theories of depression have been presented through the years. The earliest discussions of depression are in the psychoanalytic literature, where depression is viewed as mourning or melancholia (Freud, 1957). According to this perspective, loss, which may be conscious or unconscious, is central to both mourning and melancholia. Mourning is qualitatively different from melancholia in that the external world becomes impoverished and empty in mourning, and the internal world, including one's ego, feels the loss in melancholia. Psychoanalysts believe that the person experiences ambivalent feelings toward the lost object, which results from high dependency needs. Because the expression of dependency needs has the potential for destroying relationships with others, feelings of dependency, frustration, and hostility are repressed. When the loss of the loved object occurs, negative feelings of anger and hostility are unleashed against oneself.

Peplau's interpersonal theory in nursing describes depression as a painful experience occurring as a way of managing anxiety when an individual's self-esteem is threatened. The energy of anxiety is displayed as anger turned inward toward the self, and the individual experiences feelings of overwhelming guilt, hopelessness, and suicidal ideation. Thus, depression can be a life-threatening illness and a serious concern for health care providers for older adults because of the potential for suicide.

Behavioral theories of depression emphasize social learning and environmental responses or stimuli that cause or maintain feelings of sadness. For learning theorists, the concept of reduction in reinforcement is central. Reinforcement is defined by the quality of one's interactions with the environment so that, when one is faced with a loss, behaviors previously reinforced by the lost object or person decrease. This theory is relative for elderly persons, who suffer a multitude of losses in their later years. Depression therefore is attributed to a reduction in activity due to a decrease in positive reinforcement that comes from significant others. Feelings of depression are elicited when a behavior receives little or no reinforcement. In addition, lower levels of behavioral activity result in a further reduction of positive reinforcement from the environment. Therefore, both activities and rewards decrease. Behavior theorists believe that changing a person's behavior directly through positive social interactions is the best way of reducing depressive symptoms.

The self-control model of depression is a behavioral perspective from which people are viewed as capable of exercising control over their behavior (Rehm, 1997): they do not merely react to external influences but exert control over the environment. This theory of depression includes cognitive aspects because depressed persons are believed to have deficits in self-monitoring (reflected in pessimism and hopelessness), self-evaluation (reflected in low self-esteem), and self-reinforcement (reflected in excessive self-punishment and negative self-statements).

Cognitive theories of depression postulate that depressive symptoms are experienced because of disturbances in thinking that lead to false beliefs and ideas. Cognitive and behavioral theories of depression are sometimes closely related, especially when thought processes are instrumental in self-reinforcing and self-evaluating activities. The original learned helplessness theory of depression postulated that the belief that one has no control over outcomes in one's life is the basis for depression (Seligman, 1975).

The attributional theory is similar to Beck's cognitive theory of depression, which proposes that depression is primarily a result of the tendency to view the self, the future, and the world in an unrealistically negative manner. This distorted, negative view of self, world, and future has been referred to as the "negative cognitive triad" (Beck, 1978). According to this theory, depressed persons regard themselves as unworthy, incapable, and undesirable; they expect failure, rejection, and dissatisfaction and perceive most experiences as confirming these negative expectations. The major symptoms of depression (affective, behavioral, somatic, and motivational) are viewed as direct consequences of this negative cognitive set.

Most recently, biochemical theories of depression have emerged and attained credibility. Electrolyte disturbances, including increases in intracellular sodium and decreases in intracellular potassium, have been reported to occur with depression. In addition, neurophysiological alterations have been identified through electrophysiological studies of evoked potential and electroencephalography, demonstrating increased right hemisphere activity and decreased left hemisphere activity in the brain of depressed persons. Hormonal or neuroendocrine factors also have been related to depression, including decreases in estrogen, hypothyroidism, and hyperadrenalism. Finally, the neurochemical changes in the neurotransmitters, especially in the biogenic amines that act as central nervous system and peripheral neurotransmitters, have been documented in cases of depression. The biogenic amines, including catecholamines (dopamine, norepinephrine, and epinephrine), serotonin, and acetylcholine, have been hypothesized to be causally related to depression.

Specific biochemical theories have been proposed. The catecholamine hypothesis states that some, if not all, depressions are associated with an absolute or relative deficiency of catecholamines, particularly norepinephrine, at functionally important receptor sites in the brain. A competing explanation for the etiology of depression lies in the serotonin hypothesis, which specifies that there is a deficiency in serotonin in persons with depression. Empirical evidence of deficits in either norepinephrine or serotonin or both has provided an important rationale for the usefulness of antidepressant medications that are specifically designed to increase the concentration of norepinephrine, serotonin, or both, in the brain.

However, the precise etiology of depression remains unknown; that is, no single theoretical explanation is sufficient from a holistic nursing perspective. In fact, there is mounting evidence that there is probably multiple causation, including genetic, biochemical, and psychosocial factors that contribute to one's vulnerability to depression. Evidence for this model of depression lies in the success of multimodal treatment approaches for depression that may include antidepressant medication, psychotherapy, diet therapy, light therapy, and electroconvulsive therapy.

Depression severely affects quality of life in older persons because of the nature of the symptoms, which can lead to total inability of the individual to care for self and to relate to others. There is a potential for persons with depression to negatively affect family members and others around them. Not surprisingly, only 2% to 4% of elders in the community seek mental health services. Most depressed elders are seen by general practitioners for psychosomatic complaints. Part of the symptomatology of depression is a focus on physical problems and requires the practitioners to carefully assess for depressive symptoms. Suicide is a factor in the depressed older adult. The suicidal rate for individuals aged 80 and over is twice that of the general population and is particularly high in older White males. Interestingly, most suicidal elders had recently visited a general practitioner prior to their suicidal act. Direct assessment of suicidal potential should be a routine part of any assessment of dementia in elders.

Although depression follows a finite course and will eventually dissipate unless the person commits suicide, the life of the individual can be particularly miserable. For some time there was reluctance on the part of psychiatric practitioners to treat depression aggressively in older adults. This attitude was partially based on Freud's notion that individuals could not benefit from psychotherapy after age 50. However, we have learned that older adults will respond favorably to antidepressant medications and the psychotherapies. Electroconvulsive therapy, once disregarded because of the crude method of application, is now seen more favorably as a mode of treatment for depressed older adults who do not respond to medications. Due to modern technology electroconvulsion therapy is believed to be a safe and effective treatment for depression in older adults when other therapies fail. Additional therapies that are found to be useful by nurses are life review, guided imagery, and family and group therapy.

Research in depression among older adults has been ignored in the past and is a neglected area, where much more nursing research is needed. It is critical that nurses assume a leadership role in disseminating information about the outcomes of a variety of treatments that can be used for depression in later life. There is a particular need to examine suicide in late life and to develop better assessment instruments for the purpose of detecting sources of suicide ideation in elders.

MAY L. WYKLE
JACLENE A. ZAUSZNIEWSKI

See also
COGNITIVE DISORDERS
PEPLAU'S THEORETICAL MODEL
SUICIDE

DEPRESSION IN FAMILIES

Depression is a major mental health problem affecting 25 million Americans and their families. By 2020, the WHO predicts depression will be the third leading cause of disability worldwide. Most people suffering from depression live with their families, usually their spouses and children, and the negative impact of depression on families has been well documented (Coyne et al., 1987; Miller et al., 1992). Nursing has traditionally viewed families as a context for caring for the individual with depression and only recently has focused on the whole family.

Depression is a rather vague descriptive term with a broad and varied meaning ranging from normal sadness and disappointment to severe incapacitating psychiatric illness. William Styron (1990) describes in *Darkness Visible* the unsatisfactory descriptive nature of the term depression: "a noun with bland tonality and lacking any magisterial presence, used indifferently to describe the economic decline or rut in the ground, a true wimp of a word for such a major illness" (p. 37).

Depression is a universal mood state with all people experiencing lowered mood or transient feelings of sadness. For most, the feelings of sadness resolve with time and normal functioning resumes. In contrast, the symptoms associated with the psychiatric illness of depression disrupt normal functioning, influence mortality and morbidity, and cause a myriad of problems within the family (Badger, 1996a; Billings & Moos, 1985). The psychiatric illness of major depressive disorder (MDD) is diagnosed if five of the following nine symptoms are present for a minimum of 2 weeks most of the day, nearly every day: (1) depressed mood; (2) loss of interest or pleasure in all activities; (3) decrease or increase in appetite or significant weight change; (4) insomnia or hypersomnia; (5) psychomotor retardation or agitation; (6) fatigue or loss of energy; (7) feelings of worthlessness or excessive guilt; (8) difficulty concentrating or indecisiveness; and (9) recurrent thoughts of death, recurrent suicide ideation or suicide attempt (American Psychiatric Association (APA), 1994). One of the five symptoms must be depressed mood or loss of interest or pleasure. Together, these symptoms cause significant functional impairment. In addition to MDD, depression is further classified in the Diagnostic and Statistical Manual of Mental Disorders (DSM-IV) (APA, 1994) into other diagnostic subtypes such as minor depression or dysthymia by signs, symptoms, onset, course, duration, and outcomes.

Family refers to any group that functions together to perform tasks related to survival, growth, safety, socialization, or health of the family. Family members can be related by marriage, birth, adoption, or can self-identify themselves as family. This definition is sufficiently broad to be inclusive of all types of families, however, it is recommended researchers provide specific definitions of family appropriate to their research.

Genetic-biological research of depression in families includes genetic and biological marker studies (Flaskerud, 2000; Viguera & Rothschild, 1996). The four approaches used in genetic studies are: (1) familial loading studies (e.g., comparing families with depression to families without the disease); (2) studies evaluating the inheritability of mood disorders (e.g., twin studies); (3) studies of the incidence of the risk for, but not yet ill from, mood disorders to determine biological or psychological antecedents; and (4) in theory, studies using genetic probes to determine which relatives and which phenotypes are associated with the genetic contributants to mood disorders (Suppes & Rush, 1996). The results of the familial loading studies are clear whether the approach used is the "top-down" (i.e., studies of children with depressed parents) or the "bottom-up" approach (i.e., studies with parents of depressed children) (Birmaher, Ryan, & Williamson, 1996). Children with depressed parents have a significantly greater risk of developing depressive disorders and other psychiatric disorders than do children with parents without depression (Buckwalter, Kerfooot, & Stolley, 1988). First-degree relatives of children with MDD have significantly higher lifetime rates of depression and other psychiatric disorders (Birmher et al., 1996). Biological marker studies have focused on growth hormone, serotonergic and other neurotransmitter receptors, sleep, and the hypothalamic-pituitary axis (Keltner, 2000; Viguera & Rothschild, 1996). Despite evidence from genetic studies about the strong support for the genetic inheritance of depression, and that abnormalities in biological markers persist throughout the lifespan, the relationship between genetic-biological predisposition and environment remains unclear.

Psychosocial research of depression in families has focused on communication, marital problems and dissatisfaction, expressed emotion, problem-solving, coping, and family functioning (Beach, Sandeen, & O'Leary, 1990; Biglan et al., 1985; Keitner, Miller, Epstein, Bishop, & Fruzzetti, 1987). The evidence strongly supports that families who contain members with depression have greater impairment in all areas than matched control families, and than families whose members are diagnosed with alcohol dependence, adjustment disorders, schizophrenia, or bipolar disorders (Coyne et al., 1987; Keitner, Miller, & Ryan, 1993). It is not surprising depression has its most negative impact on families during acute depressive episodes (Miller et al., 1992), yet families with depressed members consistently experience more difficulties than matched control families even 1 year after initial treatment (Billings & Moos, 1985). Family members living with a depressed member also report increased health problems, with about 40% of adults reporting sufficient distress to require therapeutic intervention (Coyne et al., 1987). The majority of recent studies of families with members with depression have used primarily inpatient samples, have focused on women as the identified patient, have often excluded parents with depression, and have been quantitative in nature (Schwab, Stephenson, & Ice, 1993). Few studies have used qualitative approaches to understand family members' perspectives and treatment needs. Badger (1996a) used a grounded theory method to describe the social psychological process of families living with members with depression. The process, *family transformations*, refers to the cognitive and behavioral changes that occur within the family from the time that the member with depression initially exhibits symptoms through recovery and at remission. As family members move through the three stages (acknowledging the strangers within, fighting the battle, gaining a new perspective), all family members are transformed and family functioning forever altered. These results support findings from previous studies and provide perspectives of family members not normally included in depression research.

Despite identifying the multiple problems in these families, the role of the family in the treatment process has received less attention. Systematic family interventions have only begun to be developed and modeled after programs used with people with other psychiatric disorders and their families (Holder & Anderson, 1990). To date, few clinical trials have validated the effectiveness of these interventions. Families have identified the need for information about how to facilitate communication, decrease negative interactions, handle stigma, gain a new perspective, care for self and redesign their relationships (Badger, 1996b). In theory, education, support, and partnering interventions could move family members more quickly through the stages to prevent depression from becoming a recurrent and chronic illness for the entire family. Future research should develop and test psychoeducational and support interventions with families. Although a common concern with research with families remains the unit of analysis (individual, dyad, or family as a whole), research representing all three perspectives is needed to more fully understand and treat depression in families.

TERRY A. BADGER

See also
CHRONIC MENTAL ILLNESS
MENTAL DISORDERS PREVENTION

DRUG ABUSE

Drug abuse is a subcategory of psychiatric illnesses known as substance-related disorders according to the DSM-IV (American Psychiatric Association [APA], 1994) and categorized by the specific drug used. Drugs of abuse include alcohol, amphetamines, caffeine, cannabis (marijuana), cocaine, hallucinogens, inhalants, nicotine, opioids, phencyclidine (PCP), sedatives, hypnotics, and anxiolytics (antianxiety agents). Abuse or addiction to several substances, including alcohol, is common.

According to the DSM-IV, there are two categories of substance-related disorders: abuse and dependence. Substance abuse is diagnosed when a pattern of hazardous or maladaptive use continues in spite of serious health, social, economic, or psychological consequences but symptoms do not meet the criteria for substance dependence. Substance dependence meets the criteria for substance abuse but is a more severe form of the disorder and is characterized by increasing dosages and frequency of dosages, tolerance, and the manifestation of withdrawal symptoms when the amount of substance is reduced or stopped.

Alcohol is the most widely used and abused drug in this country; its abuse and dependence are reported elsewhere in this text. Nursing research with other drugs of abuse and dependence are reported here.

Drugs of abuse also may be categorized as legal or illegal according to cultural and societal determinations. The use of some drugs is legal in America but illegal elsewhere (e.g., alcohol in Saudi Arabia) and vice versa (e.g., peyote in South America). Designating a drug as illegal makes its use criminal and results in devastating consequences to individual users, their families, communities, and even innocent bystanders.

Some categories of drugs that have medicinal uses (e.g., opioids, sedative-hypnotics) are controlled by the Drug Enforcement Agency, and their dispensation is restricted to licensed pharmacists, physicians, and registered nurses. Use of other drugs, such as heroin, is illegal regardless of how they are used. Furthermore, legal drugs may be used illicitly. For example, prescription drugs may be misused by their intended client or sold for misuse by others.

Nursing research has been slow to recognize the serious health and social problems of drug abuse and dependence. Although sparse, early studies primarily addressed alcohol problems; but when drug abuse was studied, the focus was on nurses' attitudes toward drug abusers, the incidence of drug addiction among nurses, or characteristics of nurses addicted to drugs. Studies addressing nursing care of the drug-abusing client were virtually nonexistent until recently, when some empirical intervention studies have appeared in the literature (Barton, 1991; Lindenberg, Gendrop, Nencioli, & Adames, 1994; Nyamathi, 1991; Zauszniewski, 1995).

Recognizing the need for information about alcohol and drug abuse and dependence, the federal government initiated two programs to meet that need. First, curriculum model grants were offered by the National Institute on Drug Abuse (NIDA), the National Institute on Alcohol Abuse and Alcoholism (NIAAA), and the Office of Substance Abuse Prevention (now known as the Center for Substance Abuse Prevention). Three model projects are complete and available for nursing schools. Second, the three agencies offered training grants for faculty selected from a variety of specialty clinical areas in schools of nursing to acquire expertise in substance abuse disorders. More than 60 faculty from 13 schools of nursing have been prepared through these grants, and some are now funded by NIDA or NIAAA to conduct research in drug abuse, although results of this work are not yet available in the literature.

Drug abuse and dependence are serious health and social problems in this country. Nurses have the potential to intervene with substance-abusing clients and improve outcomes, but research is needed to determine appropriate and effective nursing interventions. The health and well-being of clients, their families, and their communities depend on improved care in substance abuse nursing.

ELEANOR J. SULLIVAN

See also
ALCOHOLISM
VIOLENCE AS A NURSING AREA OF INQUIRY

EATING DISORDERS

In the fourth edition of the Diagnostic and Statistical Manual (DSM-IV) (American Psychiatric Association, 1994), three eating disorder (ED) diagnoses are identified as mental disorders, anorexia nervosa (AN), bulimia nervosa (BN), and ED not otherwise specified (ED-NOS). Anorexia nervosa is a clinical syndrome characterized by three types of symptoms: (1) disordered attitudes toward body weight/shape; (2) failure to maintain body weight at a level of at least 85% of ideal; and (3) amenorrhea or the absence of a menstrual period for at least 3 consecutive months. In contrast to the AN diagnostic criteria that focus on attitudes and biological outcomes of disordered eating behaviors, criteria for the BN diagnosis are attitudinal and behavioral and include: (1) bingeing or ingesting objectively large quantities of food in a short period of time; (2) compensatory purging (self-induced vomiting, laxative, or diuretic use) or nonpurging (dieting, fasting, or excessive exercise) weight loss behaviors in response to the binge at least twice weekly for a period of at least 3 months; and (3) disordered attitudes about body weight/shape. ED-NOS refers to ED symptomatology that falls below the threshold identified for the AN and BN diagnoses and atypical patterns of disordered eating behaviors. A fourth diagnosis, binge-eating disorder (BED) was considered but was included only in the appendix of DSM-IV due to insufficient empirical evidence related to defining symptoms and prevalence of the disorder.

Recent studies suggest that the prevalence of the ED in the United States is increasing (Lucas, Beard, O'Fallon, & Kurlan, 1991). Estimates show that approximately 3% of adolescent and young adult women have a diagnosable AN or BN and as many as 10% have clinically serious subthreshold levels of the disorders. Among adolescent girls, AN is the third most common chronic condition, and both disorders are occurring more frequently in females at both the younger and older ends of the lifespan (Becker, Grinspoon, Klibanski, & Herzog, 1999). Furthermore, although the prevalence of ED appears to be increasing in males, AN and BN continue to disproportionately affect females with 90% to 95% of those with the disorders being female (Anderson & Holman, 1997).

Although nursing research has made important contributions related to a number of women's mental health issues, relatively little nursing research has focused on the eating disorders. The majority of nursing research on the ED has been published within the last 5 to 7 years and can be organized in three categories: (1) descriptive studies that characterize symptom patterns across subsets of women with ED; (2) studies that focus on etiology or factors that contribute to the onset and persistence of ED symptoms; and (3) studies that examine outcomes of disordered eating behaviors.

Symptom Patterns of the Eating Disorders

One focus of nursing research is symptom patterns that characterize subsets of women with ED. Jones described eating and weight control behaviors in three nonclinical groups of college students: (1) binge eaters who correctly labeled themselves as binge eaters; (2) binge eaters who did not conceptualize themselves as a binge eater; and (3) normal eaters (Jones, Doheny, Jones, & Bradley, 1986). Surprisingly, they found that 59% of their convenience sample of college students reported binge eating. Furthermore, they found that both nonlabeled and labeled binge eaters engage in nonpurging and purging types of compensatory behaviors but differed in severity of the behaviors. More specifically, the labeled group reported higher levels of self-inducted vomiting and laxative use for weight control compared to the nonlabeled group. White and Litovitz (1998) examined differences that distinguish inpatient and outpatient samples of eating disordered persons and found that persons with a previous history of hospitalization, more physical symptoms, and higher levels of feelings of ineffectiveness were more likely to be hospitalized. However, since no outcome measures such as rate of remission or indicators of level of recovery were included in the study, the usefulness of identifying these characteristics is unclear.

Etiology of the Eating Disorders

Nursing studies that have examined the etiology of the ED have focused on biological, cognitive, behavioral, and social factors. Studies that have addressed the biological basis of the ED have focused on BN and serotonin function as a cause of the core symptoms of binge eating and purging behaviors. Serotonin is a neurotransmitter in the central nervous system that has been shown to be related to postingestive satiety and decreased food intake (Wolfe, Metzger, & Jimerson, 1997). Wolfe and her colleagues have tested the hypothesis that abnormalities in serotonin transmission, particularly blunted responsitivity of the serotonin system, may contribute to the binge eating behavior (Jimerson et al., 1997; Wolfe et al., 2000). In these studies, women with current BN, remitted BN, and normal controls were given fenfluramine, a pharmacological agent known to increase serotonin transmission, and changes in serotonin levels was monitored using an indirect measure. Results suggest that women with current BN experience smaller increases in serotonin after receiving fenluramine compared to controls, thus supporting the hypothesis of impaired serotonin function in women with BN. In addition, results suggest that serotonin responsivity is negatively correlated with frequency of binging and vomiting behaviors. In a second study, women with remitted BN did not differ from controls in serotonin responsitivity (Wolfe et al., 2000). Although these studies reflect only a small segment of the ongoing research on the role of serotonin function in BN and must be carefully considered within the larger context, the findings provide some evidence to suggest that serotonin abnormalities may be a product of the dysregulated eating behaviors associated with BN rather than a biological predisposition. Furthermore, they point to the importance of interventions to extinguish binging and purging behaviors as quickly as possible since the behaviors themselves contribute to their persistence.

Other nursing studies have focused on the role of self-related cognitions in the formation of the eating disorders. Using the schema model of the self-concept as the theoretical framework, Stein has shown that by middle adolescence, girls have stable and enduring conceptions of themselves related to body weight and shape and these self-cognitions predict disordered eating behaviors and emotional well-being across the junior high to high school transition (Stein & Hedger, 1997). Subsequently, Stein extended this work using a sample of women with clinically diagnosed AN and BN. Results showed that an impoverished self-concept, that is a self-concept comprised of few positive and more negative self-conceptions, was predictive of defining oneself as fat, which in turn predicted disordered eating behaviors and attitudes (Stein & Nyquist, 2000). These findings were replicated in a longitudinal study of a sample of college-aged women engaging in subthreshold eating disordered behaviors. In this study, the self-concept variables measured during the freshman year predicted disordered eating behaviors in the sophomore year (Corte & Stein, 2000). These findings highlight the importance of nonweight related self-conceptions in the formation of the eating disorders and suggest that developing positive domains of self-definition may be an important focus for interventions to promote recovery.

Nursing studies that have addressed behavioral determinants of the eating disorders have focused on AN and BED. As part of their program of research focused on the health consequences of long-distance running, Estok and Rudy (1996) found that women who are high intensity runners (>30 miles/per week) were more likely to be at risk for AN compared to women who exercise at more moderate levels. Timmerman (1998) found that BED women experience extreme fluctuations in daily caloric intake and that the number of consecutive days in which caloric intake varied by at least 1000 calories was highly correlated with binge-eating severity. Furthermore, she found that caloric intake was lower on days preceding a binge-day but was not in the range consistent with physiological deprivation. Based on these findings Timmerman concluded that chaotic patterns of eating might disrupt appetite regulation and contribute to perceived deprivation that triggers a binge-eating episode.

Social context has been identified as an important factor in the etiology of the eating disorders (Striegel-Moore, Silberstein, & Rodin, 1986). Nursing studies have focused on the family environment as an important dimension of the social context and retrospectively examined characteristics that distinguish families of eating disordered women. Stuart found that women with BN described their families as more conflicted and less warm compared to women with a major depression and normal controls (Stuart, Laraia, Ballenger, & Lydiard, 1990). Similarly, women with BED reported lower levels of family cohesion and higher conflict compared to normal women (Hodges, Cochrane, & Brewerton, 1998). Finally, women with symptoms of AN were more likely to describe their mothers' lives as unsatisfying and not desirable for themselves compared to controls (Korb, 1994). These findings are consistent with a large body of research that suggests that characteristics of the family environment may put one at risk for an eating disorder. However, as a group, these studies are limited by the retrospective design and reliance on only the eating disordered woman's perspective in assessing family function.

Physical Outcomes of Disordered Eating

Only two nursing studies have addressed health consequences of disordered eating behaviors, and these studies have focused on biological outcomes. Clark (1997) tested the hypothesis that the co-occurrence of alcohol misuse and disordered eating behaviors is associated with lower bone mineral density in a sample of 25 women hospitalized for alcohol dependence. However, contrary to her prediction, women in the disordered eating group had higher mineral bone-density than women in her non-eating disordered group. This unexpected finding is probably due to problems with the criteria used to determine group membership and the fact that the majority of her sample had no current disordered eating behaviors. In the second study focused on outcomes, Timmerman and Stevenson (1996) found that age and the number of episodes of weight change greater than 20 pounds predicted percent body fat in women who engage in nonpurging binge-eating.

Summary and Conclusion

As a discipline, nursing is relatively new to the area of ED research. While in the last decade nurse scientists have begun to address a diverse array of types and levels of eating disorder symptomatology, sources, and consequences, relatively few programs of nursing research on the eating disorders have been established. To date, the majority of nursing research on the ED are single studies that raise interesting and important questions for further research but do not contribute to a coherent body of knowledge that can be used to guide nursing practice. Continued exploration of important topics such the biological, cognitive, behavioral, and social factors that contribute to the formation of the ED is critical not only for the development of effective approaches to treatment intervention but also for the development of effective strategies for primary prevention.

KAREN FARCHAUS STEIN
MONICA WHITE

See also
STRESS
STRESS MANAGEMENT

HEALTH CONCERNS OF WOMEN WITH SEVERE AND PERSISTENT MENTAL ILLNESS

Persons with psychiatric conditions have concomitant high rates of physical health problems (Felker, Yazel, & Short, 1996; Vogt, Pope, Mullooly, & Hollis, 1994) that are largely undiagnosed and untreated (e.g., Berren, Hill, Merikle, & Gonzalez, 1994). In addition to general disease risks such as respiratory ailments and cardiovascular compromise, persons with severe and persistent mental illness (SPMI) have high rates of sexually transmitted diseases and other infectious diseases. In particular, persons with SPMI have a frequency of physical health problems that is 50% to 90% higher than general psychiatric outpatients (e.g., Felker et al., 1996). Furthermore, Dembling, Chen, and Vachon (1999) report that the seriously mentally ill lose 8.8 more life years as compared with the general population. A recent study found that a greater number of current medical problems independently contribute to move severe psychosis and depression and a greater likelihood of a history of a suicide attempt in individuals with schizophrenia (Dixon, Postrado, Delahanty, Fischer, & Lehman, 1999). Their study, one of the first to measure the link between physical and mental health status in persons with SPMI, underscores the need to further attend to somatic health problems to provide optimal mental and physical outcomes.

Severe and persistent mental illnesses include schizophrenia, schizoaffective disorder, recurrent major depression, and bipolar disorder (Johnson, 1997). About 2.8% of the adult population in the United States (or 5 million people) experience one of these disorders in a 1-year period (National Institute of Mental Health, 1994). SPMIs are characterized by persistent symptoms that can be functionally disabling, disrupting life tasks and requiring periods of hospitalization. Women with SPMI have a high prevalence of medical illnesses and a higher mortality rate than women in general. In a cross-sectional mortality linkage study, Dembling, Chen, and Vachon (1999) found that women with SPMI lost 5.7 more years of potential life than decedents in the general population. The excess mortality resulted from infectious and respiratory disorders and "external" causes, which included accidents, homicides, suicides, and unexplained injury. Deaths from external causes were nearly four times higher than for women in the general population. In a earlier study of mortality in persons with schizophrenia, Allebeck (1989) also found that excess mortality was due to suicide for both genders and increased "natural" causes (e.g., circulatory disorders) and undetermined causes for females with schizophrenia.

For women with SPMI, gender-related health concerns such as unplanned pregnancy, poor gynecologic health, lack of preventative health-care, sexually transmitted diseases, and intimate partner violence are largely ignored. These conditions compound the generally unhealthy lifestyle that many individuals with SPMI have that consists of little exercise, a diet high in fat and low in fiber, and excess smoking (Brown, Birtwistle, Roe, & Thompson, 1999). The "women's heath care" movement that swept the nation in the 1990s did not include women with chronic psychiatric problems. As such, women with SPMI comprise a vulnerable group that deserves greater attention by psychiatric nurse researchers and clinicians. In this paper, we will review the major health problems faced by women with SPMI and discuss the presumed etiology and contributing factors related to poor health status in this vulnerable group.

Intimate Partner Violence

Many women with SPMI have difficulty establishing stable relationships and, consequently, they are prone to coercive or exploitative interpersonal relationships. As such, the majority of women with SPMI have experienced violent victimization (Goodman, Rosenberg, Mueser, & Drake, 1997). In addition to being at an increased risk for physical injury or death, victims of intimate partner violence are also at risk for anxiety disorders and suicide, chronic irritable bowel syndrome, pelvic inflammatory disease, depression, posttraumatic stress disorder (PTSD), sexually transmitted diseases, and complications of pregnancy (low birth weight infants). Physically abused women are also eight times more likely to be alcohol dependent. These conditions, resulting from intimate partner violence, in turn, adversely affect health promotion and disease prevention.

Sexual Risks

Women with schizophrenia have higher rates of unplanned pregnancy, more abortions, and more violence during pregnancy than women in the general population (Miller & Finnerty, 1996). In a recent matched comparison of women with schizophrenia with women without mental illness, Miller and Finnerty (1996) found that women with schizophrenia had more lifetime sexual partners and were more likely to have had coerced or unwanted sexual relations than women without mental illnesses. Within the SPMI population, women are more likely than men to report engaging in unprotected sex (Otto-Salaj, Kelly, & Stevenson, 1998). Sexual relations with multiple partners and inconsistent condom use are common behaviors (Carey, Carey, Weinhardt, & Gordon, 1997; Knox, Boaz, Friedrich, & Dow, 1994).

Lifetime sexual abuse is also elevated in this population. Among women hospitalized in a state facility, 51% reported that they had been sexually abused as children or adolescents (Craine, Henson, Colliver, & MacLean, 1988). In a sample of 64 women with schizophrenia, Darves-Bornoz, Lemperiere, Degiovanni, and Gaillard (1995) found that 36% had experienced childhood sexual abuse with frequent repetition. As childhood sexual and physical abuse is strongly associated with HIV-related risk behavior in women with SPMI (Goodman & Fallot, 1998), assessment for sexual abuse should be included in prevention programs.

Social/Economic Risks

In addition to elevated behavioral risks, the majority of women with SPMI face economic and social inequalities due to their marginal status. Because of their economic and social vulnerabilities, unsafe sexual activity is prevalent among women with SPMI, particularly sexual activities involving the exchange of money or drugs, otherwise known as "survival sex." The frequency of survival sex may in part explain why in contrast to the larger HIV epidemic in the United States in which males comprise the largest percentage of total HIV/AIDS cases, in most HIV seroprevalance studies of persons with SPMI, women were as likely as men to be infected (Cournos & McKinnon, 1997). In addition to multiple psychological and social risks, women have a greater physiologic vulnerability to HIV transmitted via sexual routes than men: male-to-female transmission is approximately eight times more efficient than female-to-male

Health Risks Related to Mental Illness

The cognitive changes associated with SPMI may lead to delay in recognition of, or attention to, symptoms of physical illness that may contribute to seeking medical care late in the course of an illness or condition. In addition, the cognitive deficits and disordered thought processes related to SPMI may lead to difficulty in making plans and engaging in preventative health and safety behaviors. For example, poor physical fitness and poor nutritional status are prevalent in this group. In a study of 22 outpatients with schizophrenia, Holmberg and Kane (1999) found that over half of their sample was overweight and had physical conditions requiring medical management. While a large empirical literature about improving health through diet, exercise, and general preventative health care exists, there is almost no literature regarding providing these programs for individuals with severe mental illness (Faulkner & Sparkes, 1999). There is no reason to believe, however, that persons with SPMI cannot enjoy the health benefits associated with preventative wellness-related activities. In one of the few studies focused on a sample of persons with schizophrenia, individualized aerobic exercise programs resulted in increased aerobic fitness and psychological benefits such as increased sense of well-being, increased sense of self-efficacy, and an increase in social interaction (Pelham & Campagna, 1991).

Organizational-Level Factors

Traditionally, there has been a divide between mental and physical disease care for persons with SPMI, perhaps due to the Freudian belief that separation of the psyche from the body was a necessary attribute for developing therapeutic relationships. In addition to the theoretical divide between mental and physical health care, historically there has been a division of public mental health from general health care that stems from the separation of funding streams for these activities (Kane & Ennis, 1996). As a result, for many persons with SPMI access to primary health care may be limited by a lack of integration of mental health treatment with primary care services.

Conclusion

In summary, women with SPMI have higher rates of sexually transmitted disease, more unplanned pregnancies and abortions, in addition to a higher prevalence of medical illnesses and a higher mortality rate than women from the general population. Further, the majority of women with SPMI have experienced violent victimization (Goodman et al., 1997). In addition to gender-related risks, women with SPMI have excess mortality from natural causes, suicide, homicide, and unexplained deaths. Although women with SPMI have multiple documented health risks, there has been little focus on this vulnerable group by nurse researchers. Consequently, future research incorporating both mental and physical health and illness variables is needed to address medical comorbidities and premature death in women with SPMI.

Debra E. Lyon
Catherine Kane
Barbara J. Parker

See also
CHRONIC MENTAL ILLNESS
DEPRESSION IN FAMILIES

HIV SYMPTOM MANAGEMENT AND QUALITY OF LIFE

Public discourse on quality of life has made health care providers keenly aware of client choices in therapy decisions. Scholarly endeavors on quality of life have broadened conceptualizations of outcomes of care, ultimately changing standards of care. The literature on quality of life is expansive, with a recent emphasis on refining and measuring the meaning and dimensions of quality of life for persons with human immunodeficiency virus (HIV) (Holzemer & Wilson, 1995). A recent trend has been the focus on symptom identification and management in persons living with acquired immunodeficiency syndrome (AIDS). Holzemer (2000) noted that people with HIV experience a decrease in quality of life as the severity of symptoms increase. These symptoms may be related to HIV medications, HIV disease, comorbidities, and life conditions such as poverty, or combinations of these. The purpose of this brief is to present selected articles that address symptom management as a correlate of quality of life in persons with HIV disease.

The good news is that the number of AIDS cases decreased 18% between 1996 and 1997, and 11% the following year. These data demonstrate the incidence of AIDS cases is slowing. The bad news is that the rate of new infections has increased in certain risk groups; women, ethnic minorities and adolescents, and therefore, the number of people living with HIV has never been higher (Centers for Disease Control, CDC, 1999). Reasons postulated for the initial decrease in number of cases was the advent of combination antiretroviral therapy and better management of opportunistic infections. The slowing rate of decline may indicate that much of the benefit of new therapies has been realized.

HIV disease is now conceptualized as a chronic illness (Holzemer et al., 1999). While there is an overall decline in morbidity, it is clear that persons with more advanced disease experience shorter periods of benefit from HIV medications and increased symptoms than those with better immune function (CDC, 1999). Because of the resurgence in the incidence and prevalence of HIV disease, enhancing quality of life is of paramount importance. Concepts of quality of life for people with HIV include, but are not limited to, functional, physical, and emotional status; symptom management; social support; spirituality; sexual functioning; and economic well-being. Quality of life is an omnibus concept. Although quality of life research in people with HIV disease has been multidimensional, there is still a paucity of published work regarding quality of life in certain segments of the population, including women, ethnic minorities, intravenous drug users, and transgendered persons.

Literature Review Process

Searches were conducted to identify studies that examined quality of life and HIV/AIDS that were available in the English language. The searches included all combinations of "quality of life," "AIDS," and "HIV" as exact subject key words and title words. The literature regarding quality of life in persons with HIV disease is abundant. A total of 461 articles were cited in MEDLINE/HealthSTAR database from 1995 to 2000. Major categories that were identified through this search process included symptom management, social support, adherence (medication and treatment), coping, self-care, instrument validation, combination antiretroviral treatment, complementary therapies, and economic factors. Because of the extensiveness of the categories and the experience of the authors, this paper will present selected articles that address symptom management in persons with HIV disease.

Symptom Management

In a multidimensional model of health-related quality of life (HRQOL), Wilson and Cleary (1995) defined a symptom as "a patient's perception of an abnormal physical, emotional, or cognitive state" (p. 61). Hegyvary (1993) defined symptoms as "the perceived indicators of change in normal functioning as experienced by patients" (p. 146). The University of California, San Francisco School of Nursing Symptom Management Faculty Group (1994) defined symptoms as "subjective experiences reflecting changes in a person's biopsychosocial function, sensation, or cognition" (Holzemer, 2000, p. 1). Several researchers have examined symptom status and quality of life (Cunningham et al., 1998; Linn, Monning, Cain, & Usoh, 1993; Souza, Holzemer, Henry, & Slaughter, 1999; Valente, Saunders, & Uman, 1993; Vogl et al., 1999). According to Holzemer et al. (1999), the relationship between increased symptoms and decreased quality of life has been demonstrated. Three studies are reviewed which confirm this relationship.

Using secondary analysis, Sousa et al. (1999) empirically tested the influence of biological and physiological variables, symptom and functional status, general health perceptions, and sociodemographic and environmental characteristics on overall quality of life in 142 people with AIDS. Path analysis, using multiple linear regression, was used to examine the fit between the study sample and Wilson and Cleary's (1995) HRQOL theoretical model. Symptoms were measured with the HIV-SSC (Holzemer et al., 1999). Thirty-two percent of the variance in overall quality of life was explained by the model, with symptom status having the greatest influence ($\beta = -0.237$, $R^2 = 5\%$). They found that symptom status, functional status, and perception of general health were key dimensions of HRQOL. Concentrating on HRQOL allows nursing to target concerns and issues that are appropriate to the patient. The study addressed some conceptual and operational issues surrounding the dimensions of HRQOL. The findings confirmed that the overall data were consistent with the conceptual model and increased symptoms were linked to decreased quality of life. The authors noted that the results did not account for as much variance in overall quality of life as expected.

Vogl et al. (1999) assessed the symptoms and symptom distress associated with AIDS in 504 ambulatory patients. Quality of life was assessed by the Karnofsky Scale, which measured primarily functional status, and symptoms were measured by the Memorial Symptom Assessment Scale Short Form, focusing on physical and psychological symptom distress. Patients with Karnofsky performance scores less than 70 had more symptoms and higher symptom distress scores compared to patients with totals greater than 70. The number of symptoms and symptom distress scores were highly associated with psychological distress and poorer quality of life ($r = -0.69$, $p < .0001$). Neither gender nor disease status (measured by CD4 counts) was associated with symptom number or distress. The authors concluded that symptom assessment provides information that may be valuable in developing strategies to improve quality of life.

Cunningham et al. (1998) assessed the severity of six constitutional symptom complexes (myalgias, exhaustion, anorexia/nausea/vomiting, night sweats, fever, and weight loss) in relation to quality of life in 205 (145 outpatients, 60 inpatients) HIV-infected subjects. Quality of life was measured by MOS short form health survey (Wachtel et al., 1992) and symptoms were measured by 1–5 and 1–6 Likert scales. All symptoms except weight loss were strongly related to measures of quality of life. On 0- (worst) to 100- (best) point scales, mean scores ranged from 34 (for individuals having all five symptoms other than weight loss) to 78 (for those with no symptoms) for physical function, 43 to 79 for emotional well-being, and 36 to 73 for social function. They concluded that the presence, number, and severity of symptoms in HIV disease are strongly associated to HRQOL. Identifying and treating these common symptoms has the potential to improve quality of life.

Summary and Future Directions

Cunningham et al. (1998), Sousa et al. (1999), and Vogl et al. (1999) all confirmed that increased symptoms are related to decreased quality of life for persons with HIV disease. While not reviewed here, there have also been some qualitative research reported that also supports this relationship. Bunch (1999) interviewed 19 Norwegians living with HIV disease and Wilson, Hutchinson, and Holzemer (1997) interviewed 38 persons living with HIV and both grounded theory studies support the conclusion of this relationship of decreased quality of life with increased symptoms. As people with HIV disease are living longer and represent more diverse ethnic and gender groups, more qualitative research could help us to better understand the relationship between quality of life and symptoms throughout the life span (Holzemer & Wilson, 1995).

Future research is needed to understand the symptom experience of women living with HIV disease, particularly symptoms related to gynecological issues. In addition, there is very little data on ethnic and gender differences with the symptom experience and how these differences might relate to quality of life. Finally, self-care behaviors related to symptom management are just being recognized as significant initially due to their potential harmful interaction with HIV medications. Ongoing work of this team is focusing on self-care behaviors that moderate the impact of HIV-related symptoms.

KENN M. KIRKSEY
ANGELA L. HUDSON
ELI HAUGEN BUNCH
WILLIAM L. HOLZEMER

Drs. Kirksey and Hudson were supported during the preparation of this manuscript by postdoctoral fellowships from the National Institute of Nursing Research, NIH, HIV/AIDS Nursing Care and Prevention (T32 NR07081), William L. Holzemer, RN, PhD, FAAN, Project Director.

See also
QUALITY OF LIFE
RESOURCEFULNESS

HOMELESS HEALTH

Prevalence of Homelessness in the United States

Since the 1980s homelessness has been a growing national problem. The number of homeless individuals is estimated at between 350,000 and 2.5 million (Clark,

Williams, Percy, & Kim, 1995). Every day an unknown number of individuals move into the state of homelessness due to personal crises (illness, loss of job, loss of transportation, domestic violence, eviction) and other conditions (release from prison, substance abuse, mental disorders). At the same time, others move out of the defined ranks by "doubling up" with relatives or friends or attaining employment, welfare approval, or low-income housing. Because membership in this group is continuously changing, obtaining a precise number of the homeless is impossible.

In 1987 the Stewart B. McKinney Homeless Assistance Act (PL 100-77) defined the homeless person as (a) an individual who lacks a fixed, regular, and adequate nighttime residence or (b) an individual who has a primary nighttime residence that is a shelter, including welfare hotels, congregate shelters, and transitional housing for the mentally ill; an institution that provides a temporary residence for individuals intended to be institutionalized; or a public or private place not designated for nor ordinarily used as a regular sleeping accommodation.

The profile of the homeless has changed dramatically in the past 30 years, from the stereotypical elderly alcoholic transient male to the current one of young White men and women from 25 to 39 years of age. Nationally, single men make up approximately 75% of the homeless. Although women represent only 25% of the homeless population, they generally enter homelessness accompanied by their preschool children. Women with children are the fastest-growing subgroup of the homeless nationally (Clark et al., 1995).

In large metropolitan areas, many homeless live on the street, in abandoned cars, or in cardboard "homes" because of insufficient numbers of shelter beds, fear of bodily harm in shelters, or mental disorders. Many urban homeless also reside in shelters operated by public and private agencies that serve various subgroups of the homeless, such as battered women, substance abusers, single males, families. These shelters have varying residency rules regarding clientele served, length of stay allowed, requirements for program participation, and daytime lockout. They offer a variety of social services in addition to shelter and food. Few shelters offer on-site access to health care.

Homeless Health

The state of homelessness affects health in three major ways: health problems, such as schizophrenia, may contribute to becoming homeless; homelessness may contribute to becoming ill or may exacerbate chronic illness; and being homeless may make any illness almost impossible to treat (Institute of Medicine, 1988). The homeless environment predisposes residents to a variety of health risks, including trauma, communicable and weather-related disorders, and mental health and substance abuse problems (Lindsey, 1995). Traumatic and weather-related injuries (frostbite, sunburn) are most common in the homeless living on the street. Communicable respiratory, dermatological, and gastrointestinal health problems are common due to crowded living conditions in shelters, irregular mealtimes, and questionable personal hygiene practices. Hypertension, increased incidence of mental health disorders, and high rates of tobacco, drug, and alcohol abuse are also reported in studies of shelter residents (Vredevoe, Brecht, Shuler, & Woo, 1992).

Obtaining adequate food and shelter are daily challenges for the homeless. Many spend their days walking from a nighttime shelter to a soup kitchen and then wait for the nighttime shelter to open in order to find a bed. The food available at soup kitchens and shelters is generally nutritionally adequate but high in fat and low in various minerals such as iron and calcium. Mineral deficiencies are particularly important when considering preventive health practices for women and children.

Compared to the general population, homeless males have been reported to have more respiratory ailments, skin disorders, infectious diseases, dental problems, and mental health and substance abuse problems than the general population. Homeless women have greater prevalence of mental illness, unwanted pregnancies, adverse birth outcomes, and histories of domestic abuse. Homeless children exhibit increased incidence of physical, mental, emotional, behavioral, learning, and immunization delays (Aday, 1994).

Health Care

Lack of insurance, transportation, and finances are barriers the homeless encounter in seeking health care. They generally seek health care, from emergency rooms and free clinics, for acute conditions after they have become severe. The care they receive is episodic, delivered by a variety of practitioners, and focused on the immediate acute problem. Secondary health problems and chronic problems do not receive attention or necessary routine surveillance. Because of the lifestyle of the homeless and their lack of addresses, follow-up is difficult if not impossible.

Medications prescribed for homeless individuals are often unobtainable due to costs. Many free clinics dispense donated medications or samples, which may not be the drug of choice but will provide some pharmacological assistance for the problem. The homeless have special problems in complying with prescribed medication regimens. They may not understand the directions for appropriate medication use because of their limited reading levels or their mental status. They may not have access to food at required times to accompany the medication or may discontinue medications (e.g., antibiotics) as soon as they feel better and save them for a future illness. They may also use them to trade for drugs, money, or cigarettes. Their medications are often lost or stolen because there is no safe place to store them, or they may be rendered inactive due to lack of refrigeration.

Monitoring and tracking the health and health care of the homeless are very difficult. Homeless clients generally do not have a stable source of health care, one record, or any personal record of their health care visits, treatments, or prescriptions. They may seek health care from a variety of providers for a variety of problems and may use several different names on records. They must rely on their memories or the interviewing skills of a practitioner to elicit their health and medication histories at each health visit.

Research

Studies about the health and health care of the homeless are increasing (Lindsey, 1995). Nurse practitioner– and nurse-managed clinics have been in the forefront of delivering health care for the homeless and initiating research studies of this population (Stanhope, 1990). However, most of the reported research on the homeless and their health problems, concerns, and care has been descriptive, with data gathered from clinics or emergency room record reviews, convenience sample interviews, on-site surveys, and self-reports from clinic visits. Few studies have used comparative groups, been theory-based, or used standardized instruments. Intervention studies using control groups have not been widely reported (Lindsey, 1995). Research in the areas of health promotion and disease prevention with this population are not reported.

Directions for Future Research

For research to add substantively to the body of knowledge related to homeless health and health care, researchers must design interventions studies that use the same theory or conceptual base and accepted standardized instruments. Studies should also be intervention- and outcome-focused. The same conceptual, theoretical base will allow researchers to build on knowledge gained in previous studies.

Due to the great heterogeneity of this population, intervention studies should focus on particular subgroups of the homeless (e.g., battered women, women with children, single males, families, substance abusers, pregnant women, adolescents, or new homeless vs. chronic homeless) or on other common factors, such as length of homelessness (marginal, new, chronic). This would improve the homogeneity of the groups.

Research designs to yield more generalizable results should include random selection of subjects. Because of the transient nature of the homeless, this may require the development and coordination of projects at multiple sites in order to attain sufficient numbers of subjects. Intervention studies of a longitudinal nature could add valuable information about the health problems and outcomes of the homeless and provide guidance for future interventions. Qualitative studies identifying the important themes related to health in this population could add substantively to our knowledge about this group. Research focused on health promotion and disease prevention strategies, though difficult in this population, is needed. To obtain adequate follow-up with this population, research designs that incorporate creative incentives to motivate the homeless to participate and to continue participation will be required.

MARY J. MCNAMEE
ADA M. LINDSEY

See also
CHRONIC MENTAL ILLNESS
VIOLENCE AS A NURSING AREA OF INQUIRY

HOMELESSNESS AND RELATED MOOD DISORDERS

While the causes of homeless are complex, mood disorders and related mental illnesses continue to contribute to the problem. *Mood disorders* are classified as feeling states reported by clients that can vary with external and internal changes and are characterized in the DSM-IV (1994). Approximately 20 to 25% of the single adult homeless population suffers from some form of severe and persistent mental illness (Koegel, Burnam, & Baumohl, 1996). According to the Federal Task Force on Homelessness and Severe Mental Illness, only 5 to 7% of homeless persons with mental illness require institutionalization, while most can live in the community with supportive housing options (Federal Task Force on Homelessness and Severe Mental Illness, 1992). Surveys of homeless populations during the 1980s found high rates of addiction (Koegel et al., 1996). Mental illness such as mood disorders often are accompanied with drug addiction as people attempt to cope with their mental illness without appropriate drug treatment. People experiencing homelessness also share certain basic needs, including lack of affordable housing and inadequate incomes, as well as limited mental health services.

Two growing trends that are increasingly responsible for the rise in homelessness over the past 15 to 20 years are (1) growing shortage of affordable rental housing and (2) a simultaneous increase in poverty (National Coalition for Homeless, 1999). In 1998, the U.S. Conference of Mayors' survey of homelessness in 30 cities found that children under the age of 18 accounted for 25% of the urban homeless population. This same study found that unaccompanied minors comprised 3% of the urban homeless. Most studies of the homeless show that single adults are more likely to be male and comprise 45% while 14% are single women (U.S. Conference of Mayors, 1998). Families with children are among the fastest growing segments of the homeless population, representing approximately 40% of people who become homeless (Shinn & Weitzman, 1996).

According to the Stewart B. McKinney Act (1994), a person is considered *homeless* who "lacks a fixed, regular, and adequate night-time residence and; . . . has a primary night residency that is: (A) a supervised publicly or privately operated shelter designed to provide temporary living accommodations; (B) an institution that provides temporary residence for individuals intended to be institutionalized, or (C) a public or private place not designed for, or ordinarily used as, a regular sleeping accommodations for human beings" (42 U.S.C. 11302). This definition is interpreted also usually to include those persons who are literally homeless, that is they live on the streets and have no subsequent residence or resources to obtain housing (U.S. Department of Agriculture, 1996).

The homeless population varies demographically according to geographic location. The U.S. Conference of Mayors (1998) found that 49% are African Americans, 32% Caucasian, 12% Hispanic, 4% Native American, and 3% Asian. Approximately 22% of the homeless population left their last place of residence because of domestic violence (Homes for the Homeless, 1998). The homeless population report common signs of mood disorders, such as ongoing sadness and anxiety, lack of energy, loss of interest in ordinary activities, sleep problems, excessive weight loss or gain, aches and pains, difficulty concentrating, hopelessness, and thoughts of suicide and death (McMurray-Avila, 1997). One of the mood disorders, depression is one of the most treatable of all mental illnesses. About 60 to 80% of depressed people can be successfully treated outside a hospital with psychotherapy alone or with special drugs. Unfortunately drug therapies often take at least 6 to 19 weeks before there are real signs of progress, and their continues to be a reluctant to receive treatment due side effects of the drugs (McMurray-Avila, 1997) and the continuing stigma of mental illness in our society.

Obstacles

The homeless population face many barriers in breaking the cycle of homelessness and accompanying mood disorders. Some of the obstacles described include lack of awareness of services available, lack of financial resources and health insurance, language or cultural barriers, poor attitudes of some providers of services, lack of transportation, scheduling and keeping appointment difficulties, fear or distrust of institutions, and fragmented community services (McMurry-Avila, 1997).

Advocacy

Advocacy is critical to ending homelessness. *Advocacy* means working with homeless persons to bring about positive change in policies and programs on local, state, and federal levels. Organizations that offer information and assistance with depression and treatment include The National Institute of Mental Health's special Depression/Awareness, Recognition, and Treatment Program (2000); The National Depressive and Manic-Depressive Association (2000); The National Alliance for the Mentally Ill (2000) and also a branch organization available in each state; and The National Mental Health Association, which publishes information on a variety of mental health issues (2000).

There is a paucity of nursing research related to the role that professional nurses play as advocate in improving the care for homeless persons with mental illness and related mood disorders. Due to the fact that primary health care for the homeless population is often provided by nurses, there is an excellent opportunity to do beginning research in this area as well as assist those with mental illness to get the care required so that they may function at a higher level in our society.

Interventions

Interventions are defined as action plans taken to attempt to break the cycle of homelessness. Project Achieve (*www.homelessness.net*, 2000) began a process to break the cycle of homelessness and describes the process on their web site. Decycling is defined by Project Achieve as a strategy for breaking the cycle of homelessness for individuals and families. Decycling also includes ending the continuous cycle of accessing social services and emergency shelters only then to return to homelessness. Project Achieve includes shelter services to meet basic needs, program services to prepare individuals for successful independent living, and case management services to provide counseling, assistance with employment, and housing placement.

Strengthening the family unit of individuals with chronic mental illness is identified as important by community-based case management programs. A longitudinal study of family support among homeless mentally ill persons in community-based housing programs was studied (Wood, Hurburt, Hough, & Hoffstetter, 1998). This study (Wood et al., 1998) was one of the first to look at strength of family relationships overtime with homeless individuals. As contact with family members increased, so did their mental health, with greater satisfaction reported in their relationships and housing.

The most useful strategy for professionals working with homeless mentally ill individuals and families include: setting a tone of mutual respect using observational, listening, and interviewing skills that quickly identify problems, locating existing resources, making timely and appropriate referrals, and functioning as an advocate when needed (Williams, 1994).

Conclusions

There has been an increase in research related to problems and needs of the homeless over the past decade. However, there continues to be a paucity of nursing research related to the important roles that professional nurses play and the interventions they use to provide care for the homeless mentally ill with chronic mental illness and related mood disorders. There are a limited number of studies on methodology of homelessness research despite long-standing concerns about applying methods and instruments developed for nonhomeless populations to homeless populations especially those with a mental illness (Koegel & Burnam, 1992). Past research has not sufficiently investigated the validity of mood disorders, psychiatric symptoms, and substance abuse among homeless mentally ill individuals (Herman, Stuening, & Barrow, 1993). Self-report measures studied look at self-esteem, client satisfaction, psychiatric symptoms (Calsyn et al., 1993), alienation and interpersonal adjustment (Morse, 1984), substance abuse (Fureman, Parikh, Bragg, & McLellah, 1990), and service utilization (Calsyn et al., 1997).

Case management of the homeless mentally ill was studied (Wood et al., 1998) and documents the weak family relationships of the homeless mentally ill. When no services are offered, many individuals are unable to maintain consistent housing (Koegel et al., 1996). Case management was identified as important in initiating change in family support, but long-term case management did not further improve family relationships. Findings of the study by Wood et al. (1998) support the need to connect more mentally ill homeless persons with supportive communities, beginning with the family as a significant way of decreasing homelessness. Both qualitative and quantitative nursing research is needed that may be built around the research done by other disciplines to clearly document the important role and interventions used by the professional nurse in providing care to mentally ill individuals and families with major mental illness and related mood disorders.

ALICE R. KEMPE

See also

CHRONIC MENTAL ILLNESS
HOMELESS HEALTH

MENTALLY ILL ADULTS WITH COEXISTING SUBSTANCE DISORDERS: DUAL DIAGNOSIS

Substance use disorders frequently coexist with psychiatric illness. Reports from a variety of mental health emergency, inpatient, and community settings in the 1980s reported high levels of comorbid substance abuse in psychiatric patients. The Epidemiologic Catchment Area (ECA) study, a large, multisite study of the prevalence of mental disorders, confirmed that this was not merely a result of selection bias in treated samples. Presence of any mental illness significantly increased the risk of substance use disorder (SUD), and persons with the most severe psychiatric disorders had the highest rates. Forty-seven percent of persons with schizophrenia had SUDs, as did 56% of people with bipolar disorder and 84% of people with antisocial personality disorder (Regier et al., 1990).

Comorbid psychiatric and substance use disorders, often referred to as "dual diagnosis" or "dual disorders," are associated with an array of negative consequences. These include noncompliance with treatment; increased frequency of relapse and rehospitalization; depression and suicidality; violence; legal problems; difficulty managing finances; homelessness; and HIV infection (Drake et al., 1998). The high prevalence of psychiatric/substance abuse comorbidity, especially in treatment settings, and the disastrous consequences associated with this combination makes it imperative that psychiatric nurses familiarize themselves with the existing knowledge base on assessment and treatment of dual disorders, and that nurse researchers continue to expand this knowledge base. Although the nursing literature contains several descriptions of nursing interventions for dual disorders, only one study of a nursing intervention was found (Pollack, Steubben, & Sobhan, 1997).

This review will address key issues in recent research literature on the assessment and treatment of dual disorders, with an emphasis on severe mental illnesses such as schizophrenic and bipolar disorders. The New Hampshire-Dartmouth Psychiatric Research Center (Dr. Robert Drake, Director) has played an especially prominent role in dual disorder research. Although research on nicotine dependence and smoking cessation efforts in psychiatric populations is increasing, space limitations preclude discussion of this literature.

Assessment

Substance use disorders often go undetected in psychiatric settings (Ananth et al., 1989) since the effects of substances of abuse can be similar to the symptoms of mental illness and since mental health personnel are often not trained in substance abuse detection and treatment. In addition, persons with coexisting mental disorders often experience substance-related problems at much lower levels of consumption than substance abusers who are not mentally ill (Drake et al., 1990). For this reason, substance abuse screening instruments used in other populations, such as the CAGE or the MAST, have poor classification accuracy in psychiatric populations (Rosenberg et al., 1998).

In a comparison of six different methods of identifying psychiatric inpatients in need of substance abuse treatment, Dixon and colleagues (1993) found that a brief screen for recent regular use of substances was superior to a DSM-III-R admitting or treatment diagnosis in identifying patients likely to benefit from substance abuse services. Rosenberg and coworkers (1998) developed a brief screen for SUD specific to mentally ill adults with classification accuracy of 83% for alcohol disorders and 90% for cocaine or cannabis disorders in a psychiatric inpatient sample.

For patients in ongoing treatment, Drake and colleagues (1990) developed the Case Manager Rating Scale for Alcohol Use Disorder (CMRS). This 5-point scale rates the severity of alcohol problems in people with schizophrenia, with specific criteria for each point on the scale. It is designed for use by a provider who works closely with the patient and can elicit data from multiple sources such as family, friends, and other treatment providers.

Integrated Treatment

Experts in dual disorder treatment have long advocated providing substance abuse and mental health interventions in the same programs, referred to as integrated treatment (Drake, Bartels, Teague, Noordsy, & Clark, 1993; Minkoff, 1989). Such programs combine mental health interventions, such as psychotropic medication and assertive case management, with substance abuse interventions, such as 12-step groups and addiction education. Although there have been no controlled studies comparing integrated treatment to parallel treatment (simultaneous treatment in mental health and substance abuse treatment systems) or sequential treatment (treatment of one disorder follows treatment of the other), studies of integrated models have often shown significant reductions in substance use (Drake, McHugo, & Noordsy, 1993; Ho et al., 1997; Minkoff & Regner, 1999) and hospitalization (Ho et al., 1997) from baseline levels.

Group Interventions

A recent review of group interventions in the context of integrated treatment for dual disorders (Meuser & Noordsy, 1996) summarized 11 studies of dual-diagnosis group treatment. These authors note that, in pre and post study designs, group treatment shows better retention of clients and improved outcomes compared to standard care. However, they also note a number of limitations in the research literature on dual-diagnosis groups: paucity of controlled studies; brief intervention periods; small sample sizes; sporadic group attendance by research subjects; and difficulty in distinguishing the unique contribution of group interventions from the effects of other program components, such as case management or family interventions.

Meuser and Noordsy (1996) identify four basic types of dual disorder group intervention: 12-step; educational-supportive; social skills; and stagewise treatment. They note, however, that most group interventions contain elements of several approaches, so it is difficult to compare the efficacy of different modalities. Pollack and Steubben (1998) describe the use of addiction education groups, an educative-supportive group intervention for psychiatric inpatients. An evaluation study (Pollack et al., 1997) found that patients generally perceived the experience as beneficial, were able to focus on recovery issues as a group, and utilized feedback from each other. However, patient satisfaction was the only outcome variable examined.

Assertive Community Treatment

Experts consider assertive community treatment (ACT), a comprehensive service approach including assertive outreach, in vivo service delivery, and long-term treatment, to be an essential component of treating severely ill dually diagnosed individuals (Drake et al., 1993). A retrospective case study of all clients who received services from an integrated ACT program for dually diagnosed homeless individuals over a 4-year period (Meisler, Blankertz, Santos, & McKay, 1997) found high rates of retention in treatment and housing stability and reductions in incarceration and psychiatric hospitalization. However, only 24% of the sample achieved abstinence.

A clinical trial comparing integrated dual disorder ACT to standard case management (SCM) in New Hampshire over a 3-year period (Drake et al., 1998) found greater improvements in alcohol use, substance abuse treatment progression, overall life satisfaction, and adequacy of financial support in the ACT group. Failure to find group differences on measures of community tenure, psychiatric symptoms, and remission of substance use disorder were explained by the high quality of existing SCM services and the diffusion of ACT innovations into the SCM condition.

Stagewise Treatment

Osher and Kofoed (1989) identified four stages in the process of treating dual disorder clients (engagement, persuasion, active treatment, and relapse prevention) and recommended tailoring treatment strategies to the client's stage of change. Data from 13 National Institute of Mental Health demonstration projects for dually diagnosed young adults (Mercer-McFadden & Drake, 1995) indicated that clients with comorbid disorders typically take several years to move through these stages. Typically, the early phases of treatment focus on engaging clients in integrated services and educating them about the role of substance use in their current difficulties, as well as its likely impact on attainment of goals. Reduction in substance use usually does not take place until clients have achieved some psychosocial stability (stable housing, medication compliance, etc.), and abstinence may not occur until after clients have been stable for some time.

Since abstinence is not a sensitive measure of treatment success in dually diagnosed individuals, researchers developed a scale to measure progression through the stages of integrated treatment (McHugo, Drake, Burton, & Ackerson, 1995). The Substance Abuse Treatment Scale (SATS) divides each of Osher and Kofoed's (1989) four treatment stages into early and late phases, with specific descriptors for each stage. Interrater and test-retest reliability were high (.90 and .91), and SATS ratings correlated well with other measures of substance use and functional status.

Recovery

Kasten's (1997) study focused on how dually diagnosed outpatients experience recovery. In addition to engagement in integrated treatment services, informants cited a number of strategies to resist substance use and increase well-being. These included avoiding people who use; engaging in structured activity, particularly physical exercise, prayer and meditation; anticipating consequences of use; and participation in 12-step groups. Informants generally preferred dual-disorder self-help groups to traditional 12-step groups, but those who had been in recovery for longer periods of time often found 12-step groups rewarding. Noordsy, Schwab, Fox, and Drake (1996) also found that dually diagnosed clients in the later stages of treatment, as well as those with better social skills, were more likely to participate in 12-step groups.

Directions for Further Research

Although some studies have been done on gender differences in dual disorders and response to treatment (Brunette & Drake, 1997; Comtois & Ries, 1995; Watkins, Shaner, & Sullivan, 1999; Westreich, Guedj, Galanter, & Baird, 1997), few studies have examined ethnic differences (Jerrell & Wilson, 1997). There is also a need for more rigorous research comparing different dual diagnosis treatment modalities with careful monitoring of program fidelity to insure valid comparisons (Teague, Drake, & Ackerson, 1995: Ridgely & Jerrell, 1996). Further development and testing of nursing interventions for dually diagnosed clients will also be important.

BETHANY J. PHOENIX

See also
ALCOHOLISM
DRUG ABUSE

SCHIZOPHRENIA NURSING RESEARCH

The term *schizophrenia* evokes the most identifiable picture of a psychiatric illness. Of all the major mental disorders, schizophrenia probably exacts the most stigma, cost, family burden, and controversy. Over time, debate regarding the exact definition and presentation of schizophrenia has been a catalyst for research and innovation in treatment approaches. Various methods for diagnosis and treatment have been pursued over the years, changing to fit emerging technology and a better understanding of treatment effectiveness.

The contemporary focus for research in schizophrenia has become increasingly biological in nature, with a concomitant increase in inventive approaches that involve psychiatric rehabilitation and consumer-oriented programs. Nursing research in schizophrenia mirrors those changing paradigms. Historically, one of the early pioneers of psychiatric mental health nursing, Hildegard Peplau, wrote extensively on the nature of the one-to-one relationship and the helping model for psychiatric care, particularly inpatient care. Current nursing research on the understanding and treatment of schizophrenia reflects a variety of treatment settings, including acute inpatient care, partial hospitalization, outpatient groups, psychosocial rehabilitation, family and consumer education, and medication management. Increasingly, nursing research involves a better understanding of the broad place of health and illness for persons with a diagnosis of schizophrenia.

Review of major studies, researchers, and methodology in schizophrenia reveals a medley of foci. Nursing researchers have contributed to the understanding of symptoms and symptom self-monitoring by individuals with schizophrenia. In particular, nursing studies have validated or expanded findings in the area of prodromal symptoms (McClandless-Glimcher et al., 1986; O'Connor, 1991), delineation of the course of disorder (Harding, 1988), and the nature of family burden and expressed emotion (Loukissa, 1995). Nursing researchers have been forerunners in the area of understanding comorbidity issues such as the relationship between mental illness and physical health (Holmberg & Kane, 1995). In addition, because nursing interventions are directly related to knowledge of genetics and neurochemical disturbances, nursing research related to these areas has increased (Fox, 1990).

Additionally, nursing research has contributed to much of the program and policy literature in the post-deinstitutionalization era. The movement to community-based care has been advocated for, written about, and researched by nurses in federal, state, and local community agencies (Mann et al., 1993; Palmer-Erbs & Anthony, 1995).

Research appears to be important in the nursing practice arena. Review of a MEDLINE search on the topic of schizophrenia reveals 32,914 citations, only 278 with a nursing focus. Nursing specialty organizations such as the Society for Education and Research in Psychiatric Mental Health Nursing (SERPN) and the American Psychiatric Nurses Association (APNA) organize yearly conferences around research papers and innovative educational approaches. Other methods of dissemination include nursing journals specifically for or with specific features of nursing research findings. These include *Archives of Psychiatric Nursing* and *Journal of Psychiatric Nursing*. Additionally, nurse researchers are common contributors to interdisciplinary journals (i.e., *Psychiatric Services*, a journal with an interdisciplinary purpose and nurses as contributing editors and board members).

Future Directions

Scientific advances in schizophrenia, including genetic, neurobiological, cognitive, and psychosocial findings, have been increasingly integrated with nursing practice principles and interventions. Future research in treatment areas, including incorporation of ethnic and cultural differences, responses to a variety of treatments, and focus on outcome measures, seem likely. Given what we learn from the science of schizophrenia, nursing still consists of both the art and science of human responses. Therefore, gleaning from the biological sphere, nursing research must balance the need for new and improved information related to how to provide caring, supportive, and humane treatment with biopsychosocial information. How the disabilities from schizophrenia interact with physical health, family coping, and community adaptation continues to require research.

Economic concerns exist in many shapes. The decade of the 1990s has been labeled "the decade of the brain" to reflect the growing money and effort devoted to understanding the neurobiological nature of schizophrenia and other major mental illnesses. The personal and societal loss that accompanies such a persistent and disabling disorder has economic costs difficult to measure. Primary prevention research aimed at understanding earlier detection and treatment is needed.

Ethical issues in schizophrenia present a complicated picture. Informed consent issues take the forefront in both clinical and research arenas. Informed consent, the assumption that adults have the right to consent or refuse to consent to treatment, is complicated when one determines their judgment or competence to be altered by their illness. In the era of managed care, nursing research undoubtedly will explore the justice of the allocation of resources. Issues of access, quality, and cost are important variables for nursing research in the area of health care delivery systems.

SARAH P. FARRELL

See also

CHRONIC MENTAL HEALTH
COMMUNITY MENTAL HEALTH
MENTAL HEALTH IN PUBLIC SECTOR PRIMARY CARE
MENTAL HEALTH SERVICES RESEARCH

SCHIZOPHRENIA: SYMPTOM DETECTION AND SELF-MANAGEMENT

Schizophrenia is a complex disorder that typically persists for years with a course of periodic acute episodes separated by periods of remission during which many symptoms persist at a reduced level. Antipsychotic medication is a mainstay of treatment, but as Bellack and Muser (1993) point out, "Psychosocial interventions can play a critical role in a comprehensive intervention program and are probably necessary components if treatment is to improve the patient's overall level of functioning, quality of life, and compliance with prescribed treatments" (p. 318).

The experience of the disorder is poignantly communicated in the findings of an interpretive study by Baker (1996). The 15 informants described psychic *pain* varying between chronic, subacute discomfort and terrible anguish; problematic experiences with *control*, both experiencing uncontrollable feelings that determine behavior and being controlled by others; devastating *failures*, involving a perception of letting oneself down and failing to meet others' expectations; and *loss*—of a normal life and of roles and relationships that some had managed to develop. All informants watched vigilantly for intensifying distress and symptoms, because these are the signs of relapse—leading to the pain of lack of control, failure, and loss. Baker points out that self-monitoring is embedded in the illness experience of suffering. She suggests that nurses might help people with schizophrenia who are not yet good self-monitors by encouraging them to focus on their internal experiences of fluctuating distress.

To identify recent (since the early 1990s) nursing studies for this synopsis, I searched CINAHL and Medline using the terms *schizophrenia* and *symptom management* and rummaged through personal files for saved articles. My strategy likely missed qualifying studies, and unfortunate omissions may have occurred. Nonetheless, I trust that my final collection is reasonably representative of recent self-management research by nurses.

Interest in self-monitoring as the first step of relapse prevention in schizophrenia was greatly stimulated by an influential paper by Docherty, Van Kammen, Siris, and Marder in 1978. Based on earlier literature, the authors traced the predictable process of symptom exacerbation from stability to psychosis, noting that the earliest signs of destabilization are mood- and anxiety-related. In accord with this scheme, Hamera, Peterson, Handley, Plumlee, and Frank-Ragan (1991) hypothesized that individuals identifying an anxiety or mood symptom rather than a psychotic symptom as their chief predictor of impending relapse would be higher functioning. Indeed, in their sample of 51 community mental health center clients, those reporting anxiety or depression indicators had significantly higher Global Assessment of Symptoms scores than subjects who identified psychotic predictors. A year later 28 of the original 51 participants were located, and 24 again identified an indicator, almost half of which were in a different category from their choice a year earlier (Hamera, Peterson, Young, & Schaumloffel, 1992). Interestingly, two people said they no longer focused on symptoms, as it was too negative. The authors speculate that at least some individuals may reach a stage of rebuilding their lives at which a focus on wellness becomes more productive.

Three studies explored relationships among factors that influence self-monitoring, self-perception, and disorder-management behaviors. Kozuki (1999) examined the influences of symptom unawareness on neuroleptic compliance behaviors in a sample of 134 hospitalized individuals. In her sample, high symptom awareness was associated with neuroleptic compliance. Low symptom awareness or low motivation to use medications tended to lead people to adhere to medication only as long as they felt pressured by others to do so or so long as they perceived comfort effects from the medications. Talley (1999) interviewed 69 people with schizophrenia spectrum disorders to learn about the self-regulatory processes used to understand illness, manage symptoms, and maintain wellness. She identified symptom awareness, consequences, and control efforts. Subjects used early warning symptoms, stress reduction activities, and help-seeking from providers or self-help groups. Kennedy, Schepp, and O'Connor (2000) interviewed 60 hospitalized people with schizophrenia to explore relationships among four variables hypothesized to be associated with relapse in schizophrenia. Three variables, recognition of relapse symptoms, utilization of symptom self-management, and perceived effectiveness, were all positively correlated. Insight showed no relationship to the other three variables. Insight or symptom awareness is represented in each of these studies. The concept was measured in different ways and correlated with different other concepts, making direct comparisons impossible. That said, insight doesn't appear to have functioned as similarly as might be expected. Baier, Murray, and McSweeney (1998) point out that the important concept of insight is defined, measured, and scaled in very diverse ways across studies. They encourage stronger efforts toward a common definition and means of measurement, so findings across studies can be evaluated and a better knowledge base established.

Two studies explored strategies to cope with auditory hallucinations—a common symptom that is generally negative. Frederick and Cotance (1995) interviewed 33 community mental health center clients with persistent hallucinations. Responses were grouped into three categories: strategies that change level of arousal, strategies involving cognitive action, and strategies involving change in behavior. Using descriptive approaches, coping strategies were found to vary by gender and by the usual character of voices heard. Carter, Mackinnon, and Copolor (1996) interviewed 100 individuals with psychotic disorders who experienced auditory hallucinations. Subjects used a card sort strategy to indicate which strategies they had ever used, and of these, how successful (completely, partially, not at all) each had been. Total number of strategies used and mean efficacy of all methods used by each subject were calculated. A matrix of similarities of use and efficacy between all the strategies was calculated from the data and analyzed using a multidimensional scaling procedure. This procedure revealed clusters of strategies that in fact differ from the researcher-developed categories of apparently similar strategies typically used in these studies. This calls into question the notion that strategies that appear similar function similarly and can be legitimately grouped on the basis of face similarity. Interestingly, there was a gap between efficacy and frequency of use of techniques. For example humming, supported in careful laboratory research (Green & Kinsbourne, 1989), was highly rated in this study—though few subjects had tried it. The researchers point out that this finding strengthens the case for introducing coping strategies to clients as a part of treatment.

Two intervention studies were identified. Buccheri, Trygstad, Kanas, Waldron, and Dowling (1996) reviewed the literature for strategies useful for controlling auditory hallucinations. They recruited day treatment clients to participate in 12 weekly sessions. Each week, the six randomly assigned treatment group patients learned a new strategy, which they were asked to practice during the week. Subjects kept diaries. Nonparametric statistical comparisons of diary scores showed no significant differences from the comparison group in frequency, loudness, or self-control over auditory hallucinations. However, graphs of individual subjects showed some effects—emphasizing the value of using subjects as their own controls where treatment response may very across subjects. Participants described more benefit than was apparent in the quantitative analysis, suggesting that the measures may not have been sensitive to effects that in fact occurred. Data collection continued over the following year, and there was a pattern of continued use of strategies and reported benefits (Buccheri, Trygstad, Kanas & Dowling, 1997).

The other intervention study is being conducted by Karen Schepp and associates at the University of Washington School of Nursing. This program, Family Centered Program for Adolescents with Mental Illness (award title: Self Management Therapy for Youth with Schizophrenia), is a National Institute of Mental Health-funded 5-year randomized intervention study that tests the effectiveness of a family centered, community-based, 12-session, stress/symptom self-management intervention for adolescents with symptoms of schizophrenia. The primary aim is to improve the adolescents' level of functioning in role performance, thinking/cognitive processing, behavior toward others, mood, and use of substances. The secondary aim is to assess the impact on family functioning. To review the underlying concepts and pilot study, see Schepp, 1992a, 1992b.

Symptom management research has the potential to provide information for improving personal control and quality of life as well as for reducing relapses and perhaps the deterioration that often accompanies the long-term trajectory of schizophrenia. To achieve this goal, we need to build on our own and others' cross-sectional, observational studies and mount intervention studies using experimental or quasiexperimental designs and samples large enough to detect true effects. Several ideas for strengthening studies are identified in this paper. For an excellent explication of methodological considerations that are important in outcome studies, see Merwin and Mauck (1995).

FREDERICA O'CONNOR

See also
CHRONIC MENTAL ILLNESS
MENTAL ILLNESS PREVENTION

SECLUSION AND RESTRAINT

Over the past 2 years significant legislative changes have been adopted regarding the use of seclusion and restraint (S/R) in mental health facilities. These changes are largely the result of the direct involvement of patient advocacy groups' (National Alliance for the Mentally Ill and the National Mental Health Association) in championing the defense of patient rights and safety. This article will explore the uses of seclusion and restraint, the current literature, and future considerations in the use and evaluation of S/R in clinical practice.

Seclusion is a locked, protective environment used to contain a hospitalized mentally ill person when less restrictive interventions have failed or would not be considered appropriate given the aggressiveness or inappropriateness of the patient's behavior. Patients enter seclusion based on the clinical judgement of professional staff to prevent harm to themselves or others. Patients must be closely monitored by nursing staff while in seclusion and released when they regain self-control.

Restraints are the most restrictive intervention or measure on an inpatient psychiatric unit. Chemical restraint is the administration of medication to control a patient's behavior. Physical restraint involves the use of straps, usually made of leather, applied to the limbs of the patient for the purpose of securing the patient to a bed or chair. A restrained patient also must be closely monitored as the restraints leave them defenseless and vulnerable to harm from others.

Seclusion and restraint remain controversial interventions. Proponents assert that this is an effective means of intervention with an out-of-control patient and serves to prevent harm to the patient or others. Opponents believe that seclusion and restraint actions are harsh and inhumane and their ready availability has lead to their overuse. Both agree that S/R should never to be used as a method of punishment or for staff convenience.

Review of Literature

Research on the effects of seclusion and restraint is in its infancy. While a clear definition exists regarding the characteristics of these restrictive interventions, the effectiveness of S/R and how it can be implemented in a fashion that does not undermine the therapeutic relationship has yet to be established. To date, there are no controlled studies that examine the value of S/R in those with serious mental illness (Sailas & Fenton, 1999). Instead, most studies have employed exploratory and descriptive strategies focusing on the perceptions and attitudes of patients and staff toward the S/R experience.

The use of S/R has traditionally been an accepted intervention and has been described as an essential element of a therapeutic milieu (Gunderson, 1978; Plutchik, Karasu, Conte, Siegel, & Jarrett, 1978; Tooke & Brown, 1992) and a valuable component of patient treatment (Tardiff, 1984). Survey data collected from 124 state hospitals, representing 44 states, showed that rates of S/R have remained unchanged from 1991 to 1994 (Crenshaw, Cain, & Francis, 1997) and that smaller, acute care facilities had higher rates of S/R related to aggressive behaviors common in acute psychiatric crisis. A retrospective study by Plutchik et al. (1978) sampled 450 consecutive admissions to a psychiatric hospital and found that approximately 26% of this sample had been secluded during their hospitalization. This averaged out to 2.5 seclusion events, lasting an average of 4 hours for a typical 27-day hospitalization. The majority of patients secluded had a diagnosis of schizophrenia. Nurses reported that the most common reasons for secluding was out of control, agitated or disruptive behavior or violence toward self or others. Kirkpatrick (1989) found that the peak time for seclusion was within the first 24 hours after hospital admission. The prevailing conditions on individual psychiatric units in hospitals can affect seclusion use including staff training, attitude and philosophy of care, staffing ratios, and the general anxiety of the unit.

Several descriptive studies explored seclusion from the patient's perspective (Binder & McCoy, 1983; Heyman, 1987; Martinez, Grimm, & Adamson, 1999; Norris & Kennedy, 1992; Plutchik et al., 1978; Smith, 1995; Soliday, 1985; Wadeson & Carpenter, 1976). Patient perceptions of negativity and pessimism toward the seclusion experience were a consistent theme. Although patients did view seclusion as being a place to calm down, patient's expressed disgust with the unclean and stark physical condition of the seclusion room, verbalized that they often were unclear of the reason for their being placed in seclusion, and had a poor understanding of the necessary behaviors for release. Various authors have reported on the potential for the use of S/R to retraumatize patients. Blanch and Parrish (1992) report patient perceptions of coercive techniques by staff as analogous to the experience of rape. Cohen's (1994) critique of captivity as something that causes terror, helplessness, and destruction of autonomy and Chamberlain (1985), who associates seclusion with solitary confinement in jail, support this impression. Patients reported that seclusion made them dislike and distrust nursing staff (Heyman, 1987; Tooke & Brown, 1992). Patients suggested that seclusion be used rarely, for only short periods of time, and on a voluntary basis. While in seclusion, patients desired more contact with nursing staff to assist them in regaining control and objects to help them feel better such as reading materials or music (Martinez, Grimm, & Adamson, 1999; Norris & Kennedy, 1992). Patients believe that seclusion could often be prevented if more interaction or better communication occurred between the patient and the nurse (Binder & McCoy, 1983; Martinez, Grimm, & Adamson, 1999; Norris & Kennedy, 1992). Staff education and use of specialized, less restrictive interventional skills resulted in less use of S/R (Morales & Duphorne, 1995). Although the criteria for use of S/R interventions are set by regulatory agencies, there is room for considerable individual interpretation on how these guidelines will be enacted in the clinical setting. Baradell (1985) views seclusion as an intensive care experience, a clinical setting in which patients have unique emotional, biological, and psychosocial needs and advocates active engagement with the patient to facilitate a smooth transition back to the milieu.

Clinical Application

Despite growing literature cataloging the adverse experience of patients, S/R remains a commonly practiced intervention throughout the inpatient psychiatric hospital setting. Early recognition of behavioral problems and improved lower level interventional techniques to deescalate potentially volatile situations would decrease the need for S/R interventions. If S/R procedures become unavoidable, providing a setting that is less sterile or offensive to the patient and that is more calming, interactive, and aesthetically comfortable (e.g., music, reading materials, personal items) will improve the seclusion experience. More prospective and controlled studies are needed to assess innovative interventions surrounding the seclusion experience and provide administrators with the evidence-based practice protocols they will need to educate staff on the appropriate and hopefully minimal use of S/R. Nurses and other psychiatric disciplines will need to decide whether seclusion should be therapeutic or simply containment, and at what cost.

Future Research Directions

Ideally, learning alternate ways to handle dangerous behavior without the use of seclusion and restraint should be our goal. Meanwhile, it is important to study ways to effectively and safely work with patients when they exhibit aggressive behavior. Clarity is needed to distinguish ways to work with different types of aggression. For example, aggression associated with psychosis versus aggression related to someone with an axis II diagnosis might require very different lower level interventions. Identifying which patients could benefit from which interventions and why is of vital interest. Environmental factors and attitudes of the staff are major areas for future research. How can the environment be altered for each individual patient to assist in meeting the goal of treatment? How does the nurses attitude, skill level, and rapport with the patient affect the S/R outcome? Finally, more humane ways of restraining patients is needed, especially if the patient has past traumas that involved physical force.

RUBY J. MARTINEZ
MARY ADAMSON

See also
SUICIDE
WORKPLACE VIOLENCE

SUBSTANCE ABUSE AND ADDICTION AMONG REGISTERED PROFESSIONAL NURSES

Relevance to the Profession

Research on the prevalence and nature of alcohol, tobacco, and other drug use among professional nurses derives from the need for action and policy development to be based on research findings and other evidence. As workplace factors may place nurses at risk for the development and perpetuation of dysfunctional health related behaviors, the profession is obliged to advocate for change. Nursing's interest in substance use and abuse coalesced in the early 1980s as nurses and other health professionals joined specialty organization advocates to highlight the problem. A climate of social concern and the visibility of illicit drug and alcohol related problems supported these efforts and prompted state and specialty nurses associations and ultimately the American Nurses Association to promote research and policy development in this area. In 1982, the American Nurses' Association House of Delegates passed a resolution on practice by nurses whose judgement is impaired by alcoholism, drug addiction and/or mental illness; a policy statement *Addictions and psychological dysfunctions: The profession's response to the problem* followed in (ANA, 1984). This document defined impaired practice as nursing practice which does not meet the professional ethical code and standards of nursing practice because the cognitive, interpersonal, and/or motor skills of the practitioner are impaired by psychiatric illness, or excessive use of alcohol and/or other drugs. "Chemical dependency" refers to a maladaptive, compulsive pattern of alcohol and other drug use which produces physiologic dependence on at least one drug of abuse. This action nursing specialty emerged from the need to regulate practice which could endanger public health and to promote the welfare of the professional nurse in need of treatment, rehabilitation, and support for re-entry to the workforce. This issue has since generated additional research efforts dating from the 1980's and including drug use patterns, nurses' and nursing students' attitudes about impaired practice, disciplinary practices related to drug and alcohol use, and the course, recovery and relapse patterns of registered nurses with alcohol and drug problems.

Early Research Efforts

Early estimates of alcohol use by nurses were extrapolated from a small descriptive survey of health professionals (N = 407) by Bissell and Haberman. In 1984 they reported on 100 nurses self-described as alcoholics and members of Alcoholics Anonymous (AA). Given the national prevalence figures that 9% men and 5% women develop alcohol related problems (1984), they estimated that 2% or 140,000 registered nurses would experience alcohol related problems. The validity of these estimates was limited by a volunteer, self-selected, high achieving, and predominantly Caucasian sample of nurses who had abstained from alcohol use through membership in AA. While the findings were limited, the estimate quickly became used as normative. Studies of nurses in recovery by Sullivan, Bissell, and Leffler (1990) and Finke, Williams, and Stanley (1996) indicated that between 55% and 63% respectively, had used narcotics and 64%

and 20% respectively, had used marijuana in addition to alcohol. Estimates of drug and alcohol related problems among registered nurses generally, were estimated at 6–8% (ANA, 1984).

While these studies broadened the research focus and delineated patterns of drug use in addicted nurses, they provided no information on the prevalence of drug use in the profession and were limited by volunteer self-selected samples. Use of drug is the primary risk factor for addiction, so the absence of data on use limits the prediction or estimation of the prevalence of abuse and/or addiction.

Findings of earlier studies of nursing students (Engs, 1982 and Haack and Harford, 1984) coupled with research support for alcohol and drugs use habits persisting into professional life from high school and college years (McAuliffe et al., 1984) appeared to contradict high estimates of nurses' alcohol and drug use. Engs, for example, found that nursing and social work students had rates of alcohol use lower than law, medical and pharmacy students. Haack and Harford found that nursing students using alcohol similarly to other college students used fewer drugs. Billing's 1986 random sample of nurses drank less than non-nurse women in the general population.

The work of Trinkoff, Eaton, and Anthony provides the first baseline data on the prevalence alcohol and other drug use among registered professional nurses (1991). Based on data collected in the early 1980's, their work and that of Blazer and Mansfield (1995), indicated that overall substance abuse rates in nurses were similar to those of the general population. Trinkoff et al. used a sample from the Epidemiologic Catchment Area Program (ECA) sponsored by the National Institute of Mental Health, a multi-site probability sample, to identify a sample of 143 registered nurses under 65 who were currently working full or part-time. Non-nurse controls were matched to the nurses by residence tract and gender. Data was obtained from interviews on sociodemographics, drug and alcohol abuse and psychological symptoms. Alcohol abuse was defined as experiencing two or more weeks of heavy drinking (7 drinks daily). Findings indicated that both nurses and control group members had similar rates of illicit drug use (marijuana cocaine, heroin, other opiates, psychedelics, tranquilizers, amphetamines). Among nurses, 32.9% reported any illicit drug use, non-nurses, 35.1%. Non-nurses had much higher prevalence of alcohol abuse than nurses, with 3.8% of the sample reporting heavy use, and 8.8 %, pathological use. Nurses reported heavy alcohol use at the rate of 0.7% and pathological use at 4.9% (Trinkoff, Eaton, & Anthony, 1991). Findings must be interpreted cautiously given the small sample size and reliance upon retrospective self-report. The Nurses Worklife and Health Study (NWHS), an anonymous survey of 4438 registered nurses, yielded similar rates to the general population, but indicated elevated rates of prescription drug use (Trinkoff & Storr, 1998). Blazer and Mansfield's randomized descriptive survey (N = 1,525) compared 920 nurses with other female employees and found low use patterns of licit an illicit drugs and alcohol for all subjects with lowest levels of smoking among nurse subjects (1995).

Subsequent studies by Storr and others have sought to identify factors which predict or support excessive drug use, including occupational factors. Attitudes about the capacity to control drug use have been identified as "pharmacologic optimism" and linked to an illusory sense of mastery over the addictive potential of the drug (Brewster, 1994). Research also supports accessibility as a factor in the abuse of prescription drugs (Trinkoff, Storr, & Wall, 1999; Bell, McDonough, Ellison, & Fitzhugh, 1999). In an effort to identify groups of nurses who may be at higher risk for addiction, Trinkoff and Storr explored specialty practice. Among nurses working in specialties, illicit drug use (marijuana & cocaine) was significantly higher among emergency nurses, psychiatric nurses were more like to smoke, and oncology and administrative nurses were twice as likely to engage in binge drinking (1998). Plant et al. (1991) and Collins et al. (1999) also found higher smoking rates among psychiatric nurses and Collins found significantly higher cocaine use in critical care nurses. Storr, Trinkoff and Anthony found that nurses working in high strain jobs were 50–60% more likely to be non-medical drug users, whether demands were psychological or physical (1998). In the Nurses Worklife and Health study (1994) cited earlier, investigators found that nurses reported the prevalence of drinking five or more drinks per occasion in the past year at 17%, drug use at 10%, and smoking at 15.1%. Long shift hours and night or rotating shifts were associated with increased substance use (Trinkoff & Storr, 1998) related workplace factors.

Future Directions

Future directions for research must consider the methodologic limitations of these studies, including reliance on retrospective self-report, and the challenge to improve collection of such sensitive data using more technologic and fewer personal contacts (Trinkoff & Storr, 1997). Exploration of personal "at risk" characteristics of individuals in relation to workplace factors, replication of findings and comparison of data with other professional groups would provide further direction for education, research and policy development.

MADELINE A. NAEGLE

See also
ALCOHOLISM
DRUG ABUSE

SUICIDE

Suicide is defined as a death that is the result of an intentional self-destructive act. Nurses have demonstrated a great deal of clinical and theoretical interest in suicide, suicide attempts, attitudes toward suicide, and assisted suicide but have conducted very little research on these topics. A related topic that has been studied fairly extensively by nurses is suicide survivors, those family members and significant others who are bereaved by a suicide.

Suicide, Suicide Attempts, and Suicidal Thoughts

Few studies have addressed suicide specifically. Using a qualitative methodology, messages of psychiatric patients who attempted or committed suicide were compared by Valente (1994). She found that clear suicidal messages were sent by most psychiatric patients and that the messages of suicide completers and suicide attempters could be differentiated. Demi, Bakeman, Sowell, Moneyham, and Seals (1996) studied suicidality in HIV-infected women and found that suicidal thoughts were common among the women and that family cohesion moderated the effect of HIV-related symptoms on emotional distress. They also found that there were clear differences between women who neither thought about nor attempted suicide and those who thought about or attempted suicide, but there were no significant differences between those who thought about suicide and those who attempted it. Grabbe, Demi, Camann, and Potter (1997) used a national data base to assess suicidal risk factors among the elderly during their last year of life; and using logistic regression, they confirmed the traditional risk factors of age, race, gender, alcohol use, and mental illness and provided preliminary evidence that cancer is also a risk factor among the elderly.

Two studies addressed adolescent suicide. Burge, Felts, Chenier, and Parrillo (1995), using a national data base, studied suicidal behaviors among U.S. high school students and found a significant positive relationship between cocaine use and severity of outcomes of suicide attempts. They also found a significant but less strong relationship between marijuana use, alcohol use, sexual activity, and suicide attempts. Conrad (1992) explored adolescents' beliefs about the causes of adolescent suicide and found that teens identified "too much pressure" as the major cause of teen suicide.

Attitudes toward Suicide

Several studies by nurses have investigated attitudes toward suicide in diverse groups, four studies addressed nurses' attitudes, and one studied elderly persons' attitudes. Oncology nurses' knowledge and misconceptions about suicide were explored through use of a vignette depicting a suicidal cancer patient (Valente, Saunders, & Grant, 1994). Although the nurses correctly identified a number of risk factors, few knew that race, age, and gender were risk factors. Further, few nurses assessed whether patients had a specific suicide plan, and less than one third identified appropriate interventions to prevent suicide in an at-risk patient. A second study compared nurses' attitudes toward suicide based on their clinical specialty, age, and highest degrees; they found no significant differences on any of the subscales based on clinical specialty, although age and degrees were significant on only the right to die subscale (Alston & Robinson, 1992).

When Irish casualty nurses' attitudes toward attempted suicide were assessed, older and more experienced nurses had better attitudes toward suicide attempters than did younger, less experienced nurses (McLaughlin, 1994). Positive attitudes toward suicide attempters were found among psychiatric nurses working in an acute psychiatric ward (Long & Reid, 1996). The only study of nonnurses explored attitudes toward suicide among low-income, elderly, inner city residents and compared attitudes toward suicide of men and women, African Americans and Whites, finding no significant differences. The researchers suggested that social class and place of residence may be better predictors of attitudes toward suicide in the elderly than race and gender (Parker, Cantrell, & Demi, 1997).

Suicide Survivors

Many studies have been conducted on suicide survivors, including parents, spouses, children, siblings, and therapists. Most of the studies of suicide survivors have been descriptive and have found that a death by suicide produces extreme distress in the survivors, with evidence of increased guilt, stigma, and resentment and a continuing questioning of "why" the suicide occurred. Several studies have compared those bereaved by suicide with those bereaved by other modes of death and have reported conflicting findings. Recently, an attempt was made to use a quasi-experimental design to study the effects of two group interventions on outcomes among spouse survivors of suicide (Constantino & Bricker, 1996). The researchers found that participants in both the social group intervention and the bereavement intervention experienced an overall reduction in distress; however, the bereavement intervention group experienced significantly lower levels of anger or hostility and guilt.

Future Directions

The suicide rates for the elderly are rising. At the same time, there is increased interest in euthanasia and assisted suicide. Nurses are intimately involved with elderly and terminally ill patients who are contemplating suicide and assisted suicide. At the same time, suicide rates among adolescents and young adults are rising. Much more research attention should be directed to this topic. Researchers should move beyond describing attitudes toward suicide and effects of suicide on survivors and toward studying interventions to prevent suicide and to assist those coping with a death by suicide.

ALICE S. DEMI

See also

ALCOHOLISM
CHRONIC MENTAL ILLNESS
DEPRESSION AMONG OLDER ADULTS
NO SUICIDE CONTRACTS

TRAUMATIC EVENTS: INDIVIDUAL AND COLLECTIVE RESPONSES

Traumatic events are typically unexpected and uncontrollable and occur among "normal" individuals. Exposure to traumatic events includes either experiencing or being confronted with actual or threatened death or injury to self or others (American Psychiatric Association, 1994). Events that are abrupt and of brief duration, that is, lasting a few minutes or hours, are referred to as short-term (Type I) traumatic events in contrast to Type II events that are prolonged, repeated, or ongoing (Terr, 1991). This report is limited to Type I events, which include natural disasters (earthquakes, floods, and hurricanes), accidental disasters (vehicular accidents and airplane crashes), and deliberately caused human-made disasters (bombings, school massacres, and arson fires).

Traumatic events are relevant to nursing science and practice for several reasons. First, these events are far more common than previously thought. Norris (1992), in a survey of residents in four Southeastern cities, found a lifetime exposure rate of 69%. The 69% had experienced at least one traumatic event, with tragic death (homicide, suicide, or accident), robbery, and motor vehicle accidents with injuries, as the three most frequent. Second, although responses to traumatic events vary widely, adaptation to loss is of long rather than short duration and can be accompanied by serious consequences (Green, 1994; Murphy, Das Gupta, Cain, Johnson, Lohan, Wu, & Mekwa, 1999; North, Nixon, Shariat, Mallonee, McMillen, Spitznagel, & Smith, 1999).

Human Responses to Traumatic Events

A body of research findings resulting from all types of Type I traumatic events suggests four major domains of human responses following exposure to one of these events. *Emotional responses* include shock, terror, guilt, horror, irritability, anxiety, hostility, and depression. *Cognitive responses* include inability to concentrate, confusion, self-blame, intrusive thoughts (flashbacks) about the experience, decreased sense of self-efficacy, fear of losing additional control over life events, and fear of reoccurrence of the event. *Biological responses* include sleep disturbance (insomnia, nightmares), exaggerated startle response, and psychosomatic symptoms. *Behavioral responses* include avoidance, social withdrawal, interpersonal stress (decreased intimacy and lowered trust in others), and substance abuse. These responses profoundly affect individuals' coping abilities and frequently include all four domains (Green, 1994; Meichenbaum, 1994; Murphy, Braun, Tillery, Cain, Johnson, & Beaton, 1999; Shariat, Mallonee, Kruger, Farmer, & North, 1999).

Assessment, Diagnosis, and Treatment of Posttraumatic Stress Disorder

A comprehensive clinical interview is the primary assessment strategy for differentiation among preexisting psychiatric conditions, current and past levels of functioning, acute stress disorder, and posttraumatic stress disorder (PTSD) (APA, 1994). PTSD has been shown to co-occur with other psychiatric conditions about 40 to 60% of the time (Kessler, McGonagle, & Shanyang, 1994). DSM-IV diagnostic criteria include immediate exposure responses of intense fear, helplessness, or horror, symptoms in all of the following categories: reexperiencing (one or more), avoidance (three or more), arousal (two or more), with all of at least a month duration, and resulting functional impairment (APA, 1994).

No one form of treatment for PTSD has been shown to be superior to the others. Several forms of treatment are recommended and include education, social support and social integration, therapy, and combined approaches.

Professional therapies include counseling, cognitive-behavioral individual or group approaches, and medication. Cognitive behavioral strategies reduce fear, intrusive memories, flashbacks, and nightmares. Cognitive restructuring, problem-solving, and relaxation and guided imagery are also helpful (Meichenbaum, 1994; Murphy, 1998). Several medications have shown effectiveness in the treatment of PTSD symptoms, however, medications appear to be symptom specific and are rarely sufficient to provide complete remission (Vargas & Davidson, 1993).

Research Examples of Natural Disasters, Accidents, and Deliberately-Caused Human Events

Natural Disasters. Empirical findings show that natural disasters differ widely from one another, creating unique needs and demands of victims and communities.

For example, being part of a collective disaster appears to make the event appear less overwhelming and facilitates coping (Norris & Kaniasty, 1996). According to Norris and Kaniasty (1996), their hypotheses of support mobilization and deterioration were supported by longitudinal studies of Hurricane Hugo and Hurricane Andrew. Benight and his colleagues (1999) demonstrated that coping self-efficacy serves an important mediating function for how lost resources are managed and how effective coping ensues.

Hardin and her colleagues (1994), conducted the most comprehensive study to date involving adolescents. One year after Hurricane Hugo, a team of nurses and other investigators surveyed nearly 1500 South Carolina high school students. Their results showed a "dose response," that is, the greater the exposure, the greater the psychological stress. However, the researchers also noted that other stressful life events (injured by a parent or guardian, being attacked, or experiencing the death of a family member or friend), were equally strong predictors of outcomes.

Accidental Trauma. The most common accidental trauma in the United States is involvement in a motor vehicle accident (MVA). MVAs are the leading cause of death in the United States for 15 to 20 year olds. In 1997, 3336 drivers 15 to 20 years old were killed, and an additional 365,000 were injured (U.S. Bureau of the Census, 1995). Studies have involved both victims and survivors (Harvey & Bryant, 1999; Murphy, Das Gupta, et al., 1999). Harvey and Bryant (1999) noted a 16% rate of acute stress disorder (APA, 1994) in the early assessment of 62 hospitalized adults following MVA injuries. Murphy, Braun, Tillery, Cain, et al. (1999) conducted a longitudinal, prospective study of nearly 200 parents whose 12 to 28 year old children died suddenly and violently as a result of accident, homicide, or suicide. Among the parents bereaved by accident (53% of the sample), 67% of the mothers and 55% of the fathers were experiencing rates of mental distress (depression, anxiety, cognitive dysfunction) 2 years after the deaths, which was more than twice as high as a normative sample of adults in the same age range (Murphy, Das Gupta, Cain, Johnson, et al., 1999).

Deliberately Caused Human-Made Disasters. The bombing of the Alfred P. Murrah Federal Building in Oklahoma City on April 19, 1995 was the most severe incident of terrorism ever experienced in the United States and has been studied extensively (Maningas, Robison, & Mallonee, 1997; Mallonee et al., 1996; North et al., 1999; Shariat et al., 1999). Nurses were involved in several of these studies. For example, Maningas et al. (1997), documented the emergency medical response (EMS) efforts used to treat the injured (93% of those in the building at the time of the bombing).

The resulting emotional distress was profound; 45% of adult survivors experienced a postevent psychiatric disorder (preevent rates were controlled in the study design), and 34% met diagnostic criteria for PTSD. The onset of PTSD symptoms was sudden and very unusual, with 76% of those exposed reporting same day onset (North et al., 1999). In a follow-up study conducted 1.5 to 3 years after the blast, 30% of the injured sample ($n = 494$) reported being diagnosed with audiologic deficits, anxiety, and depression, with onsets of these conditions since the initial interview. These findings suggest the occurrence of both delayed and chronic PTSD and serious consequences of impaired hearing. The most frequently used health services were counseling (63%) and audiology services (48%). Total costs of these services were reportedly $5.7 million (Shariot et al., 1999).

Results of studies involving survivor-victims of recent school shootings in Colorado, Kentucky, and Oregon are not yet published, but can be expected to provide much-needed data pertaining to the responses of various age groups, differences in response according to relationships with the deceased and injured, and community response.

In the ongoing study of the author described above, parents whose 12 to 28 year old children died by homicide (18% of the sample), experienced more negative outcomes than did parents in the other two groups. In the homicide bereavement group, 21% of the mothers and 14% of the fathers met PTSD diagnostic criteria 2 years postdeath (Murphy, Braun, et al., 1999).

In summary, the study of traumatic events has become more rigorous and involved more nurse investigators over time. Some limitations remain: (a) Pre-event data is essential for research designs, but nearly impossible to obtain; (b) there are fewer data on community response than on individual responses; (c) interventions are documented less frequently than responses to events. More self-care interventions need to be developed and tested.

Future Research Directions

Major priorities include learning more about the long-term consequences of traumatic events for both victims and service providers and differences between individual and community responses.

SHIRLEY A. MURPHY

See also

STRESS
STRESS MANAGEMENT
VIOLENCE

YOUTH SUICIDE PREVENTION IN THE AMERICAN INDIAN AND ALASKA NATIVE COMMUNITY

Suicide is a major concern in American Indian and Alaska Native communities. The rates are two to three times higher than the U.S. national average (Kirmayer, 1994; May, 1987a, 1987b) and are continuing to rise (Lester, 1994; McShane, 1988). Between 1950 and 1980, the suicide rates for Indian males 15 to 24 years old increased 200 to 300% (Rosenburg, Smith, Davidson, & Conn, 1987). Suicide rates for Indian males are higher than any other ethnic group in the United States and are higher than for Indian females (May, 1987a, 1987b; Rardin, 1988). Employing both qualitative and quantitative methodologies, researchers have examined individual, family, and community risk factors. While many intervention programs have been undertaken, they have been largely demonstration in nature and have relied on process evaluations (Duran, Duran, & Tingley, 1995; Kahn, Lejero, Antone, & Francisco, 1988; Levy & Kunitz, 1987; Manson, Beals, Dick, & Duclos, 1989; May, 1987a, b; Rardin, 1988). Much additional work is needed. In this discussion, I will review major research contributions, note unanswered questions, and consider the implications for nursing research.

Review of Related Research

Research on American Indian and Alaska Native youth suicide has been largely directed toward identifying individual, family, and community risk factors (Committee of Cultural Psychiatry, 1989; Duran, Duran, & Tingley, 1995; Howard-Pitney, LaFrombroise, & Basil, 1992; Jilek-Aall, 1988; Kirmayer, 1994). In examining individual risk factors, alcohol use, depression/emotional disorders, hopelessness, and stress have received the bulk of attention (Committee of Cultural Psychiatry, 1989; Howard-Pitney et al., 1992; Kirmayer, 1994; O'Nell, 1992–93). From this research it has been found that alcohol is an important risk factor, but its pervasiveness in Indian communities makes it a poor single predictive factor. Van Winkle and May (1994) found that 97% of suicides among Indian youth were also linked to abuse, neglect, and alcohol. Depression, another risk factor that has been examined, is also difficult to isolate as a risk factor because of its pervasiveness in Indian communities. O'Nell (1992–93) noted from a study on the Flathead reservation that depression is a part of life. The mature individuals are expected to be depressed. Lack of depression is viewed as immaturity. Hopelessness and stress have been found to have a significant correlation with Indian youth suicide. Howard-Pitney et al. (1992) found a correlation vale of $r = 0.43$ for suicide attempters; this was significantly different from nonattempters ($p = .01$). They also found that stress was significantly associated with Indian youth suicide ($r = 0.26$; $p = .008$). Individual risk factors for suicide in Indian communities appear to be similar to those in non-Indian populations (Committee of Cultural Psychiatry, 1989), but the pervasiveness of depression and alcohol use in Indian communities suggests a complex interplay among the individual factors, family, and community. Kirmayer (1994) outlined a model in which the larger issues of acculturation, community, and family were linked to predisposing factors such as alcohol and depression; a sense of hopelessness; and enabling factors such as firearms, family crises, and a lowered sense of self worth and self esteem.

Major family risk factors linked to Indian youth suicide include violence, abuse, family alcohol use, previous suicide attempts, poverty, and chronic stress (American School Health Association, 1989; Duran, Duran, & Tingley, 1995; Hoff, 1984; Jilek-Aall, 1988). Hoff (1984) found that physical abuse, sexual abuse, and exposure to violence were linked to youth suicide. A study by the American School Health Association (1989) also found that family problems and stress were linked to youth suicide. Jilek-Aall (1988) noted that Indian families teach by role model and the model that many experience in families is alcoholism, anger, an abusive father or a father who is not present, coupled with neglect, hunger, physical abuse, and illness. Duran, Duran, and Tingley (1995) suggest that the root of domestic violence is intergenerational, internalized oppression.

Family deviance and instability have also been identified as risk factors for Indian youth suicide. Families who are deemed deviant within the context of the tribal communities place a youth at risk (May, 1987b; Rardin, 1988; Levy & Kunitz, 1987). Youth are at risk in families where there is violence, alcohol, and abuse. However, taking the youth from the home and placing them in non-Indian foster homes, as well as the break up of a family that results in a single family home also places the youth at risk for suicide. Family poverty has also been substantiated as an Indian youth suicide risk factor. Among Alaska Native and American Indian youth in 12 Indian Health Service (IHS) service units in the United States, Young (1990) found poverty to be positively and significantly related to youth suicide ($r = 0.65$; $p = .05$).

Community and tribal risk factors have also been linked to Indian youth suicide. In this respect, tribal economics, education, and employment have been examined (Young, 1990). Findings have been somewhat paradoxical. Poverty and unemployment, as well as wealth, increased acculturation, and education appear to be related to greater suicide risk (Young, 1990). Qualitative research has been conducted to compare tribal differences in terms of stability, social integration, and change. For example, it was found that tribes experiencing more change, little social integration, and greater tribal instability, were found to have higher rates of suicide (May, 1987a). The level of integration also poses a paradox. Communities too loosely or too tightly integrated were associated with higher rates of suicide (Committee of Cultural Psychiatry, 1989; May, 1987a). Tightly integrated communities leave little room for deviance.

Only a few suicide prevention intervention studies have been undertaken in Indian communities. These contributions have been demonstration in nature and have used process evaluations (Kahn et al., 1988; Levy & Kunitz, 1987; O'Nell, 1992–93; Rardin, 1988). I have found no evidence of controlled experimental studies aimed at measuring the impact of interventions to reduce suicide among Indian youth. Manson and associates (1989) noted 850 community-based adolescent programs and 194 carrying out suicide prevention activities, 41 of which were school-based. Some of these programs have focused on the individual youth and others have addressed family issues. It has been recognized that it is important to address prevention; have a system established to support youth in crises; follow up after a suicide attempt; and to have family involvement and, with some tribal communities, involvement of traditional healers. Some programs have been community based and wellness oriented (Duran, Duran, & Tingley, 1995; Kahn et al., 1988; Levy & Kunitz, 1987; May, 1987a, b; Rardin, 1988). In spite of all these activities, suicide rates continue to rise. Understanding of appropriate interventions to prevent American Indian and Alaska Native youth suicide is greatly needed.

Qualitative and quantitative, basic and applied research are needed to address Indian youth suicide prevention. Key research questions that deserve nursing consideration are as follows. (a) Risk assessment—Can a suicide risk explanatory model be developed that links risk factors, reflects a respect for culture, and provides insights into work with individual American Indian and Alaska Native youth? What, if any, adjustments need to be made in suicide risk assessment tools to make them more appropriate for American Indian and Alaska Native youth? (b) Family and social support—How is social support conceptualized in a tribal community and what is the relation to youth suicide? How can the paradoxes of family support be addressed? How may the wounds of oppression and the intergenerational pains related to youth suicide be healed? (c) Community factors—What explains the conflicting findings about poverty, employment, education, and acculturation related to American Indian and Alaska Native youth suicide risk and how may greater understanding contribute to interventions that address structures, policies, and community-based interventions? (d) Culture—What part does culture play and how may the traditional healers become involved in Indian youth suicide prevention? What are the cultural strengths that may be built on to reduce Indian youth suicide? A major concern is whether we can adapt interventions that have been successful in non-Indian communities to Indian youth.

Suicide among American Indian and Alaska Native youth deserves priority in nursing research and national funding. We need well-designed, culturally appropriate American Indian and Alaska Native youth suicide prevention and follow-up management programs that address individual, family, and community needs. Accurate systems of reporting and controlled evaluation studies to determine intervention efficacy is essential. Loss of any young person to suicide is a tragedy; loss of our Indian youth robs the North Americas of the valuable gifts, heritage, and wisdom of its first people.

CAROLYN J. STRICKLAND

See also
MINORITY ISSUES IN MENTAL HEALTH
SUICIDE

REFERENCES

Aday, L. (1994). Health status of vulnerable populations. *Annual Review of Public Health, 15,* 487–509.

Aiken, L., & Aiken, J. (1973). A systematic approach to the evaluation of interpersonal relationships. *American Journal of Nursing*, 73, 863–867.

Akiskal, H. S., & Pinto, O. (1999). The evolving bipolar spectrum. Prototypes I, II, III, and IV. *Psychiatric Clinics of North America, 22*(3), 517–534, vii.

Albee, G. W. (1996). Revolutions and counterrevolutions in prevention. *American Psychologist, 51,* 1130–1133.

Allebeck, P. (1989). Schizophrenia: A life-shortening disease. *Schizophrenia Bulletin, 15*(1), 81–89.

Allen, D. G., Lovell, D., & Rhodes, L. A. (2000). *Razor wire and clozapine: A University/Prisons Collaboration on mentally ill offenders.* Manuscript submitted for publication.

Allen, J., Arber, J., & Leadbeater, B. (1990). Adolescent problem behaviors: The influence of attachment and autonomy. *Psychiatric Clinics of North America, 13*(3), 306–467.

Allison, T. G., Williams, D. E., Miller, T. D., Patten, C. A., Bailey, K. R., Squires, R. W., & Gau, G. T. (1995). Medical and economic costs of psychological distress in patients with coronary artery disease. *Mayo Clinic Proceedings, 70,* 734–742.

Alspaugh, M. E., Stephens, M. A., Townsend, A. L., Zarit, S. H., & Greene, R. (1999). Longitudinal patterns of risk for depression in dementia caregivers: Objective and subjective primary stress as predictors. *Psychology & Aging, 14*(1), 34–43.

Alston, M. H., & Robinson, B. H. (1992). Nurses' attitudes toward suicide. *Omega: Journal of Death and Dying, 25,* 205–215.

Altshuler, L. L., Post, R. M., Leverich, G. S., Mikalauskas, K., Rosoff, A., & Ackerman, L. (1995). Antidepressant-induced mania and cycle acceleration: A controversy revisited. *American Journal of Psychiatry, 152*(8), 1130–1138.

American Academy of Forensic Sciences. (1989). Position statements. [online]. (Available at http://www.aafs.org).

American Academy of Pediatrics. (1993). The pediatrician and the "new morbidity." *Pediatrics, 92*(5), 731–733.

American Association for Protecting Children. (1986). *Highlights of official child Neglect and abuse reporting: 1984.* Denver, CO: American Humane Association.

American Heart Association. (1994). *Heart and stroke facts: 1994 supplement.* Dallas, TX: AHA.

American Institute for Research. (1988). Studies of intercollegiate athletics. Report Number 1: Summary. *Results from the 1987–88 national study of intercollegiate athletes.* Washington, DC: AIR.

American Nurses Association. (1984). *Addictions and psychological dysfunctions: The profession's response to the problem.* In M. A. Naegle (Ed.), *name of book.* Kansas City, MO: American Nurse Association.

American Nurses Association. (1990). *Standards of Psychiatric Consultation-Liaison Nursing*. Kansas City, MO: Author.

American Psychiatric Association. (1994). *Diagnostic and statistical manual of mental disorders* (4th ed.). Washington, DC: Author.

American Psychiatric Association. (1999). Practice guideline for the treatment of patients with delirium. (Available at http://psych.org/clin_res/pg_delirium.html).

American School Health Association (ASHA). (1989). The national adolescent student health survey: A report of the health of America's youth. Oakland, CA: Third Party Publishers.

Ananth, J., Vandewater, S., Kamal, M., Brodsky, A., Gamal, R., & Miller, M. (1989). Missed diagnosis of substance abuse in psychiatric patients. *Hospital and Community Psychiatry, 40*(3), 297–299.

Anderson, A., & Holman, J. (1997). Males with eating disorders: Challenges for treatment and research. *Psychopharmacology Bulletin, 33,* 391–397.

Andrews, M. M., & Herberg, P. (1999). Transcultural nursing care. In M. M. Andrews & J. S. Boyle (Eds.), *Transcultural concepts in nursing care* (3rd ed., pp. 23–77). Philadelphia: Lippincott.

Anthony, W. A., Cohen, M., Farkas, M., & Cohen, B. (2000). Clinical update: The chronically mentally ill. *Community Mental Health Journal, 36*(1), 97–106.

Aquilera, D. C. (1998). *Crisis intervention* (8th ed.). St. Louis: Mosby Year Books, Inc.

Arizmendi, T., & Affonso, D. (1987). Stressful events related to pregnancy and postpartum. *Psychosomatic Research, 31,* 743–756.

Arroyo, J. A. (1996). Psychotherapist bias with Hispanics: An analog study. *Hispanic Journal of Behavioral Studies, 18,* 21–28.

Assey, J. L. (1985). The suicide prevention contract. *Perspectives in Psychiatric Care, 23*(3), 99–103.

Badger, T. A. (1996a). Family members' experiences of living With members with depression. *Western Journal of Nursing Research, 18,* 149–171.

Badger, T. A. (1996b). Living with depression: Family members' experiences and treatment needs. *Journal of Psychosocial Nursing and Mental Health Services, 34,* 21–29.

Baider, L., & Kaplan De-Nour, A. K. (1984). Couples' reactions and adjustment to mastectomy. *International Journal of Psychiatry and Medicine, 14,* 265–276.

Baier, M., Murray, R. L. E., & McSweeney, M. (1998). Conceptualization and measurement of insight. *Archives of Psychiatric Nursing, XII,* 32–40.

Baker, C. (1995). The development of the self-care ability to detect early signs of relapse among individuals who have schizophrenia. *Archives of Psychiatric Nursing, 9,* 261–268.

Baker, C. (1996). Subjective experience of symptoms of schizophrenia. *Canadian Journal of Nursing Research, 28*(2), 19–35.

Baker, I. M., Espino, D. V., Robinson, B. H., & Stewart, B. (1993). Assessing depressive symptoms in African American and Mexican American elders. *Clinical Gerontologist, 14*(1), 15–29.

Baldessarini, R. J., & Tondo, L. (2000). Does lithium treatment still work? Evidence of stable responses over three decades. *Archives of General Psychiatry, 57*(2), 187–190.

Baltes, P. B., & Danish, S. J. (1980). Intervention in life-span development and aging. In R. R. Turner & H. W. Reese (Eds.), *Life-span developmental psychology* (pp. 49–78). New York: Academic Press.

Bandura, A. (1997). *Self-efficacy: The exercise of control.* New York: W. H. Freeman.

Baradell, J. G. (1985). Humanistic care of the patient in seclusion. *Journal of Psychosocial Nursing, 23*(2), 9–14.

Barak, Y., Wittenberg, N., Naor, S., Kutzuk, D., & Weizman, A. (1999). Clozapine in elderly psychiatric patients: Tolerability, safety, and efficacy. *Comprehensive Psychiatry, 40*(4), 320–325.

Barker, P. J. (1994). Locus of control in women with a diagnosis of manic-depressive psychosis. *Journal of Psychiatric & Mental Health Nursing, 1*(1), 9–14.

Barlow, D. (1995). Task force on psychological intervention guidelines. Template for developing guidelines: Interventions for mental disorders and psychosocial aspects of physical disorders. *American Psychological Association.* Washington, D.C.

Barnard, K. E., & Eyres, S. J. (1979). *Child health assessment: Part 2. The first year of life.* Hyattsville, MD: U.S. Department of Health, Education, and Welfare, Public Health Service.

Barnard, K. E., Hammond, M. A., Booth, C. L., Bee, H. L., Mitchell, S. K., & Spieker, S. (1989). Measurement and meaning of parent child interaction. In F. Morrison, C. Lord, & D. Keating (Eds.), *Applied developmental psychology* (Vol. 3, pp. 287–296). New York: Academic Press.

Barnes, D., Eribes, C., Juarbe, T., Nelson, M., Proctor, D., Sawyer, L., Shaul, M., & Meleis, A. I. (1995). Primary health care and primary care: A confusion of philosophies. *Nursing Outlook, 43*(1), 7–16.

Barnfather, J. S., & Lyon, B. L. (1993). *Stress and coping: State of the science and implications for nursing theory, research and practice.* Indianapolis, IN: Sigma Theta Tau International.

Barton, J. A. (1991). Parental adaptation to adolescent drug abuse: An ethnographic study of role formulation in response to courtesy stigma. *Public Health Nursing, 8,* 39–45.

Beach, S. R. H., Sandeen, E. E., & O'Leary, K. D. (1990). *Depression in marriage: A model for etiology and treatment.* New York: Guildford.

Bechtel, G. A., Davidhazar, R., & Tiller, C. M. (1998). Patterns of mental health care among Mexican Americans. *Journal of Psychosocial Nursing, 36*(11), 20–27.

Beck, A. T. (1978). *Cognitive therapy and emotional disorders.* New York: International Universities Press.

Becker, A., Grinspoon, S., Klibanski, A., & Herzog, D. (1999). Eating disorders. *The New England Journal of Medicine, 340,* 1092–1098.

Beisser, A. R., & Rose, G. (1972). *Mental health consultations and education.* Los Angeles: Institute Press.

Bell, D. M., McDonough, J. P., Ellison, J. S., & Fitzhugh, E. C. (1999). Controlled drug misuse by certified registered nurses anesthetists. *American Association of Nurses Anesthetists Journal, 67*(67), 133–140.

Bellack, A. S., & Mueser, K. T. (1993). Psychosocial treatment for schizophrenia. *Schizophrenia Bulletin, 19,* 317–336.

Belsky, J. (1980). Child maltreatment: An ecological integration. *American Psychologist, 33,* 320–335.

Benarroch, E. E. (1993). The central autonomic network: Functional organization, dysfunction and perspective. *Mayo Clinic Proceedings, 68,* 908–1001.

Benazzi, F. (1999). Psychotic late-life depression: A 376-case study. *International Psychogeriatrics, 11*(3), 325–332.

Benight, C. C., Ironson, G., Klebe, K., & Carver, C. S. (1999). Conservation of resources and coping self-efficacy predicting distress following a natural disaster. *Anxiety, Stress, and Coping, 12,* 106–126.

Benner, P. (1985). Quality of life: A phenomenological perspective on explanation, prediction, and understanding in nursing science. *Advances in Nursing Science, 8*(1), 1–14.

Bennett, J. A. (1995). "Methodological notes on empathy": Further considerations. *Advances in Nursing Science, 18,* 35–50.

Benoliel, J. Q. (1983). Nursing research on death dying and terminal illness: Development, present state, and prospects. In H. Werley & J. Fitzpatrick (Eds.), *Annual Review of Nursing Research* (Vol. 1, pp. 105–123). New York: Springer Publishing.

Bensley, L., Nelson, N., Kaufman, J., Silverstein, B., Kalat, J., & Walker, J. (1997). Injuries due to assaults on psychiatric hospital employees in Washington state. *American Journal of Industrial Medicine, 31,* 92–99.

Bentelspacher, C., Chitran, S., & Rahman, M. (1994). Coping and adaptation patterns among Chinese, Indian and Malay families caring for a mentally ill relative. *Families in Society, 75,* 287–294.

Bernstein, H. A. (1981). Survey of threats and assaults directed toward psychotherapists. *American Journal of Psychotherapy, 35*(4), 542–549.

Berren, M. R., Hill, K. R., Merikle, E., & Gonzalez, N. (1994). Serious mental illness and mortality rates. *Hospital & Community Psychiatry, 45*(6), 604–605.

Bickman, L., & Salzer, M. S. (1997). Measuring quality in mental health services. *Evaluation Review, 21*(3), 285–291.

Biederman, J. (1991). New developments in pediatric psychopharmacology. *Journal of the American Academy of Child and Adolescent Psychiatry, 31*(1), 14–49.

Biglan, A., Hops, H., Sherman, L., Freidman, L. S., Arthur, J., & Osteen, V. (1985). Problem-solving interactions of depressed women and their spouses. *Behavior Therapy, 16,* 431–451.

Billings, A. G., & Moos, R. H. (1985). Psychosocial processes in unipolar depression: Comparing patients with matched community controls. *Journal of Consulting & Clinical Psychology, 53,* 314–325.

Billings, C. (April, 1986). *Alcohol consumption practices of North Carolina nurses.* Paper presented at the First National Conference for Research and Study on Substance Abuse in Nursing. Atlanta, GA.

Binder, R. L., & McCoy, S. M. (1983). A study of patient attitudes toward placement in seclusion. *Hospitals and Community Psychiatry, 34*(11), 1052–1054.

Binger, C., Albin, A., Feurstein, R., Kushner, J., Zoger, S., & Mikkelson, C. (1969). Childhood leukemia. Emotional impact on patient and family. *New England Journal of Medicine, 280,* 414–418.

Birk, S. (1992). Emerging specialties: expanded opportunities. *American Nurse, 24,* 7–9.

Birmaher, B., Ryan, N. D., & Williamson, D. E. (1996). Depression in children and adolescents: Clinical features and pathogenesis. In K. I. Shulman, M. Tohen, & S. P. Kutcher (Eds.), *Mood disorders across the life span* (pp. 51–81). New York: Wiley-Liss.

Bissell, L., & Haberman, P. C. (1984). *Alcoholism in the professions.* New York: Oxford University Press.

Bjorkqvist, K., Osterman, K., & Hjelt-Back, M. (1994). Aggression among university employees. *Aggressive Behavior, 20,* 173–184.

Blanch, A. K., & Parrish, J. (1992). *Report on roundtable on alternatives to involuntary treatment.* Rockville, MD: National Institute of Mental Health.

Blatner, A., & Blatner, A. (1997). *The art of play: Helping adults reclaim imagination and spontaneity.* Philadelphia: Brunner Mazel-Taylor & Francis.

Blaum, C. S., Liang, J., & Liu, X. (1994). The relationship of chronic disease and health status to the health services utilization of older Americans. *Journal of the American Geriatric Society, 42*(10), 1087–1093.

Blazer, L. K., & Mansfield, P. K. (1995). A comparison of substance use rates among female nurses, clerical workers and blue collar workers. *Journal of Advanced Nursing, 21,* 305–313.

Blixen, C., McDougall, G. J., & Suen, L. J (1997). Dual diagnosis in elders discharged from a psychiatric hospital. *International Journal of Geriatric Psychiatry, 12,* 307–313.

Bloom, B. L. (1984). *Community mental health: A general introduction* (2nd ed.). Belmont, CA: Brooks/Cole.

Blount, A. (Ed.). (1998). *Integrated primary care: The future of medical and mental health collaboration.* New York: W. W. Norton & Company.

Bongar, B. (1991). *The suicidal patient: Clinical and legal standards of care.* Washington, DC: American Psychological Association.

Bonin, J. P. (1999). Psychosocial determinants of lithium compliance in patients with bipolar disorder. *Canadian Journal of Nursing Research, 31*(2), 25–40.

Bottorff, J. L. (1993). The use and meaning of touch in caring for patients with cancer. *Oncology Nursing Forum, 20,* 1531–1538.

Bottorff, J. L., & Morse, J. M. (1994). Identifying types of attending: Patterns of nurses' work. *Image: Journal of Nursing Scholarship, 26,* 53–60.

Boutain, D. M., & Olivares, S. A. (1999). Nurturing educational multiculturalism in psychosocial nursing: Creating new possibilities through inclusive conversations. *Archives of Psychiatric Nursing, XIII*(5), 234–239.

Bowlby, J. (1969). *Attachment and loss.* New York: Basic Books.

Braden, C. J., McGlone, K., & Pennington, F. (1993). Specific psychosocial and behavioral outcomes from the systemic lupus erythematosus self-help course. *Health Education Quarterly, 20,* 29–41.

Braden, C. J., Mishel, M. H., & Longman, A. J. (1998). Self-help intervention project: Women receiving breast cancer treatment. *Cancer Practice: A Multidisciplinary Journal of Cancer Care, 6*(2), 87–98.

Brannstrom, B., Gustafsson, Y., Norberg, A., & Winblad, B. (1989). Problems of basic nursing care in acutely confused and non-confused hip-fracture patients. *Scandinavian Journal of Caring Sciences, 3*(1), 27–34.

Brennan, P. F., Moore, S. M., & Smyth, K. A. (1995). The effects of a special computer network on caregivers of persons with Alzheimer's disease. *Nursing Research, 44,* 166–172.

Brewster, J. M. (1994). *Drug use among Canadian professionals.* Ottowa, Canada: Minister of National Health and Welfare.

Brotman, M. A., Fergus, E. L., Post, R. M., & Leverich, G. S. (2000). High exposure to neuroleptics in bipolar patients: A retrospective review. *Journal of Clinical Psychiatry, 61*(10), 68–72; quiz 73.

Brown, N. (1999). Spirituality in nursing. *Chicago Theological Seminary Register, 89*(3), 1–24.

Brown, S., Birtwistle, J., Roe, L., & Thompson, C. The unhealthy lifestyle of people with schizophrenia. *Psychological Medicine, 29*(3), 697–701.

Brunette, M. F., & Drake, R. E. (1997). Gender differences in patients with schizophrenia and substance abuse. *Comprehensive Psychiatry, 38*(2), 109–116.

Bryson, K., & Casper, L. (1998). Coresident grandparents and grandchildren, *Current Population Reports,* P23-198. Washington, DC: U.S. Bureau of the Census.

Buccheri, R., Trygstad, L., Kanas, N., & Dowling, G. (1997). Symptom management of auditory hallucinations in schizophrenia: Results of 1-year follow up. *Journal of Psychosocial Nursing and Mental Health Services, 35*(12), 20–28.

Buccheri, R., Trygstad, L., Kanas, N., Waldron, B., & Dowling, G. (1996). Auditory hallucinations in schizophrenia: Group experience in examining symptom management and behavioral strategies. *Journal of Psychosocial Nursing and Mental Health Services, 34*(2), 12–26.

Bucht, G., Gustafson, Y, & Sandberg, O. (1999). Epidemiology of delirium. *Dementia and Geriatric Cognitive Disorders, 10,* 315–318.

Buckwalter, K. C., Hartsock, J., & Gaffney, J. (1985). Music therapy. In G. M. Bulecheck & J. C. McCloskey (Eds.), *Nursing interventions: Treatments for nursing diagnoses* (pp. 58–74). Philadelphia: W. B. Saunders.

Buckwalter, K. C., Kerfoot, K. M., & Stolley, J. M. (1988). Children of affectively ill parents. *Journal of Psychosocial Nursing and Mental Health Services, 26,* 8–14.

Budin, W. C. (1998). Psychosocial adjustment to breast cancer in unmarried women. *Research in Nursing and Health, 21*(2), 155–166.

Budman, S., & Gurman, A. (1988). *Theory and practice of brief therapy.* New York: Guilford Press.

Bunch, E. H. (1999). Quality of life in people with advanced HIV/AIDS in Norway. *Western Journal of Nursing Research, 20,* 465–477.

Burge, V., Felts, M., Chenier, T., & Parrillo, A. V. (1995). Drug use, sexual activity, and suicidal behavior in U.S. high school students. *Journal of School Health, 65,* 222–227.

Burke, J., Chandy, J., Donnerbeck, A., & Watt, J. W. (1998). The parental environment cluster model of child neglect: An integrative conceptual model. *Child Welfare, 77*(4), 389–405.

Burker, E. J., Blumenthal, J. A., Feldman, M., Burnett, R., White, W., Smith, R., Croughwell, N., Schell, R., Newman, M., & Reves, J. G. (1995). Depression in male and female patients undergoing cardiac surgery. *British Journal of Clinical Psychology, 34,* 119–128.

Burnette, D. (1997). Grandmother caregivers in inner-city Latino families: A descriptive profile and informal social supports. *Journal of Multicultural Social Work, 5*(3–4), 121–137.

Burt, D. B., Zembar, M. J., & Niederehe, G. (1995). Depression and memory impairment: A meta-analysis of the association, its pattern, and specificity. *Psychological Bulletin, 117*(2), 285–305.

Byrt, R., & Reece, J. (1997). Self-harm in a medium secure unit: The contribution of social and physical environment. [online]. (Available at *http://wwnurse.colcgi-locaUforensic.pl.*).

Cain, A., Fast, I., & Erickson, M. (1964). Children's disturbed reactions to the death of a sibling. *American Journal of Orthopsychiatry, 34,* 741–752.

Cairns, N., Clark, G., Smith, S., & Lansky, S. (1979). Adaptation of siblings to childhood malignancy. *Journal of Pediatrics, 95,* 484–487.

Callahan, L., Steadman, H. J., McGreavy, M. A., & Robbins, P. C. (1991). The volume and characteristics of insanity defense pleas: An eight-state study. *Bulletin of the American Academy of Psychiatry and Law, 19,* 331–338.

Calsyn, R., Allen, G., Morse, G., Smith, R., & Tempelhoff, B. (1993). Can you trust self-report data provided by mentally ill individual? *Evaluation Review, 17,* 353–366.

Calsyn, R., Morse, G., Klingenberg, G., & Trusty, M. (1997). Reliability and validity of self-report of data of homeless mentally ill individuals. *Evaluation and Program Planning, 20,* 47–54.

Campbell, J. C., Anderson, E., Fulmer, T. L., Girourd, S., McElmurry, B., & Raff, B. (1993). Violence as a nursing priority: Policy implications. *Nursing Outlook, 41,* 89–92.

Campbell, J. C., Harris, M. J., & Lee, R. K. (1995). Violence research: An overview. *Scholarly Inquiry for Nursing Practice: An International Journal, 9,* 104–125.

Campbell, J., & Humphreys, J. (1993). *Nursing care of survivors of family violence.* St. Louis: C. V. Mosby.

Campbell, J., & Parker, B. (in press). Clinical nursing research on battered women and their children: A review. In A. S. Hinshaw, S. Feetham, & J. Shaver (Eds.), *Handbook of clinical nursing research.* Newbury Park, CA: Sage.

Campinha-Bacoate, J. (1994a). Cultural competence in psychiatric mental health nursing: A conceptual model. *Nursing Clinics of North America, 29*(1), 1–8.

Campinha-Bacoate, J. (1994b). Transcultural psychiatric nursing: Diagnostic and treatment issues. *Journal of Psychosocial Nursing, 32*(8), 42–46.

Caplan, G. (1970). *The theory and practice of mental health consultation.* New York: Basic Books.

Caplan, G., & Caplan, R. (2000). Principles of community psychiatry. *Community Mental Health Journal, 36*(1), 7–24.

Carey, M. P., Carey, K. B., Carnike, C. L., & Meisler, A. W. (1988, November). *Learned resourcefulness, drinking, and smoking.* Paper presented at the annual meeting of the Association for the Advancement of Behavior Therapy, New York, NY.

Carey, M. P., Carey, K., Weinhardt, L., & Gordon, C. (1997). Behavioral risk for HIV infection among adults with a severe and persistent mental illness: Patterns and psychological antecedents. *Community Mental Health Journal, 33*(2), 133–142

Carlson, M. C., Fried, L. P., Xue, Q. L., Bandeen-Roche, K., Zeger, S. L., & Brandt, J. (1999). Association between executive attention and physical function performance in community-dwelling older women. *Journal of Gerontology: Social Sciences, 54B*(5), S262–S270.

Carlson-Sabelli, L. (1998). Children's puppet theatre for traumatized children: A process theory approach. *International Journal of Action Methods: Psychodrama, Skill Training, and Role Playing, 51*(3), 91–112.

Carlson-Sabelli, L., & Sabelli, H. C. (1992). Interpersonal profiles: Analysis of interpersonal relations with the phase space of opposites. *Proceedings of thirty-sixth International Society for Systems Sciences,* 668–677.

Carlson-Sabelli, L., Sabelli, H. C. & Hale, A. (1994). Sociometry and sociodynamics. In P. Holmes, M. Karp, & M. Watson (Eds.), *Psychodrama since Moreno: Innovations in theory and practice* (pp. 145–185). London: Tavistock/Routledge.

Carlson-Sabelli, L., Sabelli, H. C., Patel, M., & Holm, K. (1992). The union of opposites in sociometry: An empirical application of process theory. *Journal of Group Psychotherapy, Psychodrama and Sociometry, 44*(4), 147–171.

Carmel, H., & Hunter, M. (1989). Staff injuries from inpatient violence. *Hospital and Community Psychiatry, 40*(1), 41–46.

Carmel, H., & Hunter, M. (1990). Compliance with training in managing assaultive behavior and injuries from inpatient violence. *Hospital and Community Psychiatry, 41*(5), 558–560.

Carney, R. M., Rich, M. W., Freedland, K. E., Saini, J., teVelde, A., Simeone, C., & Clark, K. (1988). Major depressive disorder predicts cardiac events in patient with coronary artery disease. *Psychosomatic Medicine, 50,* 627–633.

Carter, D. M., Mackinnon, A., & Copolov, D. L. (1996). Patients' strategies for coping with auditory hallucinations. *Journal of Nervous and Mental Disease, 184,* 159–164.

Cassidy, F., Murry, E., Forest, K., & Carroll, B. J. (1998). Signs and symptoms of mania in pure and mixed episodes. *Journal of Affective Disorders, 50*(2–3), 187–201.

Center for Mental Health Services. (1998). *Cultural competence standards in managed care mental health services for four underserved/underrepresented racial/ethnic groups.* Rockville, MD: Center for Mental Health Services.

Centers for Disease Control. (1993). Smoking-attributable mortality and years of potential life lost—United States, 1990. *Morbidity and Mortality Weekly Reports, 42,* 645–649.

Centers for Disease Control. (1994). Cigarette smoking among adults: United States, 1993. *Morbidity and Mortality Weekly Reports, 43,* 925–930.

Centers for Disease Control. (1994). Medical-care expenditures attributable to cigarette smoking, United States, 1993. *Morbidity and Mortality Weekly Reports, 43,* 469–472.

Centers for Disease Control. (1998). Suicide among black youths, United States, 1980–1995. *MMWR Morbidity Mortality Weekly Report, 47*(10), 193–196.

Centers for Disease Control. (1999). *HIV/AIDS Surveillance Report: U. S. HIV and AIDS cases reported through June 1999, 11*(1), 3–4.

Centers for Disease Control and Prevention. (2000). Tobacco use among middle and high school students—United States 1999. *Morbidity and Mortality Weekly, 49,* 49–53.

Chamberlain, J. (1985) An ex-patient's response to Soliday. *The Journal of Nervous and Mental Disease, 173,* 289–290.

Chambless, D. K., Baker, M. J., Baucom, D. H., & Beutler, L. E. (1998). Update on empirically validated therapies II. *The Clinical Psychologist, 51,* 3–16.

Chambless, D. L., Sanderson, W. C, Shohoman, V., Bennett, J. S., Pope, K. S., & Crits-Cristoph, P. (1996). An update on empirically validated therapies. *Clinical Psychologist, 49,* 5–18.

Chapman, H. A., Hobfoll, S. A., & Ritter, C. (1997). Partners' stress underestimations lead to women's distress: A study of pregnant inner-city women. *Journal of Personality and Social Psychology, 73*(2), 418–425.

Chavetz, L. (1996). The experience of severe mental illness: A life history approach. *Archives of Psychiatric Nursing, 10,* 24–31.

Chen, Y. (1990, June). Psychological and social support systems in intensive and critical care. *Intensive Care Nursing, 6*(2), 59–66.

Cheung, F. K., & Snowden, L. R. (1990). Community mental health and ethnic minority populations. *Community Mental Health Journal, 26,* 227–291.

Chlan, L. L. (1998). Music therapy. In M. Snyder & R. Lindquist (Eds.), *Alternative/complementary therapies in nursing.* New York: Springer Publishing.

Chu, J. A. (1991). *The repetition compulsion revisited: Reliving dissociated trauma.* Grad Rounds Presentation for professional education of caregivers involved with victims of abuse. Austin, Texas.

Clark, K. (1997). Disordered eating behaviors and bone-mineral density in women who misuse alcohol. *Western Journal of Nursing Research, 19*(1), 32–55.

Clark, P. N., Williams, C. A., Percy, M. A., & Kim, Y. S. (1995). Health and life problems of homeless men and women in the Southeast. *Journal of Community Health Nursing, 12,* 101–110.

Clay, M. (1984). Development of emphatic interaction skills schedule in a nursing context. *Journal of Advanced Nursing,* 9, 343–350.

Clement, J. A. (1997). Managed care and recovery: Opportunities and challenges for psychiatric nursing. *Archives of Psychiatric Nursing, XI*(5), 231–227.

Clement, M. (1996). The characteristics of women who stay married to bipolar men. *Journal of Psychosocial Nursing & Mental Health Services, 34*(3), 22–26.

Cocozza, J. (1991). *Responding to the mental health needs of youth in the juvenile justice system.* Seattle, WA: National Coalition for the Mentally Ill in the Juvenile Justice System.

Coe, C. S. G., Wiener, L. T., Rosenberg, S., & Levine, S. (1985). *The psychobiology of attachment and separation.* Orlando, FL: Academic Press.

Cohen, D. S. (1985). Pediatric cancer: Predicting sibling adjustment. *Dissertation Abstracts International, 46,* 637, (University Microfilms No. ADG 85-08044, 8505).

Cohen, J. (1986). Statistical approaches to suicidal risk factor analysis. In J. J. Mann & M. Stanley (Eds.), *Annals of the New York Academy of Science: Vol. 487. Psychobiology of suicidal behavior* (pp. 34–41). New York: New York Academy of Sciences.

Cohen, L. (1994). Psychiatric hospitalization as an experience of trauma. *Archives of Psychiatric Nursing, 8*(2), 78–81.

Cohen, M., Farkas, M., & Cohen, B. (1992). *Training technology: Assessing readiness for rehabilitation.* Boston: Center for Psychiatric Rehabilitation.

Cohen, M., & Mynks, D. (1993). *Compendium of activities for assessing and developing readiness for rehabilitation services.* Boston: Center for Psychiatric Rehabilitation.

Coie, J. D., Watt, N. F., West, S. G., Hawkins, J. D., Asarnow, J. R., Markman, H. J., Ramey S. L., Shure, M. B., & Long B. (1993). The science of prevention: A conceptual framework and some directions for a national research program. *American Psychologist, 48,* 1013–1022.

Cole, M. (1999). Delirium: Effectiveness of systematic interventions. *Dementia and Geriatric Cognitive Disorders, 10,* 406–411.

Collins, R. L., Gollnisch, G., & Morsheimer, E. T. (1999). Substance use among a regional sample of female nurses. *Drug and Alcohol Dependence, 55,* 145–155.

Committee of Cultural Psychiatry. (1989). Suicide and ethnicity in the U.S. *Group for Abnormal Psychiatry, 128,* 1–131.

Comtois, K. A., & Ries, R. K. (1995). Sex differences in dually diagnosed severely mentally ill clients in dual diagnosis outpatient treatment. *American Journal on Addictions, 4*(3), 245–253.

Conrad, N. (1992). Stress and knowledge of suicidal others as factors in suicidal behavior of high school adolescents. *Issues in Mental Health Nursing, 13,* 95–104.

Constantino, R. E., & Bricker, P. L. (1996). Nursing post intervention for spousal survivors of suicide. *Issues in Mental Health Nursing, 17,* 151–152.

Cook, J. D. (1981).The therapeutic use of music: A literature review. *Nursing Forum, 20,* 252–266.

Corless, I. B. (1994). Dying well: Symptom control within hospice care. In J. Fitzpatrick & J. Stevenson (Eds.), *Annual Review of Nursing Research* (Vol. 12, pp. 125–146). New York: Springer Publishing.

Cornman, B. J. (1997). Female adolescent response to childhood sexual abuse. *Journal of Child and Adolescent Psychiatric Nursing, 10*(2), 17–25.

Corte, C., & Stein, K. F. (2000). *Self-Concept Impairments in the Onset of the Eating Disorders.* Paper presented at the 24th Annual Midwest Nursing Research Society Conference, Dearborn, MI.

Coté, J. J., Morse, J. M., & James, S. G. (1991). The pain response of the postoperative newborn. *Journal of Advanced Nursing, 16,* 378–387.

Council on Ethical and Judicial Affairs, American Medical Association. *JAMA, 272*(23), 1861–1865.

Cournos, F., & McKinnon, K. (1997). HIV seroprevalence among people with severe mental illness in the United States: A critical review. *Clinical Psychology Review, 17*(3), 259–269.

Cowen, P. S. (1999). Child neglect: Injuries of omission. *Pediatric Nursing, 25*(4), 401–405.

Coyne, J. C., Kessler, R. C., Tal, M., Turnbull, J., Wortman, C. B., & Greden, J. (1987). Living with a depressed person. *Journal of Clinical & Consulting Psychology, 55,* 347–352.

Craft, M. J., & Willadsen, J. A. (1992). Interventions related to family. *Nursing Clinics of North America, 27,* 517–540.

Craig, W. M., & Pepler, D. J. (1998). Conduct and oppositional defiant disorders. In C. A. Essau & F. Petermann (Eds.), *Developmental psychopathology: Epidemiology, diagnostics and treatment* (pp. 97–139). Amsterdam: Harwood Academic Publishers.

Craine, L. S., Henson, C., Colliver, J., & MacLean, D. (1988). Prevalence of a history of sexual abuse among female psychiatric patients in a state hospital system. *Hospital & Community Psychiatry, 39*(3), 300–304.

Creighton, S. J., & Noyes, P. (1989). *Child abuse trends in England and Wales 1983–1987.* London: NSPCC.

Crenshaw, W., Cain, K., & Francis, P. (1997). An updated national survey on seclusion and restraint. *Psychiatric Services, 48*(3), 395–397.

Crittenden, P. M. (1992). The social ecology of treatment: Case study of a service system for maltreated children. *American Journal of Orthopsychiatry, 62*(1), 22–34.

Cunningham, W., Shapiro, M., Hays, R., Dixon, W., Visscher, B., George, W., Ettl, M., & Beck, C. K. (1998). Constitutional symptoms and health-related quality of life in patients with symptomatic HIV disease. *American Journal of Medicine, 104,* 129–136.

Czajkowski, S. M., Terrin, M., Lindquist, R., Hoogwerf, B., Dupuis, G., Shumaker, S. A., Gray, J. R., Herd, J. A., Treat-Jacobson, D., Zyzanski, S., & Knatterud, G. L. (1997). Comparison of preoperative characteristics of men and women undergoing coronary artery bypass grafting (The Post Coronary Artery Bypass Graft (CABG) Biobehavioral Study). *The American Journal of Cardiology, 79,* 1017–1024.

Dana, R. H. (1998). *Understanding cultural identity in intervention and assessment.* Thousand Oaks, CA: Sage.

Darves-Bornoz, J.-M., Lemperiere, T., Degiovanni, A., & Gaillard, P. (1995). Sexual victimization in women with schizophrenia and bipolar disorder. *Social Psychiatry & Psychiatric Epidemiology, 30*(2), 78–84

Davidson, M. W., Wagner, W. G., & Range, L. M. (1995). Clinicians' attitudes toward no-suicide agreements. *Suicide and Life-Threatening Behavior, 25,* 410–414.

de Leon Siantz, M. L. (1994). The Mexican-American migrant farmworker family: Mental health issues. *Nursing Clinics of North America, 29*(1), 65–72.

Deegan, P. (1988). Recovery: The lived experience of rehabilitation. *Psychosocial Rehabilitation Journal, 11*(4), 11–19.

Dembling, B. P., Chen, D., & Vachon, L. (1999). Life expectancy and causes of death in a population treated for serious mental illness. *Psychiatric Services, 50*(8), 1036–1042.

Demi, A., Bakeman, R., Sowell, R., Moneyham, L., & Seals, B. (1996, October). Suicidality among HIV-infected women. Paper presented at Ninth Annual Association of Nurses in AIDS Care, Chicago, IL.

Demi, A. S., & Miles, M. S. (1986). Bereavement. In H. H. Werley, J. J. Fitzpatrick, & R. L. Taunton (Eds.), *Annual Review of Nursing Research* (Vol. 4, pp. 105–123). New York: Springer.

Depression Guideline Panel. (1993). *Depression in primary care: Volume 2. Treatment of major depression. Clinical practice guideline, Number 5.* Rockville, MD. U. S. Department of Health and Human Services, Public Health Service, Agency for Health Care Policy and Research. AHCPR Publication No. 93-0551.

DeSisto, M. J., Harding, C. M., McCormick, R. V., Ashikaga, T., & Brooks, G. W. (1987). The Maine-Vermont three decade studies of serious mental illness: Longitudinal course comparisons. *British Journal of Psychiatry, 167,* 338–342.

Desjarlais, R. R. (1992). *Body and emotion.* Philadelphia: University of Pennsylvania Press.

Devine, E. C., & Cook, T. D. (1986). Clinical and cost-saving effects of psychoeducational interventions with surgical patients: A meta-analysis. *Research in Nursing and Health, 9,* 89–105.

Devine, E. C., & Reifschneider, E. (1995). A meta-analysis of the efects of psychoeducational care in adults with hypertension. *Nursing Research, 44,* 237–245.

Devine, E. C., & Westlake, S. K. (1995). The effects of psychoeducational care provided to adults with cancer: Meta-analysis of 116 studies. *Oncology Nursing Forum, 22,* 1369–1381.

Diekelmann, N. (1994–1999). Nursing Institutes for Heideggerian Hermeneutic Studies, University of Wisconsin-Madison School of Nursing.

Diers, D., & Schmidt, R. L. (1977). Interaction analysis in nursing research. In P. J. Verhonick (Ed.), *Nursing research II* (pp. 77–132). Boston: Little, Brown.

Diers, D., Schmidt, R. L., McBride, M. A., & Davis, B. L. (1972). The effect of nursing interaction on patients in pain. *Nursing Research, 21,* 419–428.

DiLima, S. N., & Painter, S. B. (Eds.) (1998). *Holistic health promotion and complementary therapies: A resource for integrated practice*. Gaithersburg, MD: Aspen.

Dionne-Proulz, J., & Pepin, R. (1993). Stress management in the nursing profession. *Journal of Nursing Management, 1*, 75–81.

Dixon, L., Dibietz, E., Myers, P., Conley, R., Medoff, D., & Lehman, A. F. (1993). Comparison of DSM-III-R diagnoses and a brief interview for substance use among state hospital patients. *Hospital and Community Psychiatry, 44*(8), 748–752.

Dixon, L., Postrado, L., Delahanty, J., Fischer, P. J., & Lehman, A. (1999). The association of medical comorbidity in schizophrenia with poor physical and mental health. *Journal of Nervous & Mental Disease, 187*(18), 496–502.

Docherty, J. P., Van Kammen, D. P., Siris, S. G., & Marder, S. R. (1978). Stages of onset of schizophrenic psychosis. *American Journal of Psychiatry, 135*, 420–426.

Doerfler, L. A., Pbert, L., & DeCosimo, D. (1997). Self-reported depression in patients with coronary heart disease. *Journal of Cardiopulmonary Rehabilitation, 17*(3), 163–170.

Doll, R., Peto, R., & Wheatley, K. (1994). *Mortality from smoking in developed countries: 1950–2000*. Oxford, UK: Oxford University Press.

Dorn, L. D., Susman, E. J., & Peterson, A. C. (1993). Cortisol reactivity and anxiety and depression in pregnant adolescents: A longitudinal perspective. *Psychoneuroendocrinology,18*(2), 19–239.

Downs, W. R., & Harrison, L. (1998). Childhood maltreatment and the risk of substance problems in later life. *Health and Social Care in the Community, 6*(1), 35–46.

Drake, R. E., Bartels, S. J., Teague, G. B., Noordsy, D. L., & Clark, R. E. (1993). Treatment of substance abuse in severely mentally ill patients. *Journal of Nervous and Mental Disease, 181*(10), 606–611.

Drake, R. E., McHugo, G. J., Clark, R. E., Teague, G. B., Xie, H., Miles, K., & Ackerson, T. H. (1998). Assertive community treatment for patients with co-occurring severe mental illness and substance use disorder: A clinical trial. *American Journal of Orthopsychiatry, 68*(2), 201–215.

Drake, R. E., McHugo, G. J., & Noordsy, D. L. (1993). Treatment of alcoholism among schizophrenic outpatients: Four-year outcomes. *American Journal of Psychiatry, 150*(2), 328–329.

Drake, R. E., Osher, F. C., Noordsy, D. L., Hurlbut, S. C., Teague, G. B., & Beaudett, M. S. (1990). Diagnosis of alcohol use disorders in schizophrenia. *Schizophrenia Bulletin, 16*(1), 57–67.

Dretske, F. (1988). *Explaining behavior: Reasons in a world of causes*. Cambridge, MA: MIT Press.

Drew, B. L. (1999a). No-suicide contracts to prevent suicidal behavior in inpatient psychiatric settings. *Journal of the American Psychiatric Nurses Association, 5*, 23–28.

Drew, B. L. (1999b). *Suicidal behavior and no-suicide contracting in inpatient psychiatric settings*. Unpublished doctoral dissertation, Case Western Reserve University, Cleveland.

Drew, N. (1990). Psychodrama in nursing education. *Journal of Group Psychotherapy, Psychodrama and Sociometry, 42*(3), 54–61

Drew, N. (1991). Combating the social isolation of chronic mental illness. *Journal of Psychosocial Nursing, 29*(6), 14–17.

Drew, N. (1993). Reenactment Interviewing: A methodology for phenomenological research. *Image, 25*(4), 345–351.

Drew, N. (1997). Expanding self-awareness through exploration of meaningful experience. *Journal of Holistic Nursing, 14*(4), 406–424.

Drummond, D. J., Sparr, L. F., & Gordon, G. H. (1989). Hospital violence reduction among high-risk patients. *Journal of the American Medical Association, 261*(17), 2531–2534.

Drye, R. C., Goulding, R. L., & Goulding, M. E. (1973). No-suicide decisions: Patient monitoring of suicidal risk. *American Journal of Psychiatry, 130,* 171–174.

Dubowitz, H., & DePanfilis, D. (2000). *Handbook for child protection practice.* London: Sage.

Dugbartey, A. T., Rosenbaum, G., Sanchez, P. N., & Townes, B. D. (1999). Neuropsychological assessment of executive function. *Seminars in Neuropsychiatry, 4*(1), 5–12.

Duits, A. A., Boeke, S., Taams, M. A., Passchier, J., & Erdman, R. A. M. (1997). Prediction of quality of life after coronary artery bypass graft surgery: A review and evaluation of multiple, recent studies. *Psychosomatic Medicine, 59,* 257–268.

Duits, A. A., Duivenvoorden, H. J., Boeke, S., Taams, M. A., Mochtar, B., Krauss, X. H., Passchier, J., & Erdman, R. A. M. (1998). The course of anxiety and depression in patients undergoing coronary artery bypass graft surgery. *Journal of Psychosomatic Research, 45,* 127–138.

Dulcan, M. K., & Bernet, W. (Eds.). (1998). Clinical practice parameters. *Journal of the American Academy of Child and Adolescent Psychiatry, 37*(Suppl.).

Duran, D. (1995). Impact of depression, psychological factors, cultural determinants, and patient/care provider relationship on somatic complaints of the distressed latina. Unpublished doctoral dissertation, University of Denver.

Duran, E., Duran, B., & Tingley, P. (1995). *Native American postcolonial psychology.* Albany, NY: State University of New York Press.

Dyckoff, D., Goldstein, L., & Schacht-Levine, L. (1996). Continuing education. The investigation of behavioral contracting in patients with borderline personality disorder. *Journal of the American Psychiatric Nurses Association, 2*(3), 71–78.

Edwards, C. H., Knight, E. M., Johnson, A. A., Oyemade, U. J., Cole, O. J., Laryea, H., Westney, O. E., & Westney, L. S. (1994). Multiple factors as mediators of the reduced incidence of low birth weight in an urban clinic population. *Journal of Nutrition, 124,* 927S–935S.

Elliott, R., & Wright, L. (1999, June). Verbal communication: What do critical care nurses say to their unconscious or sedated patients? *Journal of Advanced Nursing, 29*(6), 1412–1420.

Emerson, E. (1992). Playing for health: The process of play and self-expression in children who have experienced a sexual trauma. Doctoral Dissertation, The University of Texas at Austin, Order Number 9225571. Ann Arbor, MI: UMI Dissertation Services.

Emerson, E., & Shelton, D. (in press). Using creative arts to build coping skills to reduce domestic violence in the lives of female juvenile offenders. *Issues in Mental Health Nursing.*

England, J. E., O'Neill, J. J., & Simpson, R. K. (1996, January–February). Pragmatic assessment of communication in dementia. *American Journal of Alzheimer's Disease, 11*(1), 7–10.

Engs, R. C. (1982). Drinking patterns and attitudes toward alcoholism of Australian human service students. *Journal of Studies on Alcohol, 43,* 517–531.

Erikson, E. H. (1963). Toys and reasons. In *Childhood and society* (2nd ed.) (pp. 209–235). New York: W. W. Norton.

Estabrooks, C. A. (1989). Touch: A nursing strategy in the intensive care. *Heart and Lung, 18,* 392–401.

Estok, P., & Rudy, E. (1996). The relationship between eating disorders and running in women. *Research in Nursing & Health, 19,* 377–387.

Fagerstom, K. O. (1994). Combined use of nicotine replacement products. *Health Values, 18,* 15–20.

Faison, K. J., Faria, S. H., & Frank, D. (1999). Caregivers of chronically ill elderly: perceived burden. *Journal of Community Health Nursing, 16*(4), 243–253.

Farrell, S. P., Koch, J. R., & Blank, M. (1999). Predicting whether patients receive continuity of care after discharge from state hospitals: Policy implications. *Archives of Psychiatric Nursing, XIII,* 6, 279–285.

Faulkner, G., & Sparkes, A. (1999). Exercise as therapy for schizophrenia: An ethnographic study. *Journal of Sport & Exercise Psychology, 121*(1), 52–69.

Federal Task Force on Homelessness and Severe Mental Illness. (1992). Outcasts on Main Street: Report of the Federal Task Force on Homelessness and Severe Mental Illness. Interagency Council on the Homeless: Washington, D.C., p. 36.

Feldstein, M. A., & Gemma, P. B. (1995). Oncology nurses and chronic compounded grief. *Cancer Nursing, 18,* 228–236.

Felker, R., Yazel, J. J., & Short, D. (1996). Mortality and medical morbidity among psychiatric patients: A review. *Psychiatric Services, 47,* 1356–1363.

Ferrans, C. E., & Powers, M. J. (1992). Psychometric assessment of the quality of life index. *Research in Nursing and Health, 15,* 29–38.

Fetter, B. J., & Lowery, B. J. (1992). Psychiatric rehospitalization of the severely mentally ill: Patient and staff perspectives. *Nursing Research, 41,* 301–305.

Fincannon, J. (1995). Analysis of psychiatric referrals and interventions in an oncology population. *Oncology Nursing Forum, 22*(1), 87–92.

Fineberg, N. A., James D. V., & Shah, A. K. (1988). Agency nurses and violence in a psychiatric ward. *The Lancet, 1,* 474.

Finke, L., Williams, J., & Stanley, R. (1996). Nurses referred to a peer assistance program for drug and alcohol problems. *Archives of Psychiatric Nursing, 10*(5), 329–324.

Finkelhor, D., & Browne, A. (1985). The traumatic impact of child sexual abuse: A conceptualization. *American Journal of Orthopsychiatry, 55,* 530–541.

Finney, J. W., Riley, A. W., & Cataldo, M. F. (1991). Psychology in primary health care: Effects of brief targeted therapy on children's medical care utilization. *Journal of Pediatric Psychology, 16*(4), 447–461.

Fiore, M. C., Bailey, W. C., Cohen, S. J., et al. (1996). *Smoking cessation. Clinical Practice Guideline No. 18.* Rockville, MD: U. S. Department of Health and Human Services, AHCPR Publication No. 96-0692.

Fitch, M. I., Remus, S., & Stade, B. (1998, Fall). Communication needs of patients receiving mechanical ventilation: A pilot study. *The Official Journal of the Canadian Association of Critical Care Nurses, 9*(3), 16–23.

Fitzpatrick, J. J. (Ed.). (1998). *Encyclopedia of nursing research.* New York: Springer.

Flaskerud, J. H. (2000). Ethnicity, culture and neuropsychiatry. *Issues in Mental Health Nursing, 21,* 5–29.

Fleming, M. F., & Barry, K. L. (1992). *Addictive disorders.* St. Louis: Mosby.

Flenniken, M.C. (1997). Psychotropic prescriptive patterns among nurse practitioners in nonpsychiatric settings. *Journal of the American Academy of Nurse Practitioners, 9*(3), 117–121.

Folkman, S., & Lazarus, R. (1980). An analysis of coping in the middle-aged community sample. *Journal of Health and Social Behavior, 21,* 219–239.

Folstein, M. F., Folstein, S. E., & McHugh, P. R. (1975). Mini-Mental State: A practical method for grading the cognitive state of patients for the clinician. *Journal of Psychiatric Research, 12,* 196–198.

Fontaine, K. L. (1999). Suicide. In K. L Fontaine & J. S. Fletcher (Eds.), *Mental health nursing* (pp. 413–426). Menlo Park, CA: Addison-Wesley.

Forchuk, C. (1991). Peplau's theory: Concepts and their relations. *Nursing Science Quarterly, 4*(2), 54–60.

Forchuk, C., Beaton, S., Crawford, L., Ide, L., Vooberg, N., & Bethune, J. (1989). Incorporating Peplau's theory and case management. *Journal of Psychosocial Nursing, 27*(3), 35–38.

Forchuk, C., & Brown, B. (1989). Establishing a nurse-client relationship. *Journal of Psychosocial Nursing, 22*(2), 30–34.

Forchuk, C., & Dorsay, J. P. (1995). Hildegarde Peplau meets family systems nursing: Innovation in theory-based practice. *Journal of Advanced Nursing, 21,* 110–115.

Foreman, M., Milisen, K., Culp, K., & Neelon, V. (2000). Issues in delirium research—Toward a research agenda for nursing. Unpublished manuscript.

Foreman, M., Wakefield, B., Culp, K., & Milisen, K. (2000). Delirium in the elderly: An overview of the state of the science. *Journal of Gerontological Nursing.*

Foreman, S., & Marmar, R. (1985). Therapist actions that address initially poor therapeutic alliances in psychotherapy. *American Journal of Psychotherapy, 42,* 922–926.

Forer, L (1994) *A rage to punish: The unintended consequences of mandatory sentencing.* New York: Norton.

Fosterling, Friedrich. (1985). Attributional retraining: A review. *Psychological Bulletin, 98*(3), 495–512.

Fowler, B. A., & Padgett, J. J. (1994). Ideological shifts needed in primary care delivery: Removing barriers through reform. *American Black Nurses Foundation Journal, 5,* 126–129.

Fox, J. (1990, November). *Etiologic factors and information processing deficits associated with schizophrenia: A review of findings.* Paper presented at National Institute of Mental Health, Washington, DC.

Fox, J., Merwin, E., & Blank, M. (1995). De facto mental health services in the rural south. *Journal of Health Care for the Poor and Underserved, 6,* 434–468.

Francis, P., Merwin, E. & Fox, J. (1995). Relationship of clinical case management to hospitalization and service delivery for seriously mentally ill clients. *Issues in Mental Health Nursing, 16,* 57–274.

Franzen, M. D., & Haut, M. W. (1991). The psychological treatment of memory impairment: A review of empirical studies. *Neuropsychology Review, 2*(1), 29–63.

Frederick, J., & Cotanch, P. (1995). Self-help techniques for auditory hallucinations in schizophrenia. *Issues in Mental Health Nursing, 16,* 213–224.

Fredriksson, L. (1998, Spring). The caring conversation—talking about suffering. A hermeneutic phenomenological study in psychiatric nursing. *International Journal for Human Caring, 2*(1), 24–32.

Fremouw, W. J., Perczel, M., & Ellis, T. E. (1990). *Suicide risk: Assessment and response guidelines.* New York: Pergamon.

Freud, S. (1957). *Mourning and melancholia: Standard edition of the complete psychological works of Sigmund Freud* (Vol. 14). London: Hogarth Press.

Friedman, M., & King, K. (1994). The relationship of emotional and tangible support to psychological well-being among older women with heart failure. *Research Nursing Health, 17,* 433–440.

Frye, M. A., Ketter, T. A., Leverich, G. S., Huggins, T., Lantz, C., Denicoff, K. D., & Post, R. M. (2000). The increasing use of polypharmacotherapy for refractory mood disorders: 22 years of study. *Journal of Clinical Psychiatry, 61*(1), 9–15.

Fuller Torrey, J., Stieber, J., Ezekiel, S., Wolfe, J., Sharfstein, J., Noble, L., & Flynn (1992). *Criminalizing the seriously mentally ill: The abuse of jails as mental hospitals.* Washington, DC: Public Citizen's Research Group and the National Alliance for the Mentally Ill.

Fureman, B., Parikh, G., Bragg, A., & McLellan, A. (1990). *Addiction Severity Index.* Philadelphia, PA: The University of Pennsylvania/Veterans Administration Center for Studies of Addiction.

Gagan, J. J. (1983). Methodological notes on empathy. *Advances in Nursing Science, 5,* 65–72.

Gallagher-Thompson, D., Dal Canto, P. G., Darnley, S., Basilio, L. A., Whelan, L., & Jacobs, T. (1997, November). A feasibility study of videotaping to assess the relationship between distress in Alzheimer's disease caregivers and their interaction style. *Aging & Mental Health, 1*(4), 346–355.

Gallo, J. J., Marino, S., Ford, D., & Anthony, J. C. (1995). Filters on the pathway to mental health care, II. Scoiodemographic factors. *Psychological Medicine, 25,* 1149–1160.

Garbarino, J. (1977). The human ecology of child maltreatment: A conceptual model for research. *Journal of Marriage and the Family, 39,* 721–727.

Garcia, M., & Rodriguez, P. F. (1989). Psychological effects of political repression in Argentina and El Salvador. In D. Koslow & E. Salett (Eds.), *Crossing cultures in mental health* (pp. 64–83). Washington, DC: SIETAR International.

Garvin, B., & Kennedy, C. (1990). Interpersonal communication between nurses and patients. In J. J. Fitzpatrick, R. L. Taunton, & J. Q. Benoliel (Eds.), *Annual Review of Nursing Research* (pp. 213–234). New York: Springer.

Garza-Trevino, E. S., Ruiz, P., & Venegas-Samuels, K. (1997). A psychiatric curriculum directed to the care of the Hispanic patient. *Academic Psychiatry, 21*(1), 1–10.

Gaston, E. T. (1951). Dynamic music factors in mood change. *Music Educators Journal, 3,* 42–44.

Geffner, R. (1992). Politics, families and values. *Family Violence & Sexual Assault Bulletin, 8*(2), 1.

Gelazis, R. S., & Coombe-Moore, J. (1993). Developing a therapeutic relationship. In R. P. Rawlins, S. R. Williams, & C. K. Beck (Eds.), *Mental Health-Psychiatric Nursing* (pp. 109–133). St. Louis: Mosby Year Book, Inc.

Gelles, R. J., & Cornell, C. P. (1990). *Intimate violence in families* (2nd ed.). London: Sage.

Gibson, J. L., Love, W., Hardie, D., Bancroft, P., & Turner, A. J. (1892). Notes on lead poisoning as observed among children in Brisbane. In L. Huxtable (Ed.), *Transactions from the Third Intercolonial Medical Congress of Australasia* (pp. 76–77). Sydney, Australia: Charles Potter.

Giger, J. N., & Davidhizar, R. E. (1995). *Transcultural nursing: Assessment and intervention*. St. Louis: Mosby.

Gil, E. (1998). Understanding and responding to post-trauma play. *Association for Play Therapy, Inc. Newsletter, 17*(1), 7–10.

Gilbert, C. M. (1988). Children in women's shelters: A group intervention using art. *Journal of Child Psychiatric Nursing, 1*(1), 7–13.

Gillis, C. L. (1991). Family nursing research, theory and practice. *Image: Journal of Nursing Scholarship, 23*(1), 19–22.

Ginott, H. (1961). *Group psychotherapy with children*. New York: McGraw Hill.

Glassman, A. H., Helzer, J. E., Covey, L. S., Cottler, L. B., Stetner, F., Tipp, J. E., & Johnson, J. (1990). Smoking, smoking cessation and major depression. *Journal of the American Medical Association, 264,* 1546–1549.

Glassman, A. H., & Shapiro, P. A. (1998). Depression and the course of coronary artery disease. *American Journal of Psychiatry, 155,* 4–11.

Goldberg, E., & Bilder, R. M. (1986). Neuropsychological perspectives: Retrograde amnesia and executive deficits. In L. W. Poon (Ed.), *Clinical memory assessment of older adults* (pp. 55–68). Washington, DC: American Psychological Association.

Goldfried, M. R., & Wolfe, B. E. (1996). Psychotherapy practice and research: Repairing a strained alliance. *American Psychologist, 51*(10), 1007–1016.

Goldman, E., & Morrison, D. (1984). *Psychodrama: Experience and Process*. Dubuque, IA: Kendall Hunt.

Goleman, D., & Gurin, J. (1993). *Mind body medicine*. Yonkers, NY: Consumer Reports.

Goodman, L. A., & Fallot, R. D. (1998). HIV risk-behavior in poor urban women with serious mental disorders: Association with childhood physical and sexual abuse. *American Journal of Orthopsychiatry, 68*(1), 73–83.

Goodman, L. A., Rosenberg, S. D., Mueser, K. T., & Drake, R. E. (1997). Physical and sexual assault history in women with serious mental illness: Prevalence, correlates, treatment, and future research directions. *Schizophrenia Bulletin, 23*(4), 685–696.

Gortner, S. R., Gillis, C. L., Shinn, T. A., Sparacino, P. A., Rankin, S., Leavitt, M., Price, M., & Hudes, M. (1988). Improving recovery following cardiac surgery: A randomized clinical trial. *Journal of Advanced Nursing, 13,* 649–661.

Gortner, S. R., & Jenkins, L. S. (1990). Self-efficacy and activity level following cardiac surgery. *Journal of Advanced Nursing, 15,* 1132–1138.

Grabbe, L., Demi, A., Camann, M., & Potter, L. (1997). The health status of elderly persons in the last year of life: A comparison of deaths by suicide, injury, and natural causes. *American Journal of Public Health, 87,* 434–437.

Green, B. L. (1994). Psychosocial research in traumatic stress: An update. *Journal of Traumatic Stress, 7*(3), 341–362.

Green, M. F., & Kinsbourne, M. (1989). Subvocal activity and auditory hallucinations: Clues for behavioral treatments? *Schizophrenia Bulletin, 16,* 617–625.

Green, N. L. (1990). Stressful events related to childbearing in African-American women: A pilot study. *Journal of Nurse-Midwifery, 35*(4), 231–236.

Grob, G. N. (1992). Mental health policy in America: Myths and realities. *Health Affairs, 11*(3), 7–21.

Gross, D., Fogg, L., & Tucker, S. (1995). The efficacy of parent training for promoting positive parent-toddler relationships. *Research in Nursing and Health, 18,* 489–499.

Grossman, J. A., Clark, D. C., Gross, D., Halstead, L., & Pennington, J. (1995). Child bereavement after paternal suicide. *Journal of Child and Adolescent Psychiatric Nursing, 82*, 5–17.

Grossman, P. (1991). Respiratory mediation of cardiac function within a psychophysiological perspective. In J. G. Carlson & A. R. Seifert (Eds.), *International perspectives on self-regulation and health* (pp. 17–39). New York: Plenum Press.

Gunderson, J. (1978). Defining the therapeutic processes in psychiatric milieu. *Psychiatry, 41,* 327–335.

Guzzetta, C. E. (1988). Music therapy: Hearing the melody of the soul. In B. M. Dossey, L. Keegan, C. E. Guzzetta, & L. G. Kolkmeier (Eds.), *Holistic nursing: A handbook for practice* (pp. 263–288). Rockville, MD: Aspen.

Haack, M. R., & Harford, T. C. (1984). Drinking patterns among student nurses. *International Journal of Addictions, 19,* 577–583.

Hale, A. E. (1985). Conducting Clinical Sociometric Explorations. Roanoke, VA: Anne E. Hale.

Hall, R. G., Duhamel, M., McClanahan, R., Miles, G., Rosen, S., Schiller, P., Tao-Yonenaga, L., & Hall, S. M. (1997). Level of functioning, severity of illness, and smoking status among chronic psychiatric patients. *Journal of Nervous and Mental Diseases, 183,* 468–471.

Hamera, E. K., Peterson, K. A., Handley, S. M., Plumlee, A. A., & Frank-Ragan, E. (1991). Patient self-regulation and functioning in schizophrenia. *Hospital and Community Psychiatry, 42,* 631–634.

Hamera, E. K., Peterson, K. A., Young, L. M., & Schaumloffel, M. M. (1992). Symptom monitoring in schizophrenia: Potential for enhancing self-care. *Archives of Psychiatric Nursing, VI,* 324–330.

Haney, C (1993). "Infamous punishment: The psychological effects of isolation." *National Prison Project Journal,* Spring, 3–21.

Hardin, S. B., Weinrich, M., Weinrich, S., Hardin, T. L., & Garrison, C. (1994). Psychological distress of adolescents exposed to Hurricane Hugo. *Journal of Traumatic Stress, 7*(3), 427–440.

Harding, C. M. (1988). Course types in schizophrenia: An analysis of European and American studies. *Schizophrenia Bulletin, 14,* 633–643.

Harding, C. M., Brooks, G. W., Ashikaga, T., Strauss, J. S., & Breier, A. (1987). The ermont Longitudinal Study of persons with severe mental illness: 1. Methodology, study sample, and overall status 32 years later. *American Journal of Psychiatry, 144,* 718–726.

Harrison, E. J. (1997). Suicidal behavior. In W-S. Tseng & J. Streltzer (Eds.), *Culture and psychopathology* (pp. 157–172). New York: Brunner/Mazel.

Harrison, M. J., & Magill-Evans, J. (1996). Mother and father interactions over the first year with term and pretrem infants. *Research in Nursing and Health, 19*(6), 451–459.

Hart, E. J., & Westin, K. (1996). The effects of negotiated contracts and dietary self study on nutrition related practices. *Journal of Health Education, 27*(3), 178–181.

Hartman, N., Leong, G. B., Glynn, S. M., Wilkins, J. N., & Jarvik, M. E. (1991). Transdermal nicotine and smoking behavior in psychiatric patients. *American Journal of Psychiatry, 148,* 374–375.

Harvey, A. G., & Bryant, R. A. (1999). Predictors of acute stress following motor vehicle accidents. *Journal of Traumatic Stress, 12*(3), 519–526.

Hauenstein, E. (1992). Shifting the paradigm: Toward integrating research on mothers and children. *Journal of Child and Adolescent Psychiatric Nursing, 5*(4), 18–29.

Hauenstein, E. (1996a). A nursing practice paradigm for depressed rural women: Theoretical basis. *Archives of Psychiatric Nursing, 10,* 283–292.

Hauenstein, E. (1996b). Testing innovative nursing care: Home intervention with depressed rural women. *Issues in Mental Health Nursing, 17,* 33–50.

Hauenstein, E. (1997). A nursing practice paradigm for depressed rural women: The women's affective illness treatment program. *Archives of Psychiatric Nursing, 11,* 1–9.

Havermans, T., & Eiser, C. (1994). Siblings of a child with cancer. *Child: Care, Health & Development, 5,* 309–322.

Heffernan, S., & Zanelli, A. (1997). Behavior changes exhibited by siblings of pediatric oncology patients: A comparison between maternal and sibling descriptions. *Journal of Pediatric Oncology Nursing, 14,* 3–14.

Hegyvary, S. T. (1993). Issues in outcomes research. *Journal of Nursing Quality Assurance, 5,* 1–6.

Heijmeriks, J. A., Pourrier, S., Dassen, P., Prenger, K., & Wellens, H. J. (1999). Comparison of quality of life after coronary and/or valvular cardiac surgery in patients ≥ 75 years of age with younger patients. *American Journal of Cardiology, 83,* 1129–1132.

Helfer, R. E., & Kempe, R. S. (Eds.). (1987). *The battered child.* Chicago: University of Chicago.

Henry, J. P. (1992). Biological basis of the stress response. *Integrative Physiological and Behavioral Science, 27,* 66–83.

Herbert, T. B., & Cohen, S. (1993). Stress and immunity in humans: A meta-analytic review. *Psychosomatic Medicine, 55,* 364–379.

Herdman, R., Hewitt, M., & Laschober, M. (1993). Smoking-related deaths and financial costs. *Office of Technology Assessment estimates for 1990.* Congress of the United States. Washington, DC. Office of Technology Assessment.

Herman, D., Struening, E., & Barrow, S. (1993). Self-assessed need for mental health services among homeless adults. *Hospital and Community Psychiatry, 44,* 1181–1183.

Herman, J. (1992). *Trauma and recovery.* New York: Basic Books.

Herrera, J. A., Salmeron, B., & Hurtado, H. (1997). Prenatal biopsychosocial risk assessment and low birthweight. *Social Science Medicine, 44*(8), 1107–1114.

Herrick, C., & Brown, H. N. (1999). Mental disorders and syndromes found among Asians residing in the United States. *Issues in Mental Health Nursing, 20,* 275–296.

Herth, K. (1990). Relationship of hope, coping styles, concurrent losses, and setting to grief resolution in the elderly widow(er). *Research in Nursing and Health, 13,* 109–117.

Heyman, E. (1987). Seclusion. *Journal of Psychosocial Nursing and Mental Health Services, 25*(11), 9–12.

Hill, R. (1958). Social stresses on the family. *Social Casework, 39,* 139–150.

Hillbrand, M., Foster, H. G., & Spitz, R. T. (1996). Characteristics and costs of staff Injuries in a forensic hospital. *Psychiatric Services, 47*(10), 1123–1125.

Hilton, B. A. (1994, August). Family communication patterns in coping with early breast cancer. *Western Journal of Nursing Research, 16*(4), 366–391.

Hinton, J. (1998, Autumn). An assessment of open communication between people with terminal cancer, caring relatives, and others during home care. *Journal of Palliative Care, 14*(3), 15–23.

Ho, A. P., Tsuang, J. W., Liberman, R. P., Wang, R., Wilkins, J. N., Eckman, T. A., & Shaner, A. L. (1997). Achieving effective treatment of patients with chronic psychotic illness and comorbid substance dependence. *American Journal of Psychiatry, 156*(11), 1765–1770.

Hobbs, C. J., Hanks, H. G., & Wynne, J. M. (1999). *Child abuse and neglect: A clinician's handbook* (2nd ed.). London: Churchill Livingstone.

Hobfoll, S. E., & Leiberman, J. R. (1989). Effects of mastery and intimacy on anxiety following pregnancy: For whom is support supportive and from whom? *Anxiety Research, 1,* 327–341.

Hodges, E., Cochrane, C., & Brewerton, T. (1998). Family characteristics of binge-eating disorder patients. *International Journal of Eating Disorders, 23,* 145–151.

Hodgkinson, P., Hillis, T., & Russell, D. (1984). Assaults on staff in a psychiatric hospital. *Nursing Times, 80,* 44–46.

Hoenig, J., & Hamilton, M. (1966). The schizophrenic patient in the community and its effect on the household. *International Journal of Social Psychiatry, 12,* 165–176.

Hoff, L. A. (1984). *People in crisis: Understanding and helping.* Menlo Park, CA: Addison-Wesley.

Hogan, M. (2000). Address to Ohio Department of Mental Health Commission of the Future of the System. Columbus, Ohio.

Holder, D., & Anderson, C. (1990). Psychoeducational family interventions for depressed patients and their families. In G. I. Keitner (Ed.), *Depression in families: Impact and treatment* (pp. 159–184). Washington, DC: American Psychiatric Press.

Hollander, C. E. (1969). A process for psychodrama training: The Hollander psychodrama curve. Denver, CO: Snow Lion Press.

Holmberg, S. K., & Kane, C. F. (1995). Severe psychiatric disorder and physical health risks. *Clinical Nurse Specialist, 9,* 287–292.

Holmberg, S. K., & Kane, C. (1999). Health and self-care practices of persons with schizophrenia. *Psychiatric Services, 50*(6), 827–829.

Holmes, H., Ziemba, J., Evans, T., & Williams, C. A. (1994). Nursing model of psychoeduation for the seriously mentally ill patient. *Issues in Mental Health, 15,* 85–104.

Holmes, T. H., & Rahe, R. (1967). The social readjustment rating scale. *Journal of Psychosomatic Research, 12,* 213–218.

Holt, L. E. (1897). *Diseases of infancy and childhood.* New York: D. Appleton.

Holzemer, W. L. (in press). Symptom management research in HIV/AIDS. *Kango Kenkyu* [in Japanese].

Holzemer, W. L., Henry, S. B., Nokes, K. M., Corless, I. B., Brown, A. M., Powel-Cope, G. M., Turner, J. G., & Inouye, J. (1999). Validation of the sign and symptom check-list for person with HIV disease (SSC–HIV). *Journal of Advanced Nursing, 30,* 1041–1049.

Holzemer, W. L., & Wilson, H. S. (1995). Quality of life and spectrum of HIV infection. *Annual Review of Nursing Research, 13,* 3–29.

Homes for the Homeless. (1998). *Ten Cities: 1997–1998: A Snapshot of Family Homelessness Across America.* New York: Homes for the Homeless & the Institute for Children and Poverty.

Honig, A., Hofman, A., Rozendaal, N., & Dingemans, P. (1997). Psycho-education in bipolar disorder: Effect on expressed emotion. *Psychiatry Research, 72*(1), 17–22.

Hoskins, C. N., Baker, S., Sherman, D., Bohlander, J., Bookbinder, M., Budin, W., Ekstrom, D., Knauer, C., & Maislin, G. (1996). Social support and patterns of adjustment to breast cancer. *Scholarly Inquiry for Nursing Practice: An International Journal, 10*(2), 99–122.

Houston-Miller, N., Smith, P. M., DeBusk, R. F., Sobel, D., & Taylor, C. B. (1997). Smoking cessation in hospitalized patients. *Archives of Internal Medicine, 7,* 409–415.

Howard-Pitney, B., LaFrombroise, T., & Basil, M. (1992). Psychological and social indicators of suicide ideation and suicide attempts in Zuni adolescents. *Journal of Consulting and Clinical Psychology, 60*(3), 473–476.

Hughes, J. R. (1995). Clinical implications of the association between smoking and alcoholism. In J. Fertig & R. Fuller (Eds.), *Alcohol and tobacco: From basic science to policy.* National Institute of Alcohol Abuse and Alcoholism Research Monograph 30. Washington, DC: U.S. Government Printing Office, 171–181.

Human Rights Watch. (1997). *Cold Storage: Super-maximum security confinement in Indiana.* New York: Human Rights Watch.

Hume, A. J., Barker, P. J., Robertson, W., & Swan, J. (1988). Manic depressive psychosis: An alternative therapeutic model of nursing. *Journal of Advanced Nursing, 13*(1), 93–98.

Hurlebaus, A., & Link, S. (1997). The effects of an aggressive behavior management program on nurses' levels of knowledge, confidence, and safety. *Journal of Nursing Staff Development, 13*(5), 260–265.

Hurt, R. D., Eberman, K. M., Croghan, I. T., Offord, K. P., Davis, L. J., Morse, R. M., Palmen, M. A., & Bruce, B. K. (1994). Nicotine dependence treatment during inpatient treatment for other addictions: A prospective intervention trial. *Alcoholism: Clinical and Experimental Research, 18,* 867–872.

Hurt, R. D., Sachs, D. P. L., Glover, E. D., Offord, K. P., Johnston, J. A., Lowell, C. D., Khayrallah, M. A., Schroeder, D. R., Glover, P. N., Sullivan C. R., Croghan, I. T., & Sullivan, P. M. (1997). A comparison of sustained-release bupropion and placebo for smoking cessation. *New England Journal of Medicine, 337,* 1195–1202.

Hyman, R. B., Feldman, H. R., Harris, R. B., Levin, R. F., & Malloy, G. B. (1989). The effects of relaxation training on clinical symptoms: A meta-analysis. *Nursing Research, 38,* 216–220.

Hyman, S. E. (1999, June 21). Mental illness in the next century. Report at the Third Annual Roundtable on Mental Health. Washington DC.

Iles, P. (1979). Children with cancer: Healthy siblings' perception during the illness experience. *Cancer Nursing, 2,* 371–379.

Inch, H., Rowlands, P., & Soliman, A. (1995). Deliberate self harm in a young offenders institution. *Journal of Forensic Psychiatry, 6,* 161–171.

Indian Health Service. (1997). (Available at *http://www.his.gov/PublicInfo/Publications/trends97/trends97.asp.*).

Infantino, J. A., & Musingo, S. Y. (1985). Assaults and injuries among staff with infection. *Annual Review of Nursing Research, 13,* 3–29.

Inglehart, J. K., Hiebert-White, J., & Zuercher, A. (Eds.). (1995). Mental health in the age of managed care. *Health Affairs, 14*(3), 7–286.

Inouye, S. K., Bogardus, S. T., Jr., Charpentier, P. A., Leo-Summers, L., Acampora, D., Holford, T. R., & Cooney, L. M., Jr. (1999). A multicomponent intervention to prevent delirium in hospitalized older patients. *New England Journal of Medicine, 340,* 669–676.

Inouye, S. K., Rusing, S. T., Foreman, M. D., Palmer, R., & Pompei, P. (1998). Does delirium contribute to poor hospital outcomes? A three-site epidemiologic study. *Journal of General Internal Medicine, 13,* 234–242.

Institute of Medicine. (1988). *Homelessness, healt, and human needs.* Washington, DC: National Academy Press.

Intrieri, R., Cerdas, M., & Morse, J. M. (1994, June). *Indices of distress in the trauma patient.* Paper presented at the 2nd Qualitative Health Research Conference, Hershey, PA.

Jablensky, A. (1999). The conflict of the nosologists: Views on schizophrenia and manic-depressive illness in the early part of the 20th century. *Schizophrenia Research, 39*(2), 95–100; discussion 159.

Jackson, D. B., & Saunders, R. B. (1993). *Child health nursing: A comprehensive approach to the care of children and their families.* Philadelphia: Lippincott.

Jacobs, S. R. (1996). The grief experience of older women whose husbands had hospice care. *Journal of Advanced Nursing, 24,* 280–286.

Jalowiec, A. (1992). Multidimensional assessment of QOL in clinical studies. *Progress in Cardiovascular Nursing, 7*(2), 7–12.

Jamerson, P. A., Scheibmeir, M., Bott, M. J., Crighton, F., Hinton, R. H., & Cobb, A. K. (1996, November–December). The experiences of families with a relative in the intensive care unit. *Heart & Lung, 25*(6), 467–474.

Jarrett, M., Heitkemper, M. M., Cain, K., Tuftin, M., Walker, E., Bond, E., & Levy, R. (in press). The relationship between psychological distress and gastrointestinal symptoms in women.

Jemelka, R., Trupin, E., & Chiles, J. (1989) The mentally ill in prisons: A review. *Hospital and Community Psychiatry, 40,* 481–491.

Jendrek, M. (1994). Grandparents who parent their grandchildren: Circumstances and decisions. *The Gerontologist, 34*(2), 206–216.

Jeon, Y. H., & Madjar, I. (1998). Caring for a family member with chronic mental illness. *Qualitative Health Research, 8*(5), 694–706.

Jerrell, J. M., & Wilson, J. L. (1997). Ethnic differences in the treatment of dual mental and substance disorders: A preliminary analysis. *Journal of Substance Abuse Treatment, 14*(2), 133–140.

Jilek-Aall, L. (1988). Suicidal behavior among youth: A cross-cultural comparison. *Transcultural Psychiatric Research Review, 25*(2), 87–105.

Jimenez, A. L., Alegria, M., Pena, M., & Vera, M. (1997). Mental health utilization in depression. *Women & Health, 25*(2), 1–21.

Jimerson, D., Wolfe, B., Metzger, E., Finkelstein, D., Cooper, T., & Levine, J. (1997). Decreased serotonin function in bulimia nervosa. *Archives of General Psychiatry, 54,* 529–534.

Johnson, D. (1990). The family's experience of living with mental illness. In H. Lefley & D. Johnson (Eds.), *Families as allies in treatment of the mentally ill.* Washington, DC: American Psychiatric Press.

Johnson, D. L. (1997). Overview of severe mental illness. *Clinical Psychology Review, 17*(3), 247–257.

Johnson, D. R. (1987). The role of the creative arts therapies in diagnosis and treatment of psychological trauma. *The Arts in Psychotherapy, 14*(1), 7–13.

Johnson, J., Kerse, N. M., Wanich, C., Sullivan, E., & Chen, K. (1992). Prospective versus retrospective methods of identifying patients with delirium. *Journal of the American Geriatric Society, 40,* 316–319.

Johnson, J. E., Rice, V. H., & Endress, M. P. (1978). Sensory information, instruction in a coping strategy, and recovery from surgery. *Research in Nursing and Health, 1,* 4–17.

Johnson, J. E., Rice, V. H., Fuller, S. S., & Endress, M. P. (1978). Sensory information, instruction in coping strategy and recovery from surgery. *Research in Nursing and Health, 1,* 4–17.

Jones, M. K. (1985). Patient violence report of 200 incidents. *Journal of Psychosocial Nursing and Mental Health Services, 23*(6), 12–17.

Jones, R. N., & O'Brien, P. (1990). Unique interventions for child inpatient psychiatry. *Journal of Psychosocial Nursing, 28*(7), 29–31.

Jones, R. N., O'Brien, P., & McMahon, W. M. (1993). Contracting to lower precaution status for child psychiatric inpatients. *Journal of Psychosocial Nursing, 31*(1), 6–10.

Jones, S. (1996). The association between objective and subjective caregiver burden. *Archives of Psychiatric Nursing, 10,* 77–84.

Jones, S., Doheny, M., Jones, P., & Bradley, N. (1986). Binge eaters: A comparison of eating patterns of those who admit to binging and those who do not. *Journal of Advanced Nursing, 11,* 545–552.

Jung, M. (1980). *Chinese American family counseling: A model for clinicians.* San Francisco: Jossey-Bass.

Kahn, M. W., Lejero, L., Antone, M., & Francisco, D. (1988). An indigenous community mental health service on the Tohono O'odham (Papago) Indian reservation: Seventeen years later. *American Journal of Community Psychology, 16*(3), 369–379.

Kalil, K. M., Gruber, J. E., Conley, J., & Sytniac, M. (1993). Social and family pressures on anxiety during pregnancy. *Pre and Perinatal Psychology Journal, 8,* 113–118.

Kane, C. F., & Ennis, J. M. (1996). Health care reform and rural mental health: Severe mental illness. *Community Mental Health Journal, 32*(5), 445–462.

Kaplan, S. J., Pelcowitz, D., & Labruna, V. (1999). Child and adolescent abuse and neglect research: A review of the past 10 years: Part I: Physical and emotional abuse and neglect. *Journal of the American Academy of Child and Adolescent Psychiatry, 28*(10), 1214–1222.

Kaslow, N. J., & Thompson, M. O. (1998). Applying the criteria for empirically supported treatments to studies of psychosocial interventions for child and adolescent depression. *Journal of Clinical Child Psychology, 27,* 146–155.

Kasten, B. P. (1997). *Experience of mentally ill adults with co-occurring substance use disorders.* Unpublished doctoral dissertation, University of California, San Francisco.

Katon, W., & Gonzales, J. (1994). A review of randomized trials of psychiatric consultation-liaison studies in primary care. *Psychosomatic, 35,* 268–278.

Katon, W. J., Von Korff, M., Lin, E., Bush, T., Russo, J., Lipscomb, P., & Wagner, E. A. (1992). Randomized trial of psychiatric consultation with distressed high utilizers. *General Hospital Psychiatry, 14,* 86–98.

Katon, W., Von Korff, M., Lin, E., Walker, E., Simon, G. E., Bush, T., Robinson, P., & Russo J. (1995). Collaborative management to achieve treatment guidelines: Impact on depression in primary care. *Journal of the American Medical Association, 273*(13), 1026–1031.

Kavanagh, K. H. (1999). Transcultural perspectives in mental health. In M. M. Andrews & J. S. Boyle (Eds.), *Transcultural concepts in nursing care* (3rd ed., pp. 223–261). Philadelphia: Lippincott.

Kavanagh, K. H., Absalom, K., Beil, Jr., W., & Schliessmann, L. (1999). Connecting and becoming culturally competent: A Lakota example. *Advances in Nursing Science, 21*(3), 9–31.

Kazdin, A. E. (1993). Psychotherapy for children and adolescents: Current progress and future research directions. *American Psychologist, 48*(6), 644–657.

Kazdin, A. E. (1996). Developing effective treatments for children and adolescents. In E. D. Hibbs & P. S. Jensen (Eds.), *Psychosocial Treatments for Child and Adolescent Disorders: Empirically Based Strategies for Clinical Practice* (pp. 9–18). Washington, DC: American Psychological Association.

Keitner, G. I., Miller, I. W., Epstein, N. B., Bishop, D. S., & Fruzzetti, A. E. (1987). Family functioning and the course of major depression. *Comprehensive Psychiatry, 1,* 54–64.

Keitner, G. I., Miller, I. W., & Ryan, C. E. (1993). The role of the family in major depressive illness. *Psychiatric Annals, 23,* 500–507.

Kellam, S. G., & Rebok, G. W. (1992). Building developmental and etiological theory through epidemiologically based preventive intervention trials. In J. McCord & R. E. Tremblay (Eds.), *Preventing antisocial behavior: Interventions from birth through adolescence* (pp. 162–195). New York: Guildford Press.

Kelley, S. (1993). Caregiver stress in grandparents raising grandchildren. *IMAGE: Journal of Nursing Scholarship, 25*(4), 331–337.

Kelly, H., & Ludwig, G. (1995). Energy field disturbance. In B. Ackley et al. (Eds.), *The nursing diagnosis handbook: A guide to planning care.* St. Louis: Mosby-Year Book.

Keltner, N. L. (2000). Neuroreceptor function and psychopharmacologic response. *Issues in Mental Health Nursing, 21,* 31–50.

Kempe, A. R. (1994). *Forming Alliances: Toward a Grounded Theory of the Nurse Caring for the Family Caregiver of a Schizophrenic Member.* Detroit, MI: Wayne State University.

Kendler, K. S., Kessler, R. C., Neale, M. C., Heath, A. C., & Eaves, L. J. (1993). The prediction of major depression in women: Toward an integrated etiologic model. *American Journal of Psychiatry, 150,* 1139–1148.

Kennedy, M. G., Schepp, K. G., & O'Connor, F. W. (2000). *Symptom self-management and relapse in schizophrenia.* Manuscript submitted for publication.

Kennett, D. J., & Nisbet, C. (1998). The influence of body mass index and learned resourcefulness skills on body image and lifestyle practices. *Patient Education and Counseling, 33*(1), 1–12.

Kent-Wilkinson, A. (2000). *Forensic education page.* [online]. (Available at *http://www.forensiceducation.com.*).

Kerr, R. B. (1994). Meanings adult daughters attach to a parent's death. *Western Journal of Nursing Research, 16,* 347–365.

Kessing, L. V. (1998). Recurrence in affective disorder. II. Effect of age and gender. *British Journal of Psychiatry, 172*, 29–34.

Kessler, R. C., McGonagle, K. A., & Shanyang, Z. (1994). Lifetime and 12-month prevalence of DSM III-R psychiatric disorders in the United States: Results from the National Comorbidity Survey. *Archives of General Psychiatry, 51,* 8–19.

Kessler, R. C., McGonagle, K. A., Zhao, S., Nelson, C. B., Hughes, M., Eshleman, S., Wittchen, H., & Kendler, K. S. (1994). Lifetime and 12 month prevalence of DSM-III-R psychiatric disorders in the United States: Results from the national comorbidity survey. *Archives of General Psychiatry, 51,* 8–19.

Kihlgren, M., Kuremyr, D., Norberg, A., Brane, G., Karlson, I., Engstrom, B., & Melin, E. (1993, February). Nurse-patient interaction after training in integrity promoting care at a long-term ward: Analysis of video-recorded morning care sessions. *International Journal of Nursing Studies, 30*(1), 1–13.

Killeen, M. (1993). Parent influences on children's self-esteem in economically disadvantaged families. *Issues in Mental Health Nursing, 14,* 323–336.

Kilzieh, N., & Akiskal, H. S. (1999). Rapid-cycling bipolar disorder. An overview of research and clinical experience. *Psychiatric Clinics of North America, 22*(3), 585–607.

Kim, M. T. (1995). Cultural influences on depression in Korean Americans. *Journal of Psychosocial Nursing, 33*(2), 13–18.

King, I. M. (1981). *A theory for nursing: Systems, concepts, process.* New York: Wiley.

King, I. M. (1992). King's theory of goal attainment. *Nursing Science Quarterly, 5*(1), 19–26.

Kinzie, J. D., Leung, P. K., Boehnlein, J., Matsunga, D., Johnson, R., Manson, S., Shore, J. H., Heinz, J., & Williams, M. (1992). Psychiatric epidemiology of an Indian village. A 19-year study replication study. *Journal of Nervous and Mental Disease, 180,* 33–39.

Kipper, D. (1986). *Psychotherapy through clinical role-playing.* New York: Bruner/Mazel.

Kipper, D. A., & Har-Even, D. (1984). Role playing techniques: The differential effect of behavior simulation interventions on the readiness to inflict pain. *Journal of Clinical Psychology, 40,* 936–941.

Kirkpatrick, H. (1989). A descriptive study of seclusion: The unit environment, patient behavior, and nursing interventions. *Archives of Psychiatric Nursing, 3*(1), 3–9.

Kirmayer, L. J. (1994). Suicide among Canadian Aboriginal peoples. *Transcultural Psychiatric Research Review, 31*(1), 3–58.

Kleinman, A., & Seeman, D. (2000). Personal experience of illness. In G. Albrecht, R. Fitzpatrick, & S. Scrimshaw (Eds.), *Handbook of social studies in health and medicine* (pp. 230–242). London: Sage.

Knitzer, J., & Aber, J. L. (1995). Young children in poverty: facing the facts. *American Journal of Orthopsychiatry, 65*(2), 174–176.

Knox, M. D., Boaz, T. L., Friedrich, M. A., & Dow, M. G. (1995). HIV risk factors for persons with serious mental illness. *AIDS Patient Care, 30,* 192–198.

Koch-Hattem, A. (1986). Siblings' experience of pediatric cancer: Interviews with children. *Health and Social Work, 1,* 107–117.

Koegel, P., & Burnam, M. (1992). Problems in the assessment of mental illness among the homeless: An empirical approach. In M. J. Robertson & M. Greenblatt (Eds.), *Homelessness: A national perspective* (pp. 77–99). New York: Plenum Press.

Koegel, P., Burnam, M., & Baumohl. (1996). The causes of homelessness. In J. Baumohl (Ed.), *Homelessness in America* (pp. 24–33). Washington, DC: Onyx Press.

Koger, S. M., & Brotons, M. (1999). Music therapy for dementia [online]. (Available at *skoger@willamette.edu.*). The Cochrane Database of Systematic Reviews. 2. Cochrane Dementia & Cognitive Impairment Group.

Koger, S. M., Chapin, K., & Brotons, M. (1999). Is music therapy an effective intervention for dementia? A meta-analytic review of literature. *Journal of Music Therapy, 36*(1), 2–15.

Kolcaba, K. (1994). A theory of holistic comfort for nursing. *Journal of Advanced Nursing, 19,* 1178–1184.

Kolcaba, K. (1995). The art of comfort care. *Image: Journal of Nursing Scholarship, 27,* 287–289.

Kolcaba, K., & Fisher, E. 1996). A holistic perspective on comfort care as an advance directive. *Critical Care Nursing Quarterly, 18*(4), 66–76.

Kolcaba, K., & Kolcaba, R. (1991). An analysis of the concept of comfort. *Journal of Advanced Nursing, 16,* 1301–1310.

Korb, M. (1994). Anorexia as symbolic expression of a woman's rejection of her mother's life. *Western Journal of Nursing Research, 16,* 69–80.

Kornitzer, M., Boutsen, M., Dramaix, M., Thijs, J., & Gustavsson, G. (1995). Combined use of nicotine patch and gum in smoking cessation: A placebo-controlled clinical trial. *Preventive Medicine, 24,* 41–47.

Kovarsky, R. S. (1989). Loneliness and disturbed grief: A comparison of parents who lost a child to suicide or accidental death. *Archives of Psychiatric Nursing, 3,* 86–96.

Kozuki, Y. (1999). *Symptom unawareness and neuroleptic compliance in schizophrenia spectrum disorders.* Unpublished doctoral dissertation, University of California at San Francisco.

Kramer, R. F. (1981). Living with childhood cancer: Healthy siblings' perspective. *Issues in Comprehensive Pediatric Nursing, 5,* 155–165.

Kruger, S., Braunig, P., & Young, L. T. (1996). Biological treatment of rapid-cycling bipolar disorder. *Pharmacopsychiatry, 29*(5), 167–175.

Kuo, C. L., & Kavanagh, K. H. (1994). Chinese perspectives on culture and mental health. *Issues in Mental Health, 15,* 551–567.

Kupers, T. (1999). *Prison madness: The mental health crisis behind bars and what we should do about it.* San Francisco: Jossey-Bass.

Kurlowicz, L. (1991). Psychiatric consultation-liaison nursing interventions with nurses of hospitalized AIDS patients. *Clinical Nurse Specialist, 5*(2), 124–129.

Laidlaw, J. K., Beeken, J. E., Whitney, F. W., & Reyes, A. A. (1999). Research brief. Contracting with outpatient hemodialysis patients to improve adherence to treatment. *American Nephrology Nurses Association Journal, 26,* 37–40.

Laidlaw, T. M., Falloon, I. R., Barnfathner, D., & Coverdale, J. H. (1999). The stress of caring for people with obsessive compulsive disorders. *Community Mental Health Journal, 35*(5), 443–450.

Lamb, H., & Weinberger, L. (1998). Persons with severe mental illness in jails and prisons: A review. *Psychiatric Services, 49,* 483–492.

Lancaster, J. (1980). *Community mental health nursing: An ecological perspective.* St. Louis: C. V. Mosby.

Landreth, G., Homeyer, L., Glover, G., & Sweeney, D. (1996). *Play therapy interventions with children's problems.* Northvale, NJ: Jason Aronson.

Larsen, L. S. (1999). Effectiveness of a counseling intervention to assist family caregivers of chronically ill relatives. *Journal of Psychosocial Nursing & Mental Health Services, 36*(8), 26–32.

Larson, B. A., & Martinson, D. J. (1990). Words can hurt: Dealing with verbal abuse in the operating room. *AORN Journal, 52*(6), 1238–1241.

Lawson, W. B. (1996a). The art and science of the psychopharmacotherapy of African Americans. *The Mt. Sinai Journal of Medicine, 63,* 301–305.

Layton, J. M. (1979). The use of modeling to teach empathy to nursing students. *Research In Nursing and Health, 2,* 163–176.

Lazarus, A. (1995). Preparing for practice in an era of managed competition. *Psychiatric Services, 46,* 184–185.

Lazarus, R., & Folkman, S. (1984). *Appraisal and coping.* New York: Springer.

Lederman, R. (1996). *Psychosocial adaptation in pregnancy: Assessment of seven dimensions of maternal development.* New York: Springer.

Lederman, R. P. (1995). Part I: Relationship of anxiety, stress, and psychosocial development to reproductive health. *Behavioral Medicine, 21,* 110–112.

Lederman, R. P., & Miller, D. (1998). Adaptation to Pregnancy in Three Different Ethnic Groups: Latin-, African-, and Anglo-American. *Canadian Journal of Nursing Research, 30,* 37–51.

Lee, S. S., Gerberich, S. G., Waller, L. A., Anderson, A., & McGovern, P. (1999). Work-Related Assaults Injuries among Nurses. *Epidemiology, 10*(6), 685–691.

Leff, J. (1981). *Psychiatry around the globe.* New York: Marcel Dekker.

Lefley, H. (1996). *Family caregiving in mental illness.* Thousand Oaks, CA: Sage.

LeFort, S. M., Gray-Donald, K., Rowat, K. M., & Jeans, M. E. (1998). Randomized controlled trial of a community-based psychoeducation program for the self-management of chronic pain. *Pain, 74*(2), 297–306.

Leibenluft, E. (1996).Women with bipolar illness: Clinical and research issues. *American Journal of Psychiatry, 153*(2), 163–173.

Leibenluft, E., Ashman, S. B., Feldman-Naim, S., & Yonkers, K. A. (1999). Lack of relationship between menstrual cycle phase and mood in a sample of women with rapid cycling bipolar disorder. *Biological Psychiatry, 46*(4), 577–580.

Leighton, A. H. (2000). Community mental health and information under load. *Community Mental Health Journal, 36*(1), 77–95.

Lester, D. (1994-B). Suicide rates in Native Americans by state and size of population. *Perceptual and Motor Skills, 78*(3), 954.

Levin, J. S. (1991). Triethnic differences in pregnancy outcomes: Findings from the GLOWBS life in ethnically diverse patients with advanced HIV/AIDS. *Qualitative Health Research, 7,* 75–97.

Levy, J. E., & Kunitz, S. J. (1987). A suicide prevention program for Hopi youth. *Social Science and Medicine (Oxford), 25*(8), 931–940.

Lewis, A., & Levy, J. (1982). *Psychiatric liaison nursing: The theory and clinical practice.* Reston, VA: Reston Publishing.

Lewis, D. J., & Robinson, J. A. (1986). Assessment of coping strategies of ICU nurses in response to stress. *Critical Care Nurse, 6*(6), 38–43.

Lewis, M., Woods, N. F., Hough, E. E., & Bensley, L. S. (1989). The family's functioning with chronic illness in the mother: the spouses' perspective. *Social Science and Medicine, 29,* 1261–126.

Li, H., Stewart, B. J., Imle, M. A., Archbold, P. G., & Felver, L. (2000). Families and hospitalized elders: A typology of family care actions. *Research in Nursing and Health, 23,* 3–16.

Liaschenko, J. (1997). Ethics and the geography of the nurse-patient relationship: Spatial vulnerabilities and gendered space. *Scholarly Inquiry for Nursing Practice: An International Journal, 11,* 47–59.

Lin, K., Inui, T. S., Kleinman, A. M., & Womack, W. M. (1997). Ethnic and cultural considerations in psychopharmatherapy. In D. Dunner (Ed.), *Current psychiatric therapy II* (pp. 75–81). Philadelphia: Saunders.

Linden, M., Habib, T., & Radojevic, V. (1996). A controlled study of the effects of EEG biofeedback on cognition and behavior of children with attention deficit disorder and learning disabilities. *Biofeedback and Self-Regulation, 21,* 35–49.

Lindenberg, C. S., Gendrop, S. C., Nencioli, M., & Adames, Z. (1994). Substance abuse among inner-city Hispanic women: Exploring resiliency. *Journal of Gynecologic and Neonatal Nursing, 23,* 609–616.

Lindsey, A. (1995). Physical health of homeless adults. In J. J. Fitzpatrick & J. Norbeck (Eds.), *Annual review of nursing research* (Vol. 13, pp. 31–61). New York: Springer Publishing.

Linn, J. G., Monning, R. L., Cain, V. A., & Usoh, D. (1993). State of illness, level of HIV symptoms, sense of coherence and psychological functioning in clients of community-based AIDS counseling centers. *Journal of the Association of Nurses in AIDS Care, 4,* 24–32.

Lipscomb, J. A., & Love, C. C. (1992). Violence towards health care workers: An emerging occupational hazard. *AAOHN (American Association of Occupational Health Nursing) Journal, 40,* 219–228.

Liptzin, B. (1999). What criteria should be used for the diagnosis of delirium? *Dementia and Geriatric Cognitive Disorders, 10,* 364–367.

Lobel, M. (1994). Conceptualizations, measurement, and effects of prenatal maternal stress on birth outcomes. *Journal of Behavioral Medicine, 17,* 225–272.

Lobo, M. L., Barnard, K. E., & Coombs, J. B. (1992). Failure to thrive: A parent-infant interaction perspective. *Journal of Pediatric Nursing, 7,* 251–261.

Long, A., & Reid, W. (1996). An exploration of nurses attitudes to the nursing care of the suicidal patient in an acute psychiatric ward. *Journal of Psychiatric and Mental Health Nursing, 3,* 29–37.

Loomis, M. E. (1985). Levels of contracting. *Journal of Psychosocial Nursing, 23*(3), 9–14.

Louie, K. B. (1999). Status of mental health needs of Asian elderly. In M. L. Wykle & A. B. Ford (Eds.), *Serving minority elders in the 21st century* (pp. 1478–159). New York: Springer.

Loukissa, D. (1995). Family burden in chronic mental illness: A review of research studies. *Journal of Advanced Nursing, 21,* 248–255.

Loustaunau, M. O., & Sobo, E. J. (1997). *The cultural context of health, illness, and medicine.* Westport, CT: Bergin & Garvey.

Lovell, D., Allen, D. G., & Jemelka, R. (In review) Evaluating the effectiveness of residential treatment for prisoners with mental illness. *Criminal Justice and Behavior.*

Lovell, D., & Jemelka, R. (1996). When inmates misbehave: The costs of discipline. *Prison Journal, 76,* 165–179.

Lovell, D., & Jemelka, R. (1998). Coping with mental illness in prisons. *Family and Community Health, 21*(3), 54–66.

Lovell, D., & Rhodes, L. (1997). Mobile consultation: Crossing correctional boundaries to cope with disturbed offenders. *Federal Probation, 41*(3), 40–45.

Lowenberg, J. S. (1994). The nurse-patient relationship reconsidered: An expaded research agenda. *Scholarly Inquiry for Nursing Practice: An International Journal, 8,* 167–184.

Lubar, J. (1991). Discourse on development of EEG diagnostics and biofeedback for attention deficit/hyperactivity disorders. *Biofeedback and Self-Regulation, 16,* 201–224.

Lucas, A. R., Beard, C. M., O'Fallon, W. M., & Kurlan, L. (1991). 50-year trends in the incidence of anorexia nervosa in Rochester, Minn: A population-based study. *American Journal of Psychiatry, 148,* 917–922.

Ludwick, R. (1999). Clinical decision making: Recognition of confusion and application of restraints. *Orthopaedic Nursing, 18*(1), 65–72.

Lyness, S. A., Eaton, E. M., & Schneider, L. S. (1994). Cognitive performance in older and middle-aged depressed outpatient controls. *Journal of Gerontology: Psychological Sciences, 49*(3), P129–P136.

Lyon, B. (1993). Summary and preliminary synthesis. In J. S. Barnfather & B. L. Lyon (Eds.), *Stress and coping: State of the science and implications for nursing theory, research and practice.* Indianapolis: Sigma Theta Tau.

Lyon, B. L. (1996). *Conquering stress in changing times.* Research Triangle Park, NC: Glaxo Wellcome Inc.

Lyon, B. L., & Werner, J. S. (1987). Stress. In J. J. Fitzpatrick & R. L. Taunton (Eds.), *Annual Review of Nursing Research* (Vol. 5, pp. 3–22). New York: Springer Publishing.

Lyons, J., Hanner, J., Strain, J., & Fulop, G. (1986). The timing of psychiatric consultation in the general hospital and length of hospital stay. *General Hospital Psychiatry, 8,* 159–162.

Magliano, L., Fadden, G., Economou, M., Xavier, M., Held, T., Guarneri, M., Marasco, C., Tosini, P., & Maj, M. (1998). Social and clinical factors influencing the choice of coping strategies in relatives of patients with schizophrenia: Results of the BIOMED I study. *Social Psychiatry and Psychiatric Epidemiology, 33,* 413–419.

Magyary, D. M., & Brandt, P. B. (1998). *Nursing leadership enhancement for culturally competent care: Children and adolescents with special health care needs, families, and communities.* Maternal and Child Health Bureau, Health Resource and Service Administration funded training grant. School of Nursing, University of Washington.

Magyary, D., Brandt, P., & Kovalesky, A. (1996, revised 1999). *Children with ADHD: A manual with decision tree and clinical path.* Vienna, VA: MCHB Clearinghouse.

Mahurin, R. K., DeBettignies, B. H., & Pirozzolo, F. J. (1991). Structured assessment of independent living skills: Preliminary report of a performance measure of functional abilities in dementia. *Journal of Gerontology: Psychological Sciences, 46*(2), P58–P66.

Mallonee, S. S., Kreger, E., Farmer, K., & North, C. (1999). A prospective study of long-term health outcomes among Oklahoma City bombing survivors. *Journal of the Oklahoma State Medical Association, 92*(4), 178–186.

Mallory, G., Lyons, J., Scherubel, J., & Reichelt, P. (1993). Nursing care hours of patients receiving varying amounts and types of consultation/liaison services. *Archives of Psychiatric Nursing, VII*(6), 353–360.

Maningas, P. A., Robison, M., & Mallonee, S. (1997). The EMS response to the Oklahoma City bombing. *Prehospital and Disaster Medicine, 12*(2), 80–85.

Mann, N. A., Tandon, R. J., Butler, J., Boyd, M., Eisner, W. H., & Lewis, M. (1993). Psychosocial rehabilitation in schizophrenia: Beginnings in acute hospitalization. *Archives of Psychiatric Nursing, 7,* 154–162.

Manson, S. M., Beals, J., Dick, R. W., & Duclos, C. (1989). Risk factors for suicide among Indian adolescents at a boarding school. *Public Health Reports, 104*(6), 609–614.

Martinez, R., Grimm, M., & Adamson, M. (1999). From the other side of the door: Patient views of seclusion. *Journal of Psychosocial Nursing and Mental Health Services, 37*(3), 13–22.

Martinson, I. M. (1995). Pediatric hospice nursing. In J. Fitzpatrick & J. Stevenson (Eds.), *Annual review of nursing research* (Vol. 13, pp. 195–214). New York: Springer Publishing.

Mathews, B., & Scholveldt, P. (1962). Measurement of psychosocial aspects of the nurse-patient relationship. *Nursing Research, 11,* 154–162.

Mauch, D. (1998). Mental Health Services system: What will they look like in 10 years? *The Future of Mental Health Services* Premeeting briefing papers. Washington, DC: National Technical Assistance Center.

Maurin, J., & Boyd. C. (1990). Burden of mental illness on the family: A critical review. *Archives of Psychiatric Nursing, 4,* 99–107.

May, C. (1990). Research on nurse-patient relationships: Problems of theory, problems of practice. *Journal of Advanced Nursing, 15,* 307–315.

May, C. (1991). Affect neutrality and involvement in nurse-patient relationships: Perceptions of appropriate behavior among nurses in acute medical and surgical wards. *Journal of Advanced Nursing, 16,* 552–558.

May, C. R., & Purkis, A. A. (1995). The configuration of nurse-patient relationships: A critical view. *Scholarly Inquiry for Nursing Practice: An International Journal, 9,* 283–295.

May, P. A. (1987a). Suicide among American Indian youth: A look at the issues. *Child Today, 16*(4), 22–25.

May, P. A. (1987b). Suicide and self-destruction among American Indian youth. *American Indian Alaska Native Mental Health Research, 1*(1), 52–69.

May, P. A., & Van Winkle, N. (1994). Indian adolescent suicide: The epidemiological picture in New Mexico. *American Indian Alaska Native Mental Health Research Monograph Series, 4,* 2–23.

Mayou, R., & Hawton, K. (1986). Psychiatric disorders in the general hospital. *British Journal of Psychiatry, 149,* 172–190.

McAuliffe, W. E., Wechsler, H., Rohman, M., Soboroff, S. H., Fishman, P., Toth, D., & Friedman, R. (1984). Psychoactive drug use by young and future physicians. *Journal of Health and Social Behaviors, 25,* 34–54.

McClandless-Glimcher, L., McKnight, S., Hamera, E., Smith, B. I., Peterson, K. A., & Plumlee, A. A. (1986). Use of symptoms by schizophrenics to monitor and regulate their illness. *Hospital and Community Psychiatry, 37,* 929–933.

McClement, S. E., & Degner, L. F. (1995, September). Expert nursing behaviors in care of the dying adult in the intensive care unit. *Heart & Lung: Journal of Critical Care, 24*(5), 408–419.

McClowry, S. G. (1998). The science and art of using temperament as the basis for intervention. *School Psychology Review, 27,* 551–563.

McClowry, S. G., & Galehouse, P. (in press). Planning a temperament-based parenting program for inner city school-age children. *Journal of Child and Adolescent Psychiatric and Mental Health Nursing.*

McCowan, D. E., & Davies, B. (1995). Patterns of grief in young children following the death of a sibling. *Death Studies, 19,* 41–53.

McDermott, J. F., & Dunne, J. E. (Eds.). (1997). Clinical practice parameters. *Journal of the American Academy of Child and Adolescent Psychiatry, 36*(Suppl.).

McDougall, G. J. (1994). Predictorsof metamemory in older adults. *Nursing Research, 43,* 212–218.

McDougall, G. J. (2000). *Mnemonic training to improve memory and memory self-efficacy in cognitively impaired nursing home residents.* Manuscript submitted for publication.

McDowell, I., & Newell, C. (1996). Mental status testing. In I. McDowell & C. Newell (Eds.), *Measuring health: A guide to rating scales and questionnaires* (pp. 287–334). New York: Oxford University Press.

McElroy, A., & Townsend, P. K. (1996). *Medical anthropology in ecological perspective.* Boulder, CO: Westview Press.

McEnany, G. W. (1990). Psychobiological indices of bipolar mood disorder: Future trends in nursing care. *Archives of Psychiatric Nursing, 4,* 29–38.

McGee, H. M., O'Boyle, C. A., Hickey, A., O'Malley, K., & Joyce, C. R. B. (1991). Individual quality of life in patients undergoing hip replacement. *Lancet, 339,* 1088–1091.

McGlynn, S. M. (1990). Behavioral approaches to neurposychological rehabilitation. *Psychological Bulletin, 108*(3), 420–441.

McHugo, G. J., Drake, R. E., Burton, H. L., & Ackerson, T. H. (1995). A scale for assessing the stage of substance abuse treatment in persons with severe mental illness. *Journal of Nervous and Mental Disease, 183*(12), 762–767.

McKay, B. (1989). Drama therapy with female victims of assault. *The Arts in Psychotherapy, 16*(4), 293–300.

McKay, S., & Roberts, J. (1990). Obstetrics by ear: Maternal and caregiver perceptions of the meaning of maternal sounds during second stage labor. *Journal of Nurse-Midwifery, 35,* 266–273.

McKinney, N., & Frank, D. I. (1998). Nursing assessment of adult females who are alcohol dependent and victims of sexual abuse. *Clinical Excellence for Nurse Practitioners, 2*(3), 152–158.

McLaughlin, C. (1994). Casualty nurses' attitudes toward attempted suicide. *Journal of Advanced Nursing, 20,* 1111–1118.

McMurran, M. (1996). Managing criminal risk through treatment. *Psychiatric Care, 3*(2), 51–55.

McMurray-Avila, M. (1997). *Organizing health services for homeless people.* Nashville, TN: National Health Care for the Homeless Council, Inc.

McShane, D. (1988). An analysis of mental health research with American Indian youth. Department of Psychology. Logan, UT: Utah State University.

Mechanic, D. (1987). *Improving mental health services: What the social sciences can tell us.* San Francisco: Jossey-Bass.

Meichenbaum, D. (1994). *A clinical handbook/practical therapist manual for assessing and treating adults with post-traumatic stress disorder.* Ontario, Canada: Institute Press.

Meisler, N., Blankertz, L., Santos, A. B., & McKay, C. (1997). Impact of assertive community treatment on homeless persons with co-occurring severe psychiatric and substance use disorders. *Community Mental Health Journal, 33*(2), 113–122.

Melnyk, B. M., Alpert-Gillis, L. J., Hensel, P. B., Cable-Beiling, R. C., & Rubenstein, J. S. (1997). Helping mothers cope with a critically ill child: A pilot test of the COPE intervention. *Research in Nursing and Health, 20*(1), 3–14.

Mercer-McFadden, C., & Drake, R. E. (1995). A review of 13 NIMH demonstration projects for young adults with severe mental illness and substance abuse problems. Rockville, MD: U.S. Department of Health and Human Services.

Merwin, E. (1995). Building interdisciplinary mental health services research teams: A case example. *Issues in Mental Health Nursing, 16,* 547–554.

Merwin, E., Goldsmith, H., & Manderscheid, R. (1995). Human resource issues in rural mental health services. *Community Mental Health Services, 31,* 525–537.

Merwin, E., & Mauck, A. (1995). Psychiatric nursing outcome research: The state of the science. *Archives of Psychiatric Nursing, IX,* 6, 311–331.

Methven, D., & Schlotfeldt, R. (1962). The social interaction inventory. *Nursing Research, 11,* 83–88.

Meyer, L. (1956). *Emotion and meaning in music.* Chicago: University of Chicago Press.

Miller, I. W., Kietner, G. I., Whisman, M. A., Ryan, C. E., Epstein, N. B., & Bishop, D. S. (1992). Depressed patients with dysfunctional families: Description and course of illness. *Journal of Abnormal Psychology, 101,* 637–646.

Miller, L. J., & Finnerty, M. (1996). Sexuality, pregnancy, and childrearing among women with schizophrenia-spectrum disorders. *Psychiatric Services, 47*(5), 502–506.

Minkler, M., Fuller-Thomson, E., Miller, D., & Driver, D. (1997). Depression in grandparents raising grandchildren: Results of a national longitudinal study. *Archives of Family Medicine, 6,* 445–452.

Minkoff, K. (1989). An integrated treatment model for dual diagnosis of psychosis and addiction. *Hospital and Community Psychiatry, 40*(10), 1031–1036.

Minkoff, K., & Regner, J. (1999). Innovations in integrated dual diagnosis treatment in public managed care: The Choate dual diagnosis case rate program. *Journal of Psychoactive Drugs, 31*(1), 3–12.

Mohr, W. K. (1998). Cross-ethnic variations in care of psychiatric patients: A review of contributing factors and practice considerations. *Journal of Psychosocial Nursing, 36*(50), 16–21.

Mohr, W. K., & Fanutzzo, J. W. (1998). The challenge of creating thoughtful research agendas. *Archives of Psychiatric Nursing, XII,* 21, 3–11.

Monteleone, J. A. (1998). *Child maltreatment: A clinical guide and reference* (2nd ed.). St. Louis, MO: G. W. Medical Publishing, Inc.

Montgomery, C. L. (1993). *Healing through communication: The practice of caring.* Newbury Park, CA: Sage.

Moore, K. W., & Schwartz, K. S. (1993, August). Psychosocial support of trauma patients in the emergency department by nurses, as indicated by communication. *Journal of Emergency Nursing, 19*(4), 297–302.

Morales, E., & Duphorne, P. L. (1995). Least restrictive measures: Alternatives to four-point restraints and seclusion. *Journal of Psychosocial Nursing, 33*(10), 13–16.

Moreno, J. L. (1953/1934). *Who Shall Survive?* (3rd Edition). Beacon, NY: Beacon House.

Moreno, J. L. (1977/1948) *Psychodrama, Vol. I* (4th ed.). Beacon, NY: Beacon House.

Moreno, Z. T. (1959). A survey of psychodramatic techniques. *Group Psychotherapy, 12*(1), 5–14.

Moriarty, H. J., Carroll, R., & Cotroneo, M. (1996). Differences in bereavement reactions within couples following death of a child. *Research in Nursing and Health, 19*(6), 461–469.

Morris, P. (1994). Superkids: Short-term group therapy for children with abusive backgrounds. *JCAPN, 7*(1), 25–31.

Morrison, E. F. (1992). A coercive interactive style as an antecedent to aggression and violence in psychiatric inpatients. *Research in Nursing and Health, 15,* 421–431.

Morse, G. (1984). *Homeless people: A typological analysis and gender comparison.* Unpublished doctoral dissertation. University of Missouri, St. Louis.

Morse, J. M. (1991). Negotiating commitment and involvement in the nurse-patient relationship. *Journal of Advanced Nursing, 16,* 455–468.

Morse, J. M., Anderson, G., Bottorff, J. L., Yonge, O., O'Brien, B., Solberg, S. M., & McIlveen, K. H. (1992). Exploring empathy: A conceptual fit for nursing practice. *Image: Journal of Nursing Scholarship, 24,* 173–280.

Morse, J. M., & Bottorff, J. L. (1990). The use of ethology in clinical nursing research. *Advances in Nursing Science, 12,* 53–64.

Morse, J. M., Bottorff, J. L., Anderson, G., O'Brien, B., & Solberg, S. (1992). Beyond empathy: Expanding expressions of caring. *Journal of Advanced Nursing, 17,* 809–821.

Morse, J. M., Miles, M. W., Clark, D. A., & Dobrneck, B. M. (1994). "Sensing" patient needs: Exploring concepts of nursing insight and receptivity used during nursing assessment. *Scholarly Inquiry for Nursing Practice: An International Journal, 8,* 233–254.

Morse, S. R., & Fife, B. (1998). Coping with a partner's cancer: Adjustment at four stages of the illness trajectory. *Oncology Nursing Forum, 25*(4), 751–760.

Mortimer, J. A. (1997). Brain reserve and the clinical expression of Alzheimer's disease. *Geriatrics, 52*(Suppl. 2), S50–S53.

Moschler, L., & Fincannon, J. (1992). Subspecialization within psychiatric consultation-liaison nursing. *Archives of Psychiatric Nursing, VI*(4), 234–238.

Mudd, S. A., Boyd, C. J., Brower, K. J., Young, J. P., & Blow, F. C. (1994). Alcohol withdrawal and related nursing care in older adults. *Journal of Gerontological Nursing, 20*(10), 17–26.

Mueser, K. T., & Noordsy, D. L. (1996). Group treatment for dually diagnosed clients. *New Directions for Mental Health Services, 70*(3), 33–51.

Mumford, E., Schlesinger, H. J., & Glass, G. V. (1982). The effects of psychological intervention on recovery from surgery and heart attacks: An analysis of the literature. *American Journal of Public Health, 72*(2), 141–151.

Munoz, R. F., Mrazek, P. J., & Haggerty, R. J. (1996). Institute of Medicine report on prevention of mental disorders: Summary and commentary. *American Psychologist, 51*(11), 1116–1122.

Murphy, L. N., Gass-Sternas, K., & Knight, K. (1995). Health of the chronically mentally ill who rejoin the community: A community assessment. *Issues in Mental Health Nursing, 16,* 239–256.

Murphy, M., & Moller, M. (1993). Relapse management in neurobiological disorders: The Moller-Murphy symptom management assessment tool. *Archives of Psychiatric Nursing, VII,* 4, 226–235.

Murphy, P. A., Forrester, D. A., Price, D. M., & Monaghan, J. F. (1992, January). Empathy of intensive care nurses and critical care family needs assessment. *Heart & Lung: Journal of Critical Care, 21*(1), 25–30.

Murphy, S. A. (1987). Self-efficacy and social support mediators of stress on mental health following a natural disaster. *Western Journal of Nursing Research, 9,* 58–86.

Murphy, S. A., Braun, T., Tillery, L., Cain, K. C., Johnson, L. C., & Beaton, R. D. (1999). PTSD among bereaved parents following the violent deaths of their 12- to 28-year-old children: A longitudinal prospective analysis. *Journal of Traumatic Stress, 12*(2), 273–291.

Murphy, S. A., Das Gupta, A., Cain, K. C., Johnson, L. C., Lohan, J., Wu, L., & Mekwa, J. (1999). Changes in parents' mental distress after the violent death of an adolescent or young adult child: A longitudinal, prospective analysis. *Death Studies, 23,* 129–159.

Murray, J. S. (1995). Social support for siblings of children with cancer. *Journal of Pediatric Oncology Nursing, 12,* 62–70.

Murray, J. S. (1998). The lived experience of childhood cancer: One sibling's perspective. *Issues in Comprehensive Pediatric Nursing, 21,* 217–227.

Murray, J. S. (1999a). Siblings of children with cancer: A review of the literature. *Journal of Pediatric Oncology Nursing, 16,* 25–34.

Murray, J. S. (1999b). Methodological triangulation in a study of social support for siblings of children with cancer. *Journal of Pediatric Oncology Nursing, 16,* 194–200.

Musil, C. (1998). Health, stress, coping and social support among grandmother caregivers. *Health Care for Women International, 19,* 441–455.

Musil, C. (2000). *Health of grandmothers: Comparisons by caregiver status.* Manuscript submitted for publication.

Musil, C. (2000). Grandmother caregivers: Changes in health and stress over 10 months. *Journal of Women and Aging, 12,* 129–145.

Nadler, A. (1990). Help-seeking behavior as a coping resource. In M. Rosenbaum (Ed.), *Learned resourcefulness: On coping skills, self-control, and adaptive behavior.* New York: Springer.

Naegle, M. A. (1995). Education, research, and theory development. In E. J. Sullivan (Ed.), *Nursing care of clients with substance abuse.* St. Louis: Mosby.

Najman, J. M., Morrison, J., Williams, G., Anderson, M., & Keeping, J. D. (1991). The mental health of women 6 months after they give birth to an unwanted baby: A longitudinal study. *Social Science Medicine, 32*, 241–247.

National Academy of Sciences. (1998). *Violence in families: Assessing prevention and treatment programs.* Washington, DC: National Academy Press.

National Alliance for the Mentally Ill Organization. (19xx). *Name of publication.* (Available from NAMI, 3 Colonial Place, 2107 Wilson Boulevard, Suite 300, Arlington, VA, 22201-3042; http://www.nami.org).

National Childhood Cancer Foundation. (1997). *Facts about childhood cancer.* Arcadia, CA: Author.

National Coalition for Homelessness. (1999). (Available from NCH, 1612 K. Street, NW #14, Washington, DC; http://www.ari.net.). Facts about homelessness.

National Depressive and Maniac-Depressive Association. (2000). (Available from NDMDA, P.O. Box 1939, Chicago, Illinois 60690; http://ndmda.org).

National Institute for Occupational Safety and Health. (1996). *Violence in the workplace: Risk factors and prevention strategies.* CIB#57. U.S. Department of Health and Human Services.

National Institute of Mental Health. (1991). *Caring for people with severe mental disorders: A national plan of research to improve services* (DHHS Publication No. ADM 91-1762). Washington, DC: U.S. Government Printing Office.

National Institute of Mental Health (NIMH). (1994). *Epidemiologic Catchment Area Project (ECA).* Washington, DC: Author.

National Institute of Mental Health's Special Depression Awareness, Recognition, and Treatment Program. (2000). (Available from National Institute of Mental Health, 5600 Fishers Lane, Room 15 C-06, Rockville, Maryland 30857; http://www.nimh.nih.gov/DART/).

National Institute on Alcohol Abuse and Alcoholism (NIAAA). (1993). *Eighth special report to US Congress: Alcohol and health* (DHHS Publication No. ADM 281-88-003). Alexandria, VA: Editorial Experts.

National Mental Health Association. (2000). (Available from NMHA, Information Center, 1021 Prince Street, Alexandria, VA 22314-2971; http://nmha.org).

Neal, M., & Briggs, M. (1999). *Validation therapy for dementia* [Online]. (Available from 113063.11@compuserve.com. The Cochrane Database of Systematic Reviews, 2. Cochrane Dementia & Cognitive Impairment Group).

Neelon, V. J., & Champagne, M. T. (1992). Managing cognitive impairment: The current bases for practice. In S. G. Funk, E. M. Tournquist, M. T. Champagne, & R. A. Weise (Eds.), *Key aspects for elder care: Managing falls, incontinence, and cognitive impairment* (pp. 239–250). New York: Springer.

Neighbors, H. W., & Jackson, C. S. (1996). Mental health in Black America: Psychosocial problems and help-seeking behavior. In H. W. Neighbors & J. S. Jackson (Eds.), *Mental health in Black America* (pp. 1–13). Thousand Oaks, CA: Sage.

Nelson, S. H., McCoy, G. F., Stetter, M., & Vanderwagen, W. C. (1992). An overview of mental health services for American Indians and Alaskan Natives in the 1990s. *Hospital and Community Psychiatry, 43,* 257–261.

Newell, M. (1997). Patient contracting for improved outcomes. *Journal of Care Management, 3*(4), 78–80.

Nolan, J. R., & Nolan-Haley, J. M. (Eds.) (1990). *Black's law dictionary* (16th ed.). St. Paul, MN: West.

Noordsy, D. L., Schwab, B., Fox, L., & Drake, R. E. (1996). The role of self-help programs in the rehabilitation of persons with severe mental illness and substance use disorders. *Community Mental Health Journal, 32*(3), 71–81.

Noppe, I. C., Noppe, L. D., & Hughes, F. P. (1991). Stress as a predictor of the quality of the quality of Parent-infant interactions. *The Journal of Genetic Psychology, 152*(1), 12–28.

Norbeck, J. S., & Anderson, N. J. (1989a). Life stress, social support, and anxiety in mid and late pregnancy among low income women. *Research in Nursing and Health, 12,* 281–287.

Norbeck, J. S., & Anderson, N. J. (1989b). Psychosocial predictors of pregnancy outcomes in Low income Black, Hispanic, and White women. *Nursing Research, 38,* 204–209.

Norris, F. (1992). Epidemiology of trauma: Frequency and impact of different potentially traumatic events on different demographic groups. *Journal of Consulting and Clinical Psychology, 60,* 409–418.

Norris, F., & Kaniasty, K. (1996). Received and perceived social support in times of stress: A test of the social support deterioration deterrence model. *Journal of Personality and Social Psychology, 71,* 498–511.

Norris, M., & Kennedy, C. (1992). The view from within: How patients perceive the seclusion process. *Journal of Psychosocial Nursing, 30*(3), 7–13.

North, C. S., Nixon, S. J., Shariat, S., Mallonee, S., McMillen, J. C., Spitznagel, E. L., & Smith, E. M. (1999). Psychiatric disorders among survivors of the Oklahoma City bombing. *Journal of the American Medical Association, 282*(8), 755–762.

Northouse, L. L. (1989a). A longitudinal study of the adjustment of patients and husbands to breast cancer. *Oncology Nursing Forum, 16,* 511–516.

Nyamathi, A. M. (1991). Relationship of resources to emotional distress, somatic complaints, and high-risk behaviors in drug recovery and homeless minority women. *Research in Nursing and Health, 14,* 269–277.

O'Connor, F. W. (1991). Symptom monitoring for relapse prevention in schizophrenia. *Archives of Psychiatric Nursing, 5,* 193–201.

O'Connor, F. W., Lovell, D., & Brown, L. (2000). *Implementing residential treatment for mentally ill prison inmates.* Manuscript in preparation.

O'Keefe, S. (1999). Delirium in the elderly. *Age and Ageing, 28-S2,* 5–8.

Olds, D., & Kitzmn, H. (1990). Can home visitation improve the health of women and children at environmental risk? *Pediatrics, 86,* 108–116.

Ollendick, T. H., & King, N. J. (1998). Empirically supported treatments for children with phobic and anxiety disorders: Current status. *Journal of Clinical Child Psychology, 27,* 156–167.

O'Nell, T. D. (1992–93). "Feeling worthless": An ethnographic investigation of depression and problem drinking at the Flathead reservation. *Culture Medicine and Psychiatry, 16*(4), 447–469.

Opie, N. (1992). Childhood and adolescent bereavement. In J. J. Fitzpatrick & J. S. Stevenson (Eds.), *Annual review of nursing research* (Vol. 10, pp. 127–141). New York: Springer Publishing.

Orlando, I. J. (1961). *The dynamic nurse-patient relationship.* New York: G. P. Putnam's Sons.

Osher, F. C., & Kofoed, L. L. (1989). Treatment of patients with psychiatric and psychoactive substance abuse disorders. *Hospital and Community Psychiatry, 40*(10), 1025–1030.

O'Toole, A. W., & Welt, S. (1980). *Interpersonal Theory in Nursing Practice: Selected Works of Hildegarde E. Peplau.* New York: Springer.

O'Toole, A., & Welt, S. (Eds.). (1989). *Interpersonal theory in nursing practice: Selected works of Hildegard E. Peplau.* New York: Springer Publishing.

Otto-Salaj, L. L., Kelly, J. A., & Stevenson, L. Y. (1998). Implementing cognitive-behavioral AIDS/HIV risk reduction group interventions in community mental health settings that serve people with serious mental illness. *Psychiatric Rehabilitation Journal, 21*(4), 394–404.

Paarlberg, K. M., Vingerhoets, A. J. J. M., Passchier, J., Dekker, G. A., Heinen, A. G. J. J., & van Geijn, H. P. (1999). Psychosocial predictors of low birthweight: A prospective study. *British Journal of Obstetrics and Gynaecology, 106,* 834–841.

Padgett, D. K., Patrick, C., Burns, B. J., & Schlesinger, H. J. (1995). Use of mental health services by black and white elderly. In D. K. Padgett (Ed.), *Handbook of ethnicity, aging, and mental health.* Westport, CT: Greenwood Press.

Padilla, G. V., Presant, C., Grant, M. M., Metter, G., Lipsett, J., & Heide, F. (1983). Quality of life index for patients with cancer. *Research in Nursing and Health, 6,* 117–126.

Pajarillo, E., Sers, A., Ryan, R., Headley, B., & Nalven, C. (1997). Consultation-liaison psychiatric nursing in long-term care. *Journal of Psychosocial Nursing, 35*(8), 24–30.

Palmer-Erbs, V. K., & Anthony, W. A. (1995). Incorporating psychiatric rehabilitation principles into mental health nursing. *Journal of Psychosocial Nursing and Mental Health Services, 33*(3), 36–44.

Parasuraman, R., & Haxby, J. V. (1993). Attention and brain function in Alzheimer's disease: A review. *Neuropsychology, 7*(3), 242–272.

Parker, L. D., Cantrell, C., & Demi, A. S. (1997). Older adults' attitudes toward suicide: Are there race and gender differences? *Death Studies, 21,* 289–298.

Parson, C. (1999). Managed care: The effect of case management on state psychiatric clients. *Journal of Psychiatric Nursing, 37*(10), 16–21.

Pary, R., Lippmann, S., & Tobias, C. R. (1988). A preventive approach to the suicidal patient. *The Journal of Family Practice, 26,* 185–189.

Pasacreta, J. V., & Pickett, M. (1998). Psychosocial aspects of palliative care. *Seminars in Oncology Nursing, 14*(2), 110–120.

Patterson, M. M. (1998). Child abuse assessment and intervention. *Orthopaedic Nursing, 17*(1), 49–56.

Paulk, D. (1999). Recognizing child abuse, child abusers, and individuals who are likely to abuse. *Physician Assistant, 23*(5), 38.

Pearson, J., Hunter, A., Ensminger, M., & Kellam, S. (1990). Black grandmothers in multigenerational households: Diversity in family structure and parenting involvement in the Woodlawn Community. *Child Development, 64,* 434–442.

Pelham, T. W., & Campagna, P. D. (1991). Benefits of exercise in psychiatric rehabilitation of persons with schizophrenia. *Canadian Journal of Rehabilitation, 4*(3), 159–168.

Penckofer, S. M., & Holm, K. (1990). Women undergoing coronary artery bypass surgery: Physiological and psychological perspectives. *Cardiovascular Nursing, 26,* 13–18.

Pender, N. (1985). Effects of progressive muscle relaxation training on anxiety and health locus of control among hypertensive adults. *Research in Nursing and Health, 8,* 67–72.

Pender, N. J., & Pender, A. J. (1987). *Health promotion in nursing practice.* Norwalk, CT: Appleton & Lange.

Pennebaker, J. W., Burnam, M. A., Schaeffer, M. A., & Harper, D. C. (1977). Lack of control as a determinant of perceived physical symptoms. *Journal of Personality and Social Psychology, 35,* 167–174.

Pennix, B. W., van Tilburg, T., Boekke, A. J., Deeg, D. J., Kriegsman, D. M., & van Eijk, J. T. (1998). Effects of social support and personal coping resources on depressive symptoms: different for various chronic diseases? *Health Psychology, 17*(6), 551–558.

Peplau, H. (1952). *Interpersonal relations in nursing.* New York: G. P. Putnam & Sons.

Peplau, H. (1988). The art and science of nursing: Similarities, differences, and relations. *Nursing Science Quarterly, 1,* 8–15.

Peplau, H. (1992). Interpersonal relations: A theoretical framework for application in nursing practice. *Nursing Science Quarterly, 5,* 13–18.

Peplau, H. E. (1997). Peplau's theory of interpersonal relations. *Nursing Science Quarterly, 10*(4), 162–167.

Perese, E. F. (1997). Unmet needs of persons with chronic mental illnesses: Relationship to their adaptation to community living. *Issues in Mental Health Nursing, 18,* 19–34.

Perlick, D., Clarkin, J. F., Sirey, J., Raue, P., Greenfield, S., Struening, E., & Rosenheck, R. (1999). Burden experienced by care-givers of persons with bipolar affective disorder. *British Journal of Psychiatry, 175,* 56–62.

Peterman, B. A., Springer, P., & Farnsworth, J. (1995). Analyzing job demand and coping techniques. *Nursing Management, 26*(2), 51–53.

Peternelj-Taylor, C. (1999). Care of individuals in correctional facilities. In C. Glod (Ed.), *Contemporary psychiatric-mental health nursing: The brain-behavior connection* (pp. 621–633). Philadelphia: Davis.

Petrila, J. (1998). Law and government: What's down the road and how will it impact mental health? *The Future of Mental Health Services* (pp. 13–17). Premeeting briefing papers. Washington, DC: National Technical Assistance Center.

Phelan, M., Slade, M., Thornicroft, G., Dunn, G., Holloway, F., Wykes, T., Strathdee, G., Loftus, L., McCrone, P., & Hayward, P. (1995). The Camberell Assessment of Need. *British Journal of Psychiatry, 167,* 589–595.

Phillips, E. L. (1999). *A Guide for Therapists and Patients to Short-Term Psychotherapy.* Springfield, IL: Charles C. Thomas Publisher.

Picot, S. J. F., Zauszniewski, J. A., & Delgado, C. (1997). Cardiovascular responses of African female caregivers. *Journal of National Black Nurses' Association, 9*(1), 3–21.

Pierce, J. P., Fiore, M. C., Novotny, T. E., Hatziandreu, E. J., & Davis, R. M. (1989). Trends in cigarette smoking in the United States projection to the year 2000. *Journal of the American Medical Association, 261,* 61–65.

Pike, A. W. (1990). On the nature and place of empathy in clinical nursing practice. *Journal of Professional Nursing, 6,* 235–241.

Pirraglia, P. A., Peterson, J. C., Williams-Russo, P., Gorkin, L., & Charlson, M. E. (1999). Depressive symptomatology in coronary artery bypass graft surgery patients. *International Journal of Geriatric Psychiatry, 14,* 668–680.

Plant, M. L., Plant, M. A., & Foster, J. (1999). Alcohol, tobacco, and illicit drug use amongst nurses: A Scottish study. *Drug and Alcohol Dependence, 28,* 195–202.

Plutchik, R., Karusu, T. B., Conte, H. K., Siegel, B., & Jerrett, I. (1978). Toward a rationale for the seclusion process. *The Journal of Nervous and Mental Disease, 166*(8), 571–579.

Pollack, L. E. (1996). Information seeking among people with manic-depressive illness. *Image—the Journal of Nursing Scholarship, 28*(3), 259–265.

Pollack, L. E., & Steubben, G. (1998). Addiction Education Groups for inpatients with dual diagnoses. *Journal of the American Psychiatric Nurses Association, 4,* 121–127.

Pollack, L. E., Steubben, G., & Sobhan, T. (1997). Dually diagnosed inpatients' satisfaction with addiction groups. *Journal of Psychosocial Nursing and Mental Health Services, 35*(7), 18–23.

Pratt, C., Gill, K., Barrett, N., & Roberts, M. (1999). *Psychiatric rehabilitation.* New York: Academic Press.

Price Spratlen, L. (1994). Perceived workplace mistreatment in higher education. *AAOHN Journal, 42*(11), 285–297.

Price Spratlen, L. (1995). Interpersonal conflict which includes mistreatment. *Violence and Victims, 10*(4), 295–298.

Priest, R. (1991). Racism and prejudice as negative impacts on African American clients in therapy. *Journal of Counseling and Development, 70,* 213–215.

Prochaska, J., Di Clemente, C., & Norcross, J. (1992). In search of how people change: application to addictive behaviors. *American Psychologist, 47,* 1102–1114.

Proctor, A., Morse, J. M., & Khonsari, E. S. (1996). Sounds of comfort in the trauma center: How nurses talk to patients in pain. *Social Science and Medicine, 42,* 1669–1680.

Project Achieve (2000). The Breaking Cycle of Homelessness. (Available at http://www.homelessness.net/).

Puskar, K., Lamb, J., & Tusaie-Mumford, K. (1997). Teaching kids to cope: A preventive mental health nursing strategy for adolescents. *Journal of Child and Adolescent Psychiatric Nursing, 10*(3), 18–28.

Quinn, J. (1984). Therapeutic touch as energy exchange: Testing the theory. *Advances in Nursing Science, 6*(2), 42–49.

Raaz, N., Carlson-Sabelli, L., & Sabelli, H. C. (1992). Psychodrama in the treatment of multiple personality disorder: A process-theory perspective. In E. Kluft (Ed.), *Expressive and functional therapies in the treatment of Multiple Personality Disorder* (pp. 169–188). Springfield, IL: Charles Thomas.

Rankin, S. H. (1987). Differences in recovery from cardiac surgery: A profile of male and female patients. *Heart and Lung, 19,* 481–485.

Rapp, C. G., Wakefiled, B., Kundrat, M., Mentes, J., Tripp-Reimer, T., Culp, K., Mobily, P., Akins, J., & Onega, L. L. (2000). Acute confusion assessment instruments: Clinical versus research usability. *Applied Nursing Research, 13*(1), 37–45.

Rapp, S. R., Shumaker, S., Schmidt, S., Naughton, M., & Anderson, R. (1998). Social resourcefulness: Its relationship to social support and well-being among caregivers of dementia victims. *Aging and Mental Health, 2*(1), 40–48.

Rardin, D. (1988). *Wind River health promotion program.* Lander, WY: Fremont Counseling Service.

Reed, A. (1996, August). Economies with "the truth": Professionals' narratives about lying and deception in mental health practice. *Journal of Psychiatric and Mental Health Nursing, 3*(4), 249–256.

Reed, P. (1996a). Peplau's interpersonal relations model. In J. Fitzpatrick & A. Whall (Eds.), *Conceptual models of nursing* (3rd ed., pp. 55–76). Stanford, CT: Appleton & Lange.

Reed, P. (1996b). Transforming practice knowledge into nursing knowledge: A revisionist analysis of Peplau. *Image: Journal of Nursing Scholarship, 29,* 29–33.

Regier, D. A., Farmer, M. E., Rae, D. S., Locke, B. Z., Keith, S. J., Judd, L. L., & Goodwin, F. K. (1990). Comorbidity of mental disorders with alcohol and other drug abuse: Results from the Epidemiologic Catchment Area (ECA) Study. *Journal of the American Medical Association, 264*(19), 2511–2518.

Rehm, L. P. (1977). A self-control model of depression. *Behavior Therapy, 8,* 787–804.

Reiger, D. A., Narrow, W. E., Rae, D. S., Manderscheid, R. W., Locke, B. Z., & Goodwin, F. K. (1993). The de facto US mental and addictive disorders service system. Epidemiologic Catchment Area perspective 1-year prevalence rates of disorders and services. *Archives of General Psychiatry, 50,* 85–94.

Reiss, D., & Price, R. H. (1996). National research agenda for prevention research: The National Institute of Mental Health report. *American Psychologist, 51*(11), 1109–1115.

Remer, R. (1997). Chaos theory and the Hollander psychodrama curve: Trusting the process. *International Journal of Action Methods: Psychodrama, Skill Training, and Role Playing, 50*(2), 51–70.

Remer, R., & Betts, G. R. (1998). The difference between strict analogue and interpersonal psychodramatic simulation (IPS) methods in research on human dynamical systems. *International Journal of Action Methods, 51,* 3–22.

Resnick, M. P. (1993). Treating nicotine addiction in patients with psychiatric comorbidity. In C. T. Orleans & J. Slade (Eds.), *Nicotine addiction: Principles and management* (pp. 556–563). New York: Oxford University Press.

Reynolds, W. J. (1986). Peplau's theory in practice. *Nursing Science Quarterly, 10*(4), 168–170.

Rhodes, L. (1998, Winter). Panoptical intimacies. *Public Culture, 10*(2), 285–311.

Richardson, L. A., Keller, A. M., Selby-Harrington, M. L., & Parrish, R. (1996). Identification and treatment of children's mental health problems by primary care providers: A critical review of research. *Archives of Psychiatric Nursing, 10*(5), 293–303.

Richter, J. M., Roberto, K. A., & Bottenberg, D. J. (1995, October). Communicating with persons with Alzheimer's disease: Experiences of family and formal caregivers. *Archives of Psychiatric Nursing, 9*(5), 279–285.

Riddle, C. (1994). Development of an adolescent inpatient sexual abuse group: Application of Lewin's Model of Change. *Journal of Child and Adolescent Psychiatric Nursing, 7*(1), 17–24.

Ridgely, M. S., & Jerrell, J. M. (1996). Analysis of three interventions for substance abuse treatment of severely mentally ill people. *Community Mental Health Journal, 32*(6), 561–572.

Rimon, D. (1980). *Children's assessment of self-control: Development of a scale*. Unpublished master's thesis, Tel-Aviv University: Tel-Avis, Israel.

Ripich, S., Moore, S. M., & Brennan, P. F. (1992). A new nursing medium: Computer networks for group intervention. *Journal of Psychosocial Nursing and Mental Health Services, 30*(7), 15–20.

Robb, J. C., Young, L. T., Cooke, R. G., & Joffe, R. T. (1998). Gender differences in patients with bipolar disorder influence outcome in the medical outcomes survey (SF-20) subscale scores. *Journal of Affective Disorders, 49*(3), 189–193.

Roberts, D. (1997). Liaison mental health nursing: Origins, definitions and prospects. *Journal of Advanced Nursing, 25,* 101–108.

Roberts, D. (1998). Nurses' perceptions of the role of liaison mental health nurse. *Nursing Times, 94*(43), 56–57.

Robins, L. N., & Kulbok, P. A. (1986). Methodological strategies in suicide. In J. J. Mann & M. Stanley (Eds.), *Annals of the New York Academy of Science: Vol. 487. Psychobiology of suicidal behavior* (pp. 1–15). New York: New York Academy of Sciences.

Robinson, J. H. (1995). Grief responses, coping processes, and social support of widows: Research with Roy's model. *Nursing Science Quarterly, 8,* 158–164.

Rose, L. E. (1996). Families of psychiatric patients: A critical review and future research directions. *Archives of Psychiatric Nursing, X*(2), 67–76.

Rose, L. E. (1998). Gaining control: Family members relate to persons with severe mental illness. *Research in Nursing & Health, 21*(4), 363–373.

Rosenbach, M. L., Hermann, R. C., & Dorwart, R. A. (1997). Use of electroconvulsive therapy in the Medicare population between 1987 and 1992. *Psychiatric Services, 48*(12), 1537–1542.

Rosenbaum, M. (1990). The role of learned resourcefulness in the self-control of health behavior. In M. Rosenbaum (Ed.), *Learned resourcefulness: On coping skills, self-control, and adaptive behavior.* New York: Springer.

Rosenberg, S. D., Drake, R. E., Wolford, G. E., Meuser, K. T., Oxman, T. E., Vidaver, R. M., Carrieri, K. L., & Luckoor, R. (1998). Dartmouth Assessment of Lifestyle Instrument (DALI): A substance use disorder screen for people with severe mental illness. *American Journal of Psychiatry, 155*(2), 232–238.

Rosenburg, M. L., Smith, J. C., Davidson, L. E., & Conn, J. M. (1987). The emergence of youth suicide: An epidemiological analysis and public health perspective. *Annual Review of Public Health, 8,* 417–440.

Rosswurm, M. A. (1991). Attention-focusing program for persons with dementia. *Clinical Gerontologist, 10,* 3–16.

Roth, D., Lauber, B. B., Crane-Ross, D., & Clark, J. A. (1997). Impact of state mental health reform on patterns of service delivery. *Community Mental Health Journal, 33*(6), 473–485.

Royall, D. R. (1999). Frontal systems impairment in major depression. *Seminars in Neuropsychiatry, 4*(1), 13–23.

Ruiz, P. (1995). Assessing, diagnosing and treating culturally diverse individuals: A Hispanic perspective. *Psychiatric Quarterly, 66,* 329–341.

Rundell, S. (1991, September). A study of nurse-patient interaction in a high dependency unit. *Intensive Care Nursing, 7*(3), 171–178.

Rutter, M. (1987). Psychosocial resilience and protective mechanisms. *American Journal of Orthopsychiatry, 57,* 316–331.

Sabelli, H. (1989). *Union of opposites: A comprehensive theory of natural and human processes.* Lawrenceville, VA: Brunswick.

Sabelli, H. C., & Carlson-Sabelli, L. (1995). Sociodynamics: The application of process methods to the social sciences. In A. Albert (Ed.), *Chaos and society* (pp. 117–140). Amsterdam: I. O. S. Press.

Sabourin, C. B., & Funk, M. (1999). Readmission of patients after coronary artery bypass graft surgery. *Heart and Lung, 28,* 243–250.

Sailaja, B. V., & Swaminathan, V. D. (1992). Working and nonworking pregnant women on state and trait anxiety. *Psychological Studies, 37,* 173–177.

Sailas, E., & Fenton, M. (1999). Seclusion and restraint as a method of treatment for people with serious mental illnesses (Cochrane Review). *Cochrane Library,* (3).

Samarel, N., Fawcett, J., & Tulman, L. (1997). Effect of support groups with coaching on adaptation to early stage breast cancer. *Research in Nursing and Health, 20*(1), 15–26.

Sandman, C. A., Wadhwa, P. D., Chicz-Demet, A., Dunkel-Schetter, C., & Porto, M. (1997). Maternal stress, HPA activity, and fetal/infant outcome. *Annals New York Academy of Sciences, 814,* 266–275.

Satcher, D. (1999). *Mental health: A report of the Surgeon General.* Washington, DC: U.S. Department of Health and Human Services.

Schaeffer, C. E. (1998). Play therapy: Critical issues for the next millennium. *Association for Play Therapy, Inc. Newsletter, 17*(1), 1–5.

Schepp, K. G. (1992a). A symptom management program for adolescents with psychotic illnesses: Theoretical basis. *Journal of Child and Adolescent Psychiatric Mental Health Nursing, 5*(4), 7–12.

Schepp, K. G. (1992b). A symptom management program for psychotically ill adolescents and their families: Preliminary clinical outcomes. *Journal of Child and Adolescent Psychiatric Mental Health Nursing, 5*(4), 13–17.

Schepp, K. G., O'Connor, F. W., Kennedy, M., Tsi, J. H. C., Davidson, B., Sekijima, M., Stein, J., & Chen, C. C. A. (1999). Family Centered Program for Adolescents with Mental Illness. *Communicating Nursing Research, 32.*

Schlotfeldt, R. (1975). The need for a conceptual framework. In P. Verhonic (Ed.), *Nursing research* (pp. 3–25). Boston: Little, Brown.

Schulmeister, L. (1999). Starting a nursing consultation practice. *Clinical Nurse Specialist, 13*(2), 94–100.

Schumacher, K. L. (1996). Reconceptualizing family caregiving: Family-based illness care during chemotherapy. *Research in Nursing and Health, 19*(4), 261–271.

Schwab, J. J, Stephenson, J. J., & Ice, J. F. (1993). Family research. In *Evaluating family mental health: History, epidemiology, and treatment issues* (pp. 157–226). New York: Plenum.

Seligman, M. (1975). *Helplessness: On depression, development, and death.* San Francisco: W. H. Freeman.

Seligman, M. E. P., & Csikszentmihalyi, M. (2000). Positive psychology: An introduction. Special issue on happiness, excellence, and optimal human functioning. *American Psychologist, 55*(1), 5–14.

Selye, H. (1976). *The stress of life* (2nd ed.). New York: McGraw-Hill.

Shariat, S., Mallonee, S., Kruger, E., Farmer, K., & North, C. (1999). A prospective study of long-term health outcomes among Oklahoma City bombing survivors. *Journal of Oklahoma State Medical Association, 92*(4), 178–186.

Sheehan, K. H., Sheehan, D. V., White, K., Leibowitz, A., & Baldwin, D. C. (1990). A pilot study of medical student "abuse": Student perceptions of mistreatment and misconduct in medical school. *Journal of the American Medical Association, 263,* 533–537.

Shelton, D. (1998). Estimates of emotional disorder in detained and committed youth in the Maryland juvenile justice system. *Proceedings of the Annual Systems of Care for Children, 11,* 9–15.

Shelton, D. (2000). *Aids and drug use prevention intervention for confined youthful offenders.* Manuscript submitted for publication.

Shepherd, G., & Hill, R. G. (1996). Manic depression: Do people receive adequate support? *Nursing Times, 92*(26), 42–44.

Shinn, M., & Weitzman, B. (1996). Homeless families are different. In *Homelessness in America.* Washington, DC: National Coalition for the Homeless.

Shires, B., & Tappan, T. (1992). The clinical nurse specialist as brief psychotherapist. *Perspectives in Psychiatric Care, 28*(4), 15–18.

Shorto, R. (1999). *Saints and madmen: Psychiatry opens its doors to religion.* New York: Henry Holt and Company.

Shulman, K. I., & Herrmann, N. (1999). The nature of management of mania in old age. *Psychiatric Clinics of North America, 22*(3), 649–665.

Silver, H. K., & Glicken, A. D. (1990). Medical student abuse: Incidence, severity, and significance. *Journal of the American Medical Association, 263,* 527–532.

Simmons, M. (1982). Psychiatric consultation and liaison. In D. Critchley & J. Maurin (Eds.), *The clinical specialist in psychiatrist mental health nursing: Theory, research and practice* (pp. 362–381). New York: Wiley.

Simon, G. E., & Unutzer, J. (1999). Health care utilization and costs among patients treated for bipolar disorder in an insured population. *Psychiatric Services, 50*(10), 1303–1308.

Simon, R. I. (1998). Psychiatrist awake! Suicide risk assessments are all about a good night's sleep. *Psychiatric Annals, 28*(9), 479–485.

Simpson, H. (1991). *Peplau's model in action.* London: Macmillan.

Singh, U., & Saxena, M. S. (1991). Anxiety during pregnancy and after childbirth. *Psychological Studies, 36*(2), 108–111.

Slavinsky, A. T., & Krauss, J. B. (1982). Two approaches to the management of long-term psychiatric outpatients in the community. *Nursing Research, 33,* 284–289.

Sleven, P., & Claiborne, W. (2000, March 1). First grader shoots classmate to death. *The Washington Post,* p. A01.

Sloper, P., & While, D. (1996). Risk factors in the adjustment of siblings of children with cancer. *Journal of Child Psychology, Psychiatry and Allied Disciplines, 37,* 597–607.

Smith, G. R., Rost, K., & Kashner, M. A. (1995). Trial of the effect of a standardized psychiatric consultation on health outcomes and costs in somatizing patients. *Archives of General Psychiatry, 52,* 238–243.

Smith, J. A. (1983). *The idea of health implications for the nursing professional.* New York: Columbia University.

Smith, M., Buckwalter, L., & Albanese, M. (1990). Psychiatric nursing consultation: A different choice for nursing homes. *Journal of Psychosocial Nursing and Mental Health Services, 28*(3), 23–27.

Smith, S. B. (1995). Restraints: Retraumatization for rape victims? *Journal of Psychosocial Nursing, 33*(7), 23–28.

Snowden, L. R., & Cheung, F. K. (1990). Use of inpatient mental health services by members of ethnic minority groups. *American Psychologist, 45,* 347–355.

Snyder, M. (1993). The influence of intervention on the stress-health outcome linkage. In J. S. Barnfather & B. L. Lyon (Eds.), *Stress and coping: State of the science and implications for nursing theory, research and practice* (pp. 159–170). Indianapolis, IN: Sigma Theta Tau International.

Snyder, M. (1997, April). *The influence of interventions on the stress-health outcomes linkage.* Paper presented at Midwest Nursing Research Society preconference. Minneapolis.

Sobo, E. J. (1995). *Choosing unsafe sex: AIDS-risk denial among disadvantaged women.* Philadelphia: University of Pennsylvania Press.

Soliday, S. M. (1985). A comparison of patient and staff attitudes toward seclusion. *Journal of Nervous and Mental Disease, 173,* 282–286.

Solomon, J., & Marx, J. (1999). Who cares? Grandparent/grandchild households. *Journal of Women & Aging, 11*(1), 3–25.

Solomon, P. (1997). Issues in designing and conducting randomized human service trials: Lessons from the field. *Journal of Social Service Research, 22*(4), 57–77.

Solomon, P., & Draine, J. (1995). Subjective burden among family members of mentally ill adults: Relation to stress, coping, and adaptation. *American Journal of Orthopsychiatry, 65,* 419–427.

Sousa, K. H., Holzemer, W. L., Henry, S. B., & Slaughter, R. (1999). Dimensions of health-related quality of life in persons living with HIV disease. *Journal of Advanced Nursing, 29*(1), 178–187.

Spector, A., Orrell, M., Davies, S., & Woods, B. (1999). Reality orientation for dementia [nline]. (Available at *a.spector@ucl.ac.uk.edu.*). The Cochrane Database of Systematic Reviews, 2. Cochrane Dementia & Cognitive Impairment Group.

Spilker, B., Simpson, R. L. Jr., & Tilson, H. H. (1991). Quality of life bibliography and indexes: 1991 update. *Journal of Clinical Research in Pharmacoepidemiology, 6,* 205–266.

Spinnetta, J. (1981). The siblings of the child with cancer. In J. Spinetta & P. Spinetta (Eds.), *Living with childhood cancer.* St. Louis, MO: Mosby.

Spitz, R. (1945). Hospitalism: An inquiry into the genesis of psychiatric conditions in early childhood. *Psychoanalytic Study of the Child, 1,* 52–74.

Staff. (1993, Spring). NCNR conference sets research priorities. *Southern Connections, 4.*

Stanhope, M. (1990). An innovative approach to health care for the homeless/very poor: A nurse managed clinic. Washington, DC: U.S. Department of Commerce, National Technical Information Service.

Starfield, B. (1992). *Primary care: Concept evaluation and policy.* New York: Oxford University Press.

Steadman, H., & Cocozza, J. (Eds.). (1993). *Mental illness in America's prisons.* Seattle, WA: The National Coalition for the Mentally Ill in the Criminal Justice System.

Stein, K. F., & Hedger, K. (1997). Body weight and shape self-cognitions, emotional distress and disordered eating in middle adolescent girls. *Archives of Psychiatric Nursing, 11*(5), 264–275.

Stein, K. F., & Nyquist, L. (2000). *The impoverished self: Identity disturbances and the eating disorders*. Manuscript submitted for publication.

Steptoe, A. (1991). The links between stress and illness. *Journal of Psychosomatic Research, 35*, 633–644.

Stewart, C. (1995). Cultural consideration. In D. Anatai-Otong (Ed.), *Psychiatric nursing: Biological and behavioral concepts* (pp. 47–64). Philadelphia: Saunders.

Stickney, S. (1981). Psychiatric nurse consultation: who calls and why. *Journal of Psychiatric Nursing and Mental Health Services, 19*(10), 22–26.

Storr, C. L., Trinkoff, A. M., & Anthony, J. C. (1999). Job strain and non-medical drug use. *Drug and Alcohol Dependence, 55,* 45–51.

Strawbridge, W., Wallhagen, M., Shema, S., & Kaplan, G. (1997). New burdens or more of the same? Comparing adult grandparent, spouse and adult-child caregivers. *Gerontologist, 37*(4), 505–510.

Striegel-Moore, R., Silberstein, L., & Rodin, J. (1986). Toward an understanding of risk factors for bulimia. *American Psychologist, 41*(3), 246–263.

Strober, M., Freeman, R., Rigali, J., Schmidt, S., & Diamond, R. (1992). The pharmacotherapy of depressive illness in adolescence: Effects of lithium augmentation in nonresponders to imipramine. *Journal of the Academy of Child and Adolescent Psychiatry, 31*(1), 16–49.

Stuve, P., Erickson, R. C., & Spaulding, W. (1991). Cognitive rehabilitation: The next step in psychiatric rehabilitation. *Psychosocial Rehabilitation Journal, 15*(1), 9–26.

Styron, W. (1990). *Darkness visible*. New York: Random House.

Sue, D. W., & Sue, D. (1990). *Counseling the culturally different*. New York: Wiley.

Sue, S. (1998). In search of cultural competence in psychotherapy and counseling. *American Psychologist, 53*(4), 440–448.

Sue, S., Zane, N., & Young, K. (1994). Research on psychotherapy with culturally diverse populations. In A. E. Bergin & S. L. Garfield (Eds.), *Handbook of psychotherapy and behavioral change* (4th ed., pp. 783–817). New York: Wiley.

Sullivan, E. J. (1995). *Nursing care of clients with substance abuse*. St. Louis: Mosby.

Sullivan, E. J., Bissell, L., & Leffler, D. L. (1990). Drug use and disciplinary actions among 300 nurses. *International Journal of Addictions, 25*(4), 375–391.

Sullivan-Marx, E. M. (1994). Delirium and physical restraint in the hospitalized elderly. *IMAGE: Journal of Nursing Scholarship, 26,* 295–300.

Suppes, T., & A. John Rush (1996). Evolving clinical characteristics or distinct disorders? In K. I. Shulman, M. Tohen, & S. P. Kutcher (Eds.), *Mood disorders across the life span* (pp. 3–16). New York: Wiley-Liss.

Sutherland, J. A. (1993). The nature and evolution of phenomenological empathy in nursing: An historical treatment. *Archives of Psychiatric Nursing, 7,* 369–376.

Szinovacz, M., DeViney, S., & Atkinson, M. (1999). Effects of surrogate parenting on grandparents' well-being. *Journal of Gerontology, 54B*(6), D376–D388.

Szmukler, G., Burgess, P., Herrman, H., Benson, A., Colusa, S., & Bloch, S. (1996). Caring for relatives with serious mental illness. *Social Psychiatry & Psychiatric Epidemiology, 31,* 137–148.

Tabora, B., & Flaskerud, J. H. (1994). Depression among Chinese Americans: A review of the literature. *Issues in Mental Health Nursing, 15*(6), 569–584.

Takeucchi, D. T., & Uehara, E. S. (1996). Ethnic minority mental health services: Current research and future directions. In B. L. Levin & J. Petrila (Eds.), *Mental health services: A public health perspective* (pp. 63–80). New York: Oxford University Press.

Talley, S. L. (1999). *Self-regulation activities used by individuals with schizophrenia.* Unpublished doctoral dissertation, University of Utah, Salt Lake City.

Talley, S., Davis, D., Goicoechea, N., Brown, L., & Barber, L. (1990). Effect of psychiatric liaison nurse specialist consultation on the care of medical-surgical patients with sitters. *Archives of Psychiatric Nursing, IV*(2), 114–123.

Tappen, R. M., Williams-Burgess, C., Edelstein, J., Touhy, T., & Fishman, S. (1997, October). Communicating with individuals with Alzheimer's disease: Examination of recommended strategies. *Archives of Psychiatric Nursing, 11*(5), 249–256.

Tardiff, K. (1984). *The psychiatric uses of seclusion and restraint.* Washington, DC: American Psychiatric Press.

Taylor, A., & Taylor, R. S. (1998). Neuropsychologic aspects of multiple sclerosis. *Physical Medicine & Rehabilitation Clinics of North America, 9*(3), 643–657.

Taylor, O. (1989). The effects of cultural assumptions on cross-cultural communication. In D. Koslow & E. Salett (Eds.), *Crossing cultures in mental health* (pp. 18–27). Washington, DC: SIETAR International.

Teague, G. B., Drake, R. E., & Ackerson, T. H. (1995). Evaluating use of continuous treatment teams for persons with mental illness and substance abuse. *Psychiatric Services, 46*(7), 689–695.

Terr, L. (1991). Childhood trauma: An outline and overview. *American Journal of Psychiatry, 148,* 10–20.

Tetrick, L. E., & LaRocco, J. M. (1987). Understanding, prediction and control as moderators of the relationships between perceived stress, satisfaction and psychological well being. *Journal of Applied Psychology, 72,* 538–543.

The Institute for Health & Aging, University of California, San Francisco. (1996, August). *Chronic care in America: A 21st century challenge.* Princeton: Robert Wood Johnson Foundation.

Thomas, M. D., Brandt, P. A., & O'Connor, F. W. (1999). Preparing psychosocial nurse practitioners for health care delivery. *Archives of Psychiatric Nursing, XIII*(5), 227–233.

Tilley, S., Pollock, L., & Tait, L. (1999). Discourses on empowerment. *Journal of Psychiatric and Mental Health Nursing, 6,* 53–60.

Timberlake, N., Klinger, L., Smith, P., Venn, G., Treasure, T., Harrison, M., & Newman, S. (1997). Incidence and patterns of depression following coronary artery bypass graft surgery. *Journal of Psychosomatic Research, 43*(2), 197–207.

Timmerman, G. (1998). Caloric intake patterns of nonpurge binge-eating women. *Western Journal of Nursing Research, 20*(1), 103–118.

Timmerman, G., & Stevenson, J. (1996). The relationship between binge eating severity and body fat in nonpurge binge eating women. *Research in Nursing & Health, 19,* 389–396.

Tomlinson, P. S., & Irwin, B. L. (1993). Qualitative study of women's reports of family adaptation pattern four years following transition to parenthood. *Issues in Mental Health Nursing, 14*(2), 119–138.

Tondo, L., & Baldessarini, R. J. (1998a). Rapid cycling in women and men with bipolar manic-depressive disorders. *American Journal of Psychiatry, 155*(10), 1434–1436.

Tondo, L., Baldessarini, R. J., Hennen, J., & Floris, G. (1998b). Lithium maintenance treatment of depression and mania in bipolar I and bipolar II disorders. *American Journal of Psychiatry, 155*(5), 638–645.

Tooke, S., & Brown, J. (1992). Perceptions of seclusion: Comparing patient and staff reactions. *Journal of Psychosocial Nursing, 30*(8), 23–26.

Torrance, G. W. (1987). Utility approach to measuring health-related quality of life. *Journal of Chronic Diseases, 40*, 593–603.

Torres, S. (1999). Barriers to mental-health-care access faced by Hispanic elders. In M. L. Wykle & A. B. Ford (Eds.), *Serving minority elders in the 21st century* (pp. 200–218). New York: Springer.

Travelbee, J. (1972). *Interpersonal aspects of nursing* (2nd ed.). Philadelphia: F. A. Davis.

Trinkoff, A. M., Eaton, W. W., & Anthony, J. C. (1991). *Nursing Research, 40*(3), 172–175.

Trinkoff, A. M., & Storr, C. L. (1998). Substance use among nurses: Differences between specialties. *American Journal of Public Health, 88,* 581–584.

Trinkoff, A. M., Storr, C. L., & Wall, M. P. (1999). Prescription-type drug misuse and workplace access among nurses. *Journal of Addictive Diseases, 18*(1), 9–17.

Trzepacz, P. (1999). Update on the neuropathogenesis of delirium. *Dementia and Geriatric Cognitive Disorders, 10,* 330–334.

Tucker, C., Barker, A., & Gregoire, A. (1998). Living with schizophrenia: Caring for person with a severe mental illness. *Social Psychiatry and Epidemiology, 33*, 305–309.

Turner, S. M., & Cooley-Quille, M. R. (1996). Sociological and sociocultural variables in psychopharmacological research: Methodological considerations. *Psychopharmacology Bulletin, 32,* 183–192.

U.S. Bureau of the Census. (1995). *Statistical Abstract of the United States (115th ed.).* Table 127, Deaths by Age and Leading Causes of Deaths in 1992, p. 94. Washington, DC: U.S. Government Printing Office.

U.S. Conference of Mayors. (1998). *A Status Report on Hunger and Homelessness in America's Cities*. Washington, DC: U. S. Conference of Mayors.

U.S. Department of Agriculture, Rural Economic and Community Development. *Rural Homelessness: Focusing on the Needs of the Rural Homeless* (1996). Washington, DC: U.S. Department of Agriculture, Rural Housing Service, Rural Economic and Community Development.

U.S. Department of Health and Human Services. (1991). *Healthy People 2000: National health promotion and disease prevention objectives*. Washington, DC: DHHS Publication No. 91-50212.

U.S. Department of Health and Human Services. (1994). *Preventing tobacco use among young people: A report of the surgeon general.* Atlanta: U.S. Department of Health and Human Services, Public Health Service, Centers for Disease Control and Prevention, National Center for Chronic Disease Prevention and Health Promotion, Office on Smoking and Health.

U.S. Department of Health and Human Services (USDHHS). (1999). *Mental health: A report of the Surgeon General.* Rockville, MD: US Department of Health and Human Services, Substance Abuse and Mental Health Services Administration, Center for Mental Health Services, National Institutes of Health, National Institute of Mental Health.

U.S. Department of Health and Human Services, Center for Mental Health Services. (1999). Mental health: A report of the Surgeon General. Rockville, MD: DHHS.

U.S. Department of Labor, Bureau of Labor Statistics. (1995). *Survey of occupational injuries and illnesses, work injuries and illnesses by selected characteristics, 1993.*

U.S. Health and Human Services. (1995). Double Jeopardy: Persons with mental illness in the criminal justice system. Report to Congress, Februrary 24, 1995.

U.S. Public Health Service. (1995). *Healthy people 2000: Midcourse review and 1995 revisions.* Washington, DC: U.S. Department of Health and Human Services.

University of California, San Francisco School of Nursing Symptom Management Faculty Group. (1994). A model for symptom management. *Image: Journal of Nursing Scholarship, 26,* 272–276.

Unutzer, J., Simon, G., Pabiniak, C., Bond, K., & Katon, W. (2000). The use of administrative data to assess quality of care for bipolar disorder in a large staff model HMO. *General Hospital Psychiatry, 22*(1), 1–10.

Ursano, R. J., & Fullerton, C. S. (1997). Trauma, time, and recovery. In C. S. Fullerton & R. J. Ursano (Eds.), *Posttraumatic stress disorder* (pp. 269–274). Washington, DC: American Psychiatric Press.

Valente, S. M. (1994). Messages of psychiatric patients who attempted or committed suicide. *Clinical Nursing Rsearch, 3,* 316–333.

Valente, S. M., Saunders, J. M., & Grant, M. (1994). Oncology nurses knowledge and misconceptions about suicide. *Journal of Cancer Care, 2,* 209–216.

Valente, S., Saunders, J. M., & Uman, G. (1993). Self-care, psychological distress and HIV disease. *Journal of the Association of Nurses in AIDS Care, 4,* 15–25.

Van Dongen-Melman, J., De Groot, A., Hahlen, K., & Verhulst, F. (1995). Siblings of childhood cancer survivors: How does this "forgotten" group of children adjust after cessation of successful cancer treatment? *European Journal of Cancer, 31A,* 2277–2283.

Van Riper, M. (1999). Maternal perceptions of family-provider relationships and well-being in families of children with Down Sydrome. *Research in Nursing and Health, 22*(5), 357–368.

Varcarolis, E. M. (1998). People who contemplate suicide. In E. M. Varcarolis (Ed.), *Foundations of psychiatric mental health nursing* (pp. 725–748). Philadelphia: W. B. Saunders.

Vargas, M. A., & Davidson, J. (1993). Post-traumatic stress disorder. *Psychopharmacology, 16,* 737–748.

Vartianen, H., Suonio, S., Halonen, P., & Rimon, R. (1994). Psychosocial factors, female fertility and pregnancy: A prospective study—part II: Pregnancy. *Journal of Psychosomatic Obstetrics and Gynaecology, 15,* 77–84.

Vaughn, K., Webster, D. C., Orahood, S., & Young, B. C. (1995). Brief inpatient psychiatric treatment: Finding solutions. *Issues in Mental Health Nursing, 16,* 519–531.

Vedhara, K., Cox, N. K., Wilcock, G. K., Perks, P., Hunt, M., Anderson, S., Lightman, S. L., & Shanks, N. M. (1999). Chronic stress in elderly carers of dementia patients and antibody response to influenza vaccination. *Lancet, 353*(9153), 627–631.

VenGerpen, M. W., Johnson, J. E., & Winstead, D. K. (1999). Mania in the geriatric population: A review of the literature. *American Journal Geriatric Psychiatry, 7*(3), 188–202.

Viguera, A. C., Nonacs, R., Cohen, L. S., Tondo, L., Murray, A., & Baldessarini, R. J. (2000). Risk of recurrence of bipolar disorder in pregnant and nonpregnant women after discontinuing lithium maintenance. *American Journal of Psychiatry, 157*(2), 179–184.

Viguera, A. C., & Rothschild, A. J. (1996). Depression: Clinical features and pathogenesis. In K. I. Shulman, M. Tohen, & S. P. Kutcher (Eds.), *Mood disorders across the life span* (pp. 189–215). New York: Wiley-Liss.

Vingerhoets, G. (1998). Perioperative anxiety and depression in open-heart surgery. *Psychosomatic, 39,* 30–37.

Visintainer, M., & Wolfer, J. (1979, January). Theater as therapy. How rehearsing your patients can help them cope. *RN,* 57–62.

Vogl, D., Rosenfeld, B., Breitbart, W., Thaler, H., Passik, S., McDonald, M., & Portenoy, R. (1999). Symptom prevalence, characteristics, and distress in AIDS outpatients. *Journal of Pain and Symptom Management, 18,* 253–262.

Vogt, T. M., Pope, C., Mullooly, J., & Hollis, J. F. (1994). Mental health status as a predictor of morbidity and mortality: A 15–year follow-up of members of a health maintenance organization. *American Journal of Public Health, 84*(2), 227–231.

Volicer, B. J., & Bohannon, M. W. (1975). A hospital stress rating scale. *Nursing Research, 24,* 352–359.

Von Korff, M., Burke, J. D., & Teitlebaum. (1987). Mental disorders in primary care. *Archives of General Psychiatry, 44,* 152–156.

Vredevoe, D., Brecht, M., Shuler, P., & Woo, M. (1992). Risk factors for disease in a homeless population. *Public Health Nursing, 9,* 263–269.

Wachtel, T., Piette, J., Mor, V., Stein, M., Fleishman, J., & Carpenter, C. (1992). Quality of life in persons with human immunodeficiency virus infection: Measurement by the Medical Outcomes Study instrument. *Annals of Internal Medicine, 116,* 129–137.

Waddell, K. L., & Demi, A. S. (1993). Effectiveness of an intensive partial hospitalization program for treatment of anxiety disorders. *Archives of Psychiatric Nursing, 7*(1), 2–10.

Wadeson, H., & Carpenter, W. T. (1976). Impact of the seclusion room experience. *Journal of Nervous and Mental Disease, 163,* 318–328.

Wadhwa, P. D., Dunkel-Schetter, C., Chicz-DeMet, A., Porto, M., & Sandman, C. A. (1996). Prenatal psychosocial factors and the neuroendocrine axis in human pregnancy. *Psychosomatic Medicine, 58,* 432–446.

Wadhwa, P. D., Sandman, C. A., Porto, M., Dunkel-Schetter, C., & Garite, T. J. (1993). The association between prenatal stress and infant birth weight and gestational age at birth: A prospective investigation. *American Journal of Obstetrics and Gynecology, 169,* 858–865.

Walker, C. L. (1988). Stress and coping in siblings and childhood cancer patients. *Nursing Research, 12,* 208–212.

Walker, C., Adams, J., Curry, D., Guttuso, J., Gleason-Morgan, D., Hinds, P., Kramer, R., Panzarella, C., Vogel, R., Weekes, D., & Wright, P. (1992). A Delphi study of pediatric oncology nurses' facilitative behaviors. *Journal of Pediatric Oncology Nursing, 10,* 126–132.

Wallace, L. J. D., Calhoun, A. D., Powell, K. E., O'Neil, J., & James, S. P. (1996). Homicide and suicide among Native Americans, 1979–1992. Violence Surveillance Summary Series No. 2. Atlanta, GA: CDC, National Center for Injury Prevention and Control.

Wallhagen, M. I., & Brod, M. (1997). Perceived control and well-being in Parkinson's disease. *Western Journal of Nursing Research, 19*(1), 11–25.

Wang, R., & Martinson, I. (1996). Behavioral responses of healthy Chinese siblings to the stress of childhood cancer in the family: A longitudinal study. *Journal of Pediatric Nursing, 11,* 383–391.

Warchol, G. (1998). Workplace violence 1992–1996: Report from the Bureau of Justice Statistics, National Crime Victimization Survey. Washington, DC: U.S. Government Printing Office.

Ward, A. J. (1991). Prenatal stress and childhood psychopathology. *Child Psychiatry and Human Development, 22*(2), 97–110.

Warren, B. J. (1994). Depression in African American women. *Journal of Psychosocial Nursing, 32*(3), 29–33.

Waters, C. M. (1999). Professional nursing support for culturally diverse family members of critically ill adults. *Research in Nursing and Health, 22*(2), 107–117.

Watkins, K. E., Shaner, A., & Sullivan, G. (1999). The role of gender in engaging the dually diagnosed in treatment. *Community Mental Health Journal, 35*(2), 115–126.

Webb, C., Pfeiffer, M., Mueser, K., Gladis, M., Mensch, E., DeGirolamo, J., & Levinson, D. (1998). Burden and well-being of caregivers for the severely mentally ill: The role of coping style and social support. *Schizophrenia Research, 34* 169–180.

Webb, C., Pfeiffer, M., Mueser, K., Gladis, M., Mensch, E., DeGirolamo, J., & Levinson, D. (1998). Burden and well-being of caregivers for the severely mentally ill: The role of coping style and social support. *Schizophrenia Research, 34,* 169–180.

Webster, J., & Grossberg, G. T. (1998). Late-life onset of psychotic symptoms. *American Journal of Geriatric Psychiatry, 6*(3), 196–202.

Webster-Stratton, C. (1990). Enhancing the effectiveness of self-administered videotape parent training for families with conduct-problem children. *Journal of Abnormal Child Psychology, 18,* 479–492.

Webster-Stratton, C. H. (1981). Modification of mothers' behaviors and attitudes through a videotape modeling goup discussion program. *Behavior Therapy, 12,* 634–642.

Webster-Stratton, C. H. (1982a). The long term effects of a videotape modeling parent training program: Comparison of immediate and one year follow-up results. *Behavior Therapy, 13,* 702–714.

Webster-Stratton, C. H. (1982b). Teaching mothers through videotape modeling to change their children's behavior. *Journal of Pediatric Psychology, 7,* 279–294.

Webster-Stratton, C. H. (1984). Randomized trial of two parent training programs for families with conduct disordered children. *Journal of Consulting and Clinical Psychology, 53,* 666–678.

Webster-Stratton, C. H. (1998). Preventing conduct problems in Head Start children: Strengthening parenting competencies. *Journal of Consulting and Clinical Psychology, 66*(5), 715–730.

Webster-Stratton, C. H., & Fjone, A. (1989). Interactions of mothers and fathers with conduct problem children: Comparison with a nonclinic group. *Public Health Nursing, 6*(4), 218–223.

Webster-Stratton, C. H., Kolpacoff, M., & Hollinsworth, T. (1988). Self-administered videotape therapy for families with conduct-problem children: Comparison with two cost effective treatments and a control group. *Journal of Consulting and Clinical Psychology, 56,* 558–566.

Weinberg, N. (1995). Does apologizing help? The role of self-blame and making amends in recovery from bereavement. *Health and Social Work, 20,* 292–299.

Weissman, M. M., Bland, R. C., Canino, G. J., Faravelli, C., Greenwald, S., Hwu, H. G., Joyce, P. R., Karam, E. G., Lee, C. K., Lellouch, J., Lepine, J. P., Newman, S. C., Rubio-Stipec, M., Wells, J. E., Wickramaratne, P. J., Wittchen, H., & Yeh, E. K. (1996). Cross-national epidemiology of major depression and bipolar disorder. *Journal of the American Medical Association, 276*(4), 293–299.

Weissman, M., & Olfson, M. (1995). Depression in women: Implications for health care research. *Science, 269,* 279–801.

Wells, R., & Gionnetti, V. (1990). *Handbook of brief psychotherapies.* New York: Plenum Press.

Werner, P., Yesavage, J., Becker, J., Brunsting, D., & Isaacs, J. (1983). Hostile wards and assaultive behavior on an acute inpatient psychiatric unit. *Journal of Nervous and Mental Disorders, 171,* 385–387.

Westreich, L., Guedj, P., Galanter, M., & Baird, D. (1997). Differences between men and women in dual-diagnosis treatment. *American Journal on Addictions, 6*(4), 311–317.

Wheeler, S. Q. (1993). *Telephone Triage: Theory, Practice, and Protocol Development.* Albany, NY: Delmar Publishers, Inc.

Whipple, E. E., & Webster-Stratton, C. H. (1991). The role of parental stress in physically abusive families. *Child Abuse and Neglect, 15*(3), 279–291.

White, J., & Litovitz, G. (1998). A comparison of inpatient and outpatient women with eating disorders. *Archives of Psychiatric Nursing, 12*(4), 181–194.

White, R., Tata, P., & Burns, T. (1996). Mood, learned resourcefulnes, and perceptions of control in Type 1 diabetes mellitus. *Journal of Psychosomatic Research, 40*(2), 205–212.

Widom, C. (1995). *Victims of childhood sexual abuse—later criminal consequences.* (NCJ 151525). Washington, DC: National Institute of Justice.

Williams, B. (1994). Patient Satisfaction: A valid concept? *Social Science & Medicine, 38,* 509–516.

Williams, C., & Vine, S. W. (1999). Broken past, fragile future: Personal stories of high-risk adolescent mothers. *Journal of the Society of Pediatric Nurses, 4*(1), 15–23.

Williams, M. S., Ward, S. E., & Campbell, E. B. (1986). Issues in study of confusion in older hospitalized patients (abstract). In S. M. Stinson, J. C. Kerr, P. Giovanetti, P. A. Field, & J. MacPhail (Eds.), *New frontiers in nursing research* (p. 390). Edmonton, Canada: University of Alberta.

Williams, P. D., Hanson, S., Karlin, R., Ridder, L., Liebergen, A., Olson, J., Barnard, M. U., & Tobin-Rommelhart, S. (1997). Outcomes of a nursing intervention for siblings of chronically ill children. *Journal of the Society of Pediatric Nurses, 2,* 127–137.

Wilson, H. S., Hutchinson, S. A., & Holzemer, W. L. (1997). Salvaging quality of Life in ethnically diverse patients with advanced HIV/AIDS. *Qualitative Health Research, 7,* 75–97.

Wilson, I. B., & Cleary, P. D. (1995). Linking clinical variables with health-related Quality of life. A conceptual model of patient outcomes. *Journal of the American Medical Association, 273,* 59–65.

Wing, D. M., & Thompson, T. (1995). Causes of alcoholism: A qualitative study of traditional Muscogee (Creek) Indians. *Public Health Nursing, 12,* 417–423.

Winslow, B. W. (1997). Effects of formal supports on stress outcomes in family caregivers of Alzheimer's patients. *Research in Nursing and Health, 20*(1), 27–37.

Wolf, S. (1981). Introduction: The role of the brain in bodily disease. In H. Weiner, M. A. Hofer, & A. J. Stunkard (Eds.), *Brain, behavior and bodily disease* (pp. 1–9). New York: Raven Press.

Wolfe, B., Metzger, E., & Jimerson, D. (1997). Research update on serotonin function in bulimia nervosa and anorexia nervosa. *Psychopharmacology Bulletin, 33*(2), 345–354.

Wolfe, B., Metzger, E., Levine, J., Finkelstein, D., Cooper, T., & Jimerson, D. (2000). Serotonin function following remission from bulimia nervosa. *Neuropsychopharmacology, 22*(3), 257–263.

Wolff, P. (1978). Psychiatric nursing consultation: A study of the referral process. *Journal of Psychiatric Nursing and Mental Health Services, 16*(5), 42–47.

Wood, P., Hurburt, M., Hough, R., & Hofstetter, C. (1998). Longitudinal assessment of family support among homeless mentally ill participants in a housing program. *Journal of Community Psychology, 26*(4), 327–344.

Wright, L., & Leahey, M. (1994). *Nurses and Families: A Guide to Family Assessment and Intervention* (2nd ed.). Philadelphia: F. A. Davis.

Yoest, M. (1989). The clinical nurse specialist on the psychiatric team. *Journal of Psychosocial Nursing, 27*(3), 27.

Young, T. J. (1990). Poverty and homicide among Native Americans. *Psychological Reports, 67*(3), 1153–1154.

Zandee, G. L., & Oermann, M. H. (1996). Effectiveness of contingency contracting: Component of a worksite weight loss program. *American Association of Occupational Health Nurses Journal, 44*(4), 183–188.

Zauszniewski, J. A. (1994). Health-seeking resources and adaptive functioning in depressed and nondepressed adults. *Archives of Psychiatric Nursing, 8*(3), 159–168.

Zauszniewski, J. A. (1995). Health-seeking resources in depressed outpatients. *Archives of Psychiatric Nursing, 9*(4), 179–187.

Zauszniewski, J. A. (1996). Self-help and help-seeking behavior in healthy elders. *Journal of Holistic Nursing, 14*(3), 223–236.

Zauszniewski, J. A. (1997a). Teaching resourcefulness skills to older adults. *Journal of Gerontological Nursing, 23*(2), 14–20.

Zauszniewski, J. A. (1997b). Evaluation of a measure of learned resourcefulness in older adults. *Journal of Nursing Measurement, 5*(1), 71–86.

Zauszniewski, J. A. (1998). *Personal and Social Resourcefulness Scale.* Unpublished manuscript.

Zauszniewski, K. A. (1995). Severity of depression, cognitions, and functioning among depressed inpatients with and without coexisting substance abuse. *Journal of the American Psychiatric Nurses Association, 1,* 55–60.

Zayas, L. H., & Busch-Rossnagel, N. A. (1992). Pregnant Hispanic women: A mental health study. *Family and Society, 73,* 515–521.

Zero to Three/National Center for Clinical Infant Program. (1994). *Diagnostic classification of mental health and developmental disorders of infancy and early childhood.* Arlington, VA: Zero to Three/National Center for Clinical Infant Program.

Zhang, A. Y., Snowden, L. R., & Sue, S. (1998). Differences between Asian and white Americans help-seeking behavior patterns in Los Angeles area. *Journal of Community Psychology, 26,* 317–326.

Ziedonis, D. M., & George, T. P. (1997). Schizophrenia and nicotine use: Report of a pilot smoking cessation program and review of neurogiological and clinical issues. *Schizophrenia Bulletin, 23,* 247–254.

Ziedonis, D. M., Kosten, T. R., Glazer, W. M., & Frances, R. J. (1994). Nicotine dependence and schizophrenia. *Hospital and Community Psychiatry, 45,* 204–206.

Zimmermann-Tansella, C., Bertagni, P., Siani, R., & Micciolo, R. (1994). Marital relationships and somatic and psychological symptoms in pregnancy. *Social Science Medicine, 38,* 559–564.

INDEX

Access to care, 66
Accountability, 13, 66
Activities of daily living, 110
Acupressure, 33
Acute confusion:
  assessment and diagnosis, 148–149
  implications of, 147, 171
  interventions, 149–150
  nursing education, 151
  prevention of, 150
Adaptation:
  psychosocial, 104
  siblings, childhood cancer, 160–163
Adaptiveness, 103
Addiction, among registered nurses, 224–227
Adjusted Quality of Life Years Utility Index, 112
Adjustment, 104. *See also* Psychosocial adjustment, family role in
Adolescents:
  dating violence, 130
  depression in, 41
  eating disorders in, 193–197
  juvenile justice system:
    forensic psychiatric care, 40–42
    girls, 28
  mental health inventions:
    assessment, range and design of, 11
    biopsychosocial development, model of, 10
    empirical evidence, 11–12
    incidence of, 9
    intervention protocols, 11
    preventive measures, 10
    science-practice synergy, 13–14
  sexual abuse of, 27
  substance abuse in, 40
  suicide, 228
  violent, 131
ADVANCE program, 165
Advocacy, 38, 210
Affective disorders, 70
African Americans population, mental health issues, 70
Age-associated memory impairment (AAMI), 171
Agency for Health Care Policy and Research (AHCPR), 97, 123
Agitation, 185
Aggressive behavior, 41, 131, 164. *See also* Violence
AIDS, *see* HIV, quality of life issues
  psychosocial interventions, 111
  prevalence of, 201
Alaska Native population:
  mental health issues, 72
  youth suicide prevention, 234–237
Alcohol abuse, prevalence of, 192. *See also* Alcoholism; Substance abuse
Alcoholics Anonymous (AA), 152, 225
Alcoholism:
  diagnosis, 151
  health, impact on, 151–152

Alcoholism *(continued)*
- nursing education, 153
- prevalence of, 152–153

Alcohol withdrawal syndrome, 151–152
Alliances, in family caregiving, 36–38
Alzheimer's disease (AD), 54, 111, 171–172
Alzheimer's disease and related dementias (ADRD), 171, 173
American Association of Psychology, 12
American Indians population, mental health issues, 72
American Institute for Research, 134
American Medical Association, Council on Ethical and Judicial Affairs, 133
American Nurses Association, 225
American Psychiatric Nurses Association (APNA), 217
Anorexia nervosa (AN), 14, 193–194
Anticipatory grief, 46
Antidepressants, 12, 187
Antihypertensive medications, 110
Antipsychotics, 12
Antisocial behavior, 41, 164
Anxiety:
- biofeedback and, 6
- CABG surgery and, 179
- in children, 131
- comorbid, 61
- in elderly, 105
- genetic predisposition, 11
- management of, 89–90, 186
- pregnancy and, *see* Pregnancy, anxiety and conflict levels
- psychophysiologic responses to, 94–95
- psychosocial adjustment and, 105
- in women, 138–139

Arthritis, 116
Art therapy, 32. *See also* Creative art
Asian Americans population, mental health issues, 71
Assault, *see* Violence; Workplace violence
Assertive community treatment (ACT), 214
Attachment, impaired, 6
Attention deficit hyperactivity disorder (ADHD), 8, 11–12
Attribution, 168
Attributional theory, 186–187
Auditory hallucinations, 220–221
Autogenic training, 111
Autonomy, 78
Axis I diagnosis, 182

Barriers to care, 70, 72–74, 209
BASIC intervention program, 165
Battered women:
- children of, 130–131
- dating violence, 130
- domestic violence, 130
- prevalence of, 129

Behavioral theory, 186
Bereavement, defined, 46. *See also* Grief
Bereavement Experience Questionnaire, 47
Binge eating, 194, 196
Biofeedback training:
- description of, 4–5
- goals of, 7, 32
- mechanisms of, 8–9
- psychophysiology, 5–6
- self-management and, 6–8
- success with, 7–8

Biochemical theory, 187
Bipolar disorders:
- burden of care, 155–156
- gender differences, 154
- late-onset, 156–157
- manifestation of, 153–154
- treatment concerns, 154–155
- in women, 197

Biomedical health care, 30
Biopsychosocial development, 10
Bio-psycho-social-spiritual healing, 30
Break the Cycle program, 28
Breast cancer, family adjustment research, 106–107
Breathing exercises/techniques, 111, 127
Brief Symptom Inventory, 47

Brief therapy, 50–51
Bulimia nervosa (BN), 193

Camberwell Assessment of Need, 38
Cancer, pediatric, *see* Childhood cancer
Cardiac illness, coping with, 120–122
Caregivers:
  of Alzheimer's patients, 111
  burden, 37–39, 102, 105, 155–156
  family, *see* Family caregiving; Grandmothers, as caregivers
CASE, 213
Case management, 11, 51–52, 211
Case Manager Rating Scale for Alcohol Use Disorder (CMRS), 213
Catharsis, 102
Character disorders, 41
Child abuse:
  defined, 131, 157–158
  future research directions, 159–160
  history of, 164
  theoretical models:
    cultural context, 159
    medical, 158
    psychosocial, 159
Child Abuse Prevention and Treatment Act (1974), 158
Child And Adolescent Clinical Practice Parameters, 13
Child Behavior Questionnaire, 47
Childhood cancer:
  hospice care, 47
  prevalence of, 160–161
  sibling psychosocial adaptation:
    age-related differences, 162
    generally, 161–162
    interventions, 162–163
    phenomonological studies, 162
Childhood sexual abuse, creative expression therapy, 26–27
Child neglect:
  defined, 158
  future research directions, 159–160
  grandmother caregivers and, 43–44
  theoretical models:
    cultural context, 159
    medical, 158
    psychosocial, 159
Child psychopathology:
  conduct disorder, 164
  future research directions, 166
  implications, 166
  literature review, 164–165
  statistics, 163
Children, mental health inventions:
  assessment, range and design of, 11
  biopsychosocial development, model of, 10
  empirical evidence, 11–12
  failure to thrive, *see* Failure to thrive
  family psychosocial adjustment and, 103–104
  incidence of, 9
  intervention protocols, 11
  preventive measures, 10
  science-practice synergy, 13–14
Chronically ill:
  biofeedfack and, 6
  family caregiving and, 36
  resourcefulness and, 118
Chronic fatigue, 6
Chronic mental illness:
  community health service delivery, 169
  future research directions, 170
  interventions, 168
  medication as intervention, 169
  morbidity/mortality rates, 169
  self-regulation, 168
  support and, 169–170
CINAHL, 52, 103, 125, 219
Client-centered consultation, 22
Clinical Paths, 13
Clozapine, 32
Cognitive-behavioral skills, 115
Cognitive-behavioral therapy:
  anxiety, 12
  depressed children, 12
  for depressed women, 140
Cognitive distortions, 33
Cognitive impairment:
  attention, as indicator, 171–172

Cognitive impairment *(continued)*
- Cochrane Database of Systematic Reviews:
  - music therapy, 173
  - reality orientation, 173–174
  - reminiscence therapy, 174
  - validation therapy, 174
- defined, 171
- rehabilitation outcomes, 171
- types of, generally, 8–9, 149, 170–171

Cognitive theory, generally, 186
Collaboration, 40–41, 86, 97
Comfort:
- defined, 17
- future directions, 19
- relevance to nursing, 18
- research, 18–19
- theory of, 17–18

Community care, 29
Community mental health:
- chronic mental illness, 169
- family caregiving and, 39
- historical perspective, 20–21
- legislation, 20–22
- treatment approaches, 21–22

Community Mental Health Centers Act (1963), 20
Comorbidity, 23, 61, 122, 153
Conduct disorder, in children, 131, 164
Consultation-liaison nursing (C/L nursing):
- comorbidity, 23
- defined, 22–23
- future research directions, 25
- general medical units, 23–24
- nurse's role, 23
- subspecialization in, 25

Consultee-centered consultation, 22
Coordination of care, 51–52
COPE (creating opportunities for parent empowerment), 104
Coping skills:
- creative arts and, 28–29
- development of, 11
- in elderly, 118
- family caregiving and, 37–38
- grief and, 48
- in grandmother caregivers, 45
- siblings, childhood cancer, 162–163

Coronary artery bypass graft (CABG) surgery, psychological sequelae:
- anxiety, 179
- depression, 175, 178–179
- future research directions, 180
- gender issues, 179–180

Correctional mental health:
- individual level research, 183
- institutional research, 182–183
- mentally ill:
  - background of, 182
  - identification of, 181–182
- systems research, 181

Creative arts, as nursing intervention:
- adolescent girls detained in juvenile justice, 28
- adults in community care, 29
- adult women abused as children, 27–28
- children in domestic violence shelter, 27
- child survivors of abuse, 26–27
- coping skills and, 28–29
- significance of, 26

Crisis intervention, 51
Cultural differences:
- anxiety levels during pregnancy, 93–94
- battered women, 130
- grandmother caregivers, 45
- homelessness, 209

Cultural diversity, psychosocial diversity and, 107–108
Cumulative Index to Nursing and Allied Health Literature, 125

Dating violence, 130
Death, of child, 47, 232–233. *See also* Grief
Decycling, 210
Dementia, 54, 185, 188. *See also specific types of dementia*
Deinstitutionalization, impact of, 36, 136
Delirium:

assessment and diagnosis, 148–149
implications of, 147, 171
interventions, 149–150
nursing education, 151
prevention of, 150
Dependency, 105
Depression:
in adolescents, 41
child failure to thrive, 15
defined, 189
dementia distinguished from, 185
in elderly, 105
ethnic differences, 71
etiology of, 187
in families, 188–191
genetic-biological research, 11, 189–190
maternal, 121
mood disorders distinguished from, 189–190
in older adults, 185–188
prevalence of, 97, 138
psychosocial adjustment and, 103, 105
symptoms, 184–185, 189
in young women:
cognitive-behavioral therapy, 140
exercise, therapeutic, 139–140, 200
misdiagnosis/mistreatment of, 138–139
nursing practice paradigm, 139–141
prevalence of, 138
psychosocial therapies, 140
risk factors, 139
Diagnosis, *see specific types of disorders and illnesses*
Diabetes, 116
Diagnostic and Statistical Manual of Mental Disorders (DSM IV), 32, 58, 74, 96, 98, 148, 171, 185, 189, 191, 208
Diet, major depressive disorder and, 139–140, 187. *See also* Eating disorders
Disregulatory diseases, 6
Distress, psychosocial adjustment and, 104
Dix, Dorthea Lynde, 20
Domestic violence, *see* Violence, battered women
Down's Syndrome, 103
Drake, Dr. Robert, 212
Drug abuse, *see* Substance abuse
categories of, 191
definitions, 191
significance of, 192–193
Dual disorder, *see* Comorbidity
integrated treatment, 213
stagewise treatment, 214–215
Dysthymia, 189

Eating disorders:
behavioral determinants, 195–196
etiology, 194–197
physical outcomes, 196
prevalence of, 193–194
symptom patterns, 194
types of, 193
Elder abuse, 132
Elderly:
coping skills in, 118
dementia in, generally, 188
psychosocial adjustment in, 104–106
Electroconvulsive therapy, 155, 187–188
Electroencephalographic (EEG) patterns, implications of, 4, 8
Emergency care, 70, 207
Emotional health, 31–32, 184–185
Empathy, 33–35, 110
Ethnopsychopharmacology, 74–75
Etiology, *see specific types of disorders and illnesses*
Ethnoscience, 82
Exercise, therapeutic, 139–140, 200
Experience of Caregiving Inventory (ECI), 38
Epidemiologic Catchment Area (ECA), 212, 226
Exploitation, in nurse-client relationship, 89

Factor analysis, 93
Failure to thrive:

Failure to thrive *(continued)*
classification, 14
current perspective, 16
historical perspective, 15
Family:
as caregivers, *see* Family caregiving; Grandmothers, as caregivers
depression:
genetic-biological research, 189–190
prevalence of, 188–189
psychosocial research, 190
symptoms, 189
treatment, 191
psychosocial adjustment and, *see* Psychosocial adjustment, family role in
support, for homeless, 210
Family caregiving, of mentally ill:
alliances, 36, 38
burden, 37, 39, 102, 105
community resources, 39
coping strategies, 37–38
grandmother as caregiver, *see* Grandmothers, as caregivers
Family-centered intervention, 11
Family Centered Program for Adolescents with Mental Illness, 221
Family therapy, 188
Family transformations, 190
Feil, Naomi, 174
Fenluramine, 195
Fetal alcohol syndrome, 11
Fibromyalgia, 6
Food and Drug Administration, 112
Forensic psychiatric care, juvenile justice system:
characteristics of, generally, 40–41
recovery, 41–42
rehabilitation, 41–42
Fragmentation, 209

Gender differences:
bipolar disorder, 154
coronary artery bypass graft (CABG) surgery, psychological response to, 175–180
eating disorders, 193–196
smoking behavior, 122
Generalized anxiety disorder, 70
Geriatrics, consultation-liaison nursing, 25
Global Assessment of Symptoms, 219
Goldman spiral diagram, 102
Grandmothers, as caregivers:
coping skills, 45
incidence of, 43–44
health status of grandmother, 44–45
resources for, 45
supplemental, 44
Grief:
in battered women, 130
defined, 46
research studies:
ethical issues, 48
strengths and limitations of, 48
types of, 46–48
Grief Experience Inventory, 47
Grounded theory, 47, 82, 85, 87, 130
Group therapy, 27–28, 188

Hallucinations, auditory, 220–221
Head injury, 8–9
Health Belief Models, 42
Health care utilization, 97–98
Health-related quality of life (HRQOL), 202–203
Healing touch, 33
Help-seeking behavior, 115–117
Help-seeking behavior training (HSBT), 118
Hispanic American population, mental health issues, 71–72
HIV, quality of life issues:
future research directions, 204
literature review, 202
symptom management, 202–203
Holism, 18–19, 62
Homelessness:
case management issues, 211
health:
future research directions, 207–208
health care, 206–207

health problems, types of, 205–206
respiratory ailments, 206
schizophrenia, 205–206
service delivery research, 207
weather-related injuries, 205–206
homeless, defined, 205
institutionalization and, 208
mood disorders, related:
advocacy for, 210
barriers to care, 209
interventions, 210–211
prevalence of, 204–205, 208–209
reasons for, 208–209
Homeostatis, 5–6
Hospitalism, 15
Hostility, 104
Hyperactivity, 8, 131
Hypertension:
biofeedback and, 6
resourcefulness and, 116
self-regulation, 8
Hynosis, 32

Identification, in nurse-client relationship, 89
Illness, family psychosocial adjustment and, 106–107
Imagery, 32, 111, 114, 127, 188
Immune response, 106
Impact of Events Questionnaire, 47
Indian Health Services (IHS), 235
Indian population, youth suicide prevention, 234–237
Individual nursing therapy:
brief therapy, 50–51
case management, 51–52
crisis intervention, 51
interpersonal paradigm, 49–50
INSIGHTS, 57
Institute of Medicine, 56
Institute of Mental Health, 10, 57–59
Integration, comorbidity and, 213. *See also* Primary mental health services, integration in
Interpersonal communication:
demented patients, 54
importance of, 52–53
nonpsychiatric patients vulnerable to emotional distress, 54
psychiatric patients, 53
research studies:
future directions, 55–56
methodology, 54–55
researchers, types of, 55
Interpersonal relations, *see* Nurse-patient relationship; Peplau's theoretical model
Interpersonal theory, 186
Involuntary commitment, 70, 136
Irritable bowel syndrome, 6

Jacobson, Edmund, 114
Jin shin jyutsu, 33
Journaling, 27

Karnofsky Scale, 203
Kraepelin, Emil, 153

Lamaze, 111
Learned resourcefulness training (LRT), 118
Length of stay, 19, 24, 136
Life events, stressful, 92–93
Life review, 188
Light therapy, 187
Loss, defined, 46. *See also* Grief

Major depression:
etiology, 122, 185
recurrent, 197
Major depressive disorder (MDD), 122, 138–139, 175, 189–190
Managed care, 39
Mania, 70, 154
Massage, 32–33, 114, 127
MAST, 213
Meditation, 32, 111, 127
MEDLINE, 103, 217, 219
Memorial Symptom Assessment Scale Short Form, 203

Memory:
  cognitive impairment and, 174
  loss, biofeedback and, 9
Mental disorders prevention:
  classification, 57
  future research directions, 58–59
  goals of, generally, 56–57
  interventions, types of, 57–58
  risk factors and, 56
  standardization and, 58
Mental health services research (MHSR), 66–67
Mental Health Study Act, 20
Mental Health Systems Act, 21
Mental illness, generally:
  chronic, *see* Chronic mental illness
  prevalence of, 10
  stigmatization of, 21, 71
Mind/body interface, 5–6
Mini Mental State Exam (MMSE), 148, 172
Minor depression, 189
Minority issues in mental health:
  African Americans, 70
  Alaska Native, 72
  American Indians, 72
  Asian Americans, 71
  barriers to care, 72–74
  ethnic groups, generally, 69
  ethnopsychopharmacology, 74–75
  Hispanic Americans, 71–72
  historical perspective, 67–68
  Native Americans, 72
  Native Hawaiians, 72
  nursing literature, 68–69
  Pacific Islanders, 71
  psychometric studies, 68
Misdiagnosis, 70, 73–74, 138–139
Mood disorders, 189–190
Mood stabilizers, 155
Mortality rates, 169, 198, 200
Mother-child relationship, 15
Mourning, 46, 185. *See also* Grief
Multiinfarct dementia, 171–172
Munchausen Syndrome By Proxy, 158
Music therapy:
  benefits of, generally, 32, 76–78, 173
  categories of music, 77
  future research directions, 77
  historical perspective, 76
  musical preferences, 76
  music selections, 77
  in stress reduction, 114, 127

Narcissism, 41
National Academy of Science, 157
National Alliance for the Mentally Ill Organization, 36, 38–39, 210, 221
National Co-Morbidity Study, 138
National Crime Victimization Survey (NCVS), 135
National Depressive and Manic-Depressive Association, 210
National Institute of Mental Health (NIMH), 20, 67, 96, 155, 210, 215, 226
National Institute of Nursing Research, 157
National Institute on Alcohol Abuse and Alcoholism (NIAA), 152, 192
National Institute on Drug Abuse (NIDA), 152, 192
National Mental Health Act, 20
National Mental Health Association, 210, 221
National Survey of Families and Household (NSFH), 44
Native American population, mental health issues, 72
Native Hawaiian population, mental health issues, 72
Natural disasters, response to, 120, 231–232
Neuroleptics, 32, 155
Nicotine replacement therapy (NRT), 123–124
Nonorganic failure to thrive (NOFTT), 14–16
Normal grief, 46
No-suicide contracts:

defined, 78
negotiation motives, 78–79
relevance to nursing research, 79
research studies:
future directions for, 80–81
major, 79–80
Nurse Orientation System, 84
Nurse-patient communication:
data collection methods, 83
effects of, 82–83
importance of, 81–82
nonverbal behavior, 83
seclusion and restraint and, 223
verbal behavior, 83
Nurse-patient interaction:
conversational analysis, 85
defined, 82, 86
discourse analysis, 85
documentation, 85
ethology, 85
grounded theory, 85
importance of, 84, 86
video technology and, 85
Nurse-patient relationship:
characteristics of, 86–87
complexities of, 87–88
development of, 86
empathy and, 33–35
influences on, 49–50, 87
Peplau's theoretical model:
anxiety, 89–90
future research directions, 90–91
health, defined, 89–90
in nurse education, 90
in nursing practice, 90
overview of, 88–89
phases of, 89
research, 90
significance of, 86
Nurses Worklife and Health Study (NWHS), 226–227
Nursing education:
acute confusion, 151
alcoholism, 153
delirium, 151
graduate programs, 96
nurse-patient relationship, 90
psychodrama in, 100
Nursing home placement, 105
Nursing Practice Paradigm for Depressed Women, 139
Nutritional deprivation, 15–16

Obsessive-compulsive disorder, 11–12
Occupational Safety and Health Administration (OSHA), 136, 138
Office of Substance Abuse Prevention, 152, 192
Older adults, depression in:
attributional theory, 186–187
behavioral theory, 186
biochemical theories, 187
cognitive theory, 186
diagnosis, 185
interpersonal theory, 186
quality of life and, 187
self-control model, 186
symptoms of, 184–185
theories, generally, 185–187
treatment of, 188
Oncology, *see also specific types of cancer*
consultation-liaison nursing, 25
suicide and, 228–229
Organic brain syndrome, 171
Orientation, in nurse-client relationship, 89. *See also* Reality orientation

Parental Environment Cluster Model, 159
Parent-child relationship, 15–16
PARTNERS2, 165
Pediatric oncology, *see* Childhood cancer
Pharmacological interventions, 11–12. *See also specific types of disorders and illnesses*
Play, therapeutic, 27–28
Positive psychology, 13
Posttraumatic stress disorder (PTSD), 6, 27, 131, 231, 231, 233
Posttraumatic stress symptoms, 104
Poverty, impact of, 165, 183, 235

Pregnancy:
  alcoholism and, 154
  anxiety and conflict levels:
    acceptance of pregnancy, 92
    cultural differences, 93–94
    planned pregnancy, 92
    psychophysiologic response to anxiety, 94–95
    social support and, 93
    stressful life events, 92–93
    trimester differences in anxiety levels, 91–92
    wanted pregnancy, 92
  labor and delivery, 83
  violence during, 129–130, 198
Premenstrual syndrome (PMS), 138–139
Primary care, public sector, 59–62
Primary Care Evaluation Model, 99
Primary degenerative dementia, 171
Primary mental health services, integration in:
  epidemiologic profile, 95–96
  future research directions, 98–99
  models of care, 98
  support of integration, 96–98
Primary prevention, 57
Process theory, 100
Professional Support Questionnaire for Critical Care Nurses Working with Family Members (PSQ), 107
Profile of Mood States, 47
Progressive muscle relaxation, 111, 114, 127
Project Achieve, 210
Pseudodementia, 171
Psychiatric mental health nursing:
  assessment, 30
  care environments, 32
  cognitive issues, 33
  emotional health, 31–32
  health promotion, 31
  neurological issues, 33
  normalcy throughout lifespan, 30–31
  pathologic conditions, 32
  research, priority areas of, 33
  risk reduction, 31
Psychiatric nursing research, mental health policy:
  current developments in, 64–65
  future potential for, 65–66
  influence of policy, 63–64
  policy development, 63–64
PscyhInfo, 103
Psychodrama:
  defined, 99–100
  effectiveness of, 101
  historical development, 100–101
  interpersonal psychodramatic simulation (IPS) research methods, 102
  interpersonal profile trajectory plots, 101–102
  purpose of, 100
  role-reversal, 101
Psychopathology, in children, *see* Child psychopathology
Psychosis, 70
Psychosocial adaptation, 104
Psychosocial family adjustment:
  children, 103–104
  cultural diversity and, 107–108
  elders, 104–106
  illness, 106–107
  importance of, 102–103
Psychosocial interventions:
  cancer patients, 110
  caregivers, 110
  defined, 12
  hypertensive patients, 109–110
  relaxation training, 110–111
  surgical patients, 109
  technology interventions, 111
Psychosocial therapy, for depressed women, 140
Psychostimulants, 12
Psychotropics, 32, 136, 154
PubMed, 153

Qualitative ethology, 82, 85
Quality of care, 65–66
Quality of life:
  HIV patients, 201–204

importance of, 112–113, 174, 187
serious and persistent mental illness (SMI) and, 170

Rapid cycling bipolar disorder (RCBD), 154–155
Reality orientation, 173–174
Recovery, 41–42, 130, 215
Referrals, 24–25
Reflexology, 33
Reframing, 33
Rehabilitation, 41–42, 171
Reiki, 33
Reinstitutionalization, 180
Relapse, 214–215
Relationships:
family-centered, 104
nurse-patient, 86–88
spousal, 105
Relaxation techniques:
benefits of, 113–114
complementary therapies, 114–115
historical perspective, 114
progressive muscle relaxation, 114
purpose of, 32, 110–111
in stress management, 127
Reminiscence therapy, 174
Report on Mental Health, 63–64, 95–96
Resolution, in nurse-client relationship, 89
Resourcefulness:
conceptualization, 115–117
interventions and, 117–118
operationalization, 117
Responsiveness, 103
Restraints, *see* Seclusion and restraints
Rogers, Carl, 34
Role captivity, 15
Role-reversal, 101
Role training, 99–100

Schedule of Recent Experiences (SRE), 126
Schepp, Karen, 221
Schizoaffective disorder, 197
Schizophrenia:
alcoholism and, 154
auditory hallucinations, 220–221
diagnosis, 216
ethical issues, 218
generally, 123
future research directions, 217
information resources, 217
misdiagnosis, 70
pharmacological intervention, 11
self-management, 218–220
symptom detection, 218–219
symptom management, 221
treatment, 216
in women, 197
School-based intervention, 11
School-related problems, 131
Seclusion and restraint (S/R):
clinical applications, 223–224
defined, 221–222
future research directions, 224
incidence of, 222
literature review, 222–223
reasons for, 149, 223
Secondary prevention, 57
Sedative music, 77
Selective serotonin reuptake inhibitors (SSRIs), 12
Self-care, 26, 105, 115
Self-concept, 195
Self-control, 7, 116, 186
Self-Control Schedule (SCS), 117
Self-efficacy:
cardiac recovery, 120–121
children of battered women, 130
family roles, 121
general construct, 119–120
memory aging, 121–122
natural disaster and, 120
Self-esteem, 41, 130, 211
Self-harm behavior, 80–81
Self-management, biofeedback training and, 4–5
Self-monitoring, 219
Self-regulation, 6, 8, 219

Self-Regulation Interview for Schizophrenics, 168
Senile dementia of the Alzheimer type (SDAT), 171
Serious and persistent mental illness (SMI/SPMI), *see* Chronic mental illness
  female health concerns:
    intimate partner violence, 198
    mortality rates, 198
    sexual risks, 198–199
    social/economic risks, 199
  health risks related to, 199–200
  organizational-level factors, 200
  prevalence of, 197–198
Sexual abuse, 199. *See also* Childhood sexual abuse
Sleep disturbance, 185
Sleep deprivation, major depression disorder and, 139–140
Smoking cessation:
  comorbidity and, 122
  statistics, 122
  treatment, research on, 123–124
Society for Education and Research in Psychiatric Mental Health Nursing (SERPN), 217
Social Readjustment Rating Scale (SRRS), 126
Social Science Citations, 103
Social support, importance of, 37, 93, 127
Sociodynamics, 100–101
Sociometry, 100
Specialization, 100, 227
Stereotyping, 31
Stewart B. McKinney Homeless Assistance Act, 205, 209
Stimulative music, 77
Storytelling, 27
Stress:
  chronic, 106
  defined, 125
  management of, *see* Stress management
  psychometric studies, 125–126
  psychosocial adjustment and, 104
  research studies, need for, 126–127
Stress management:
  importance of, 127
  support groups and, 127–128
Subspecialization, 25
Substance abuse:
  alcohol, 192
  defined, 191
  in the homeless, 205–206
  in juvenile offenders, 40
  parental, 160
  among registered nurses, 225–227
Substance Abuse Treatment Scale (SCAS), 215
Substance dependence, defined, 191
Substancc usc disorder (SUD), in mentally ill adults:
  assertive community treatment (ACT), 214
  assessment, 212–213
  defined, 212
  future research directions, 215–216
  group interventions, 213–214
  integrated treatment, 213
  recovery, 215
  stagewise treatment, 214–215
Subthreshold somatization syndrome, 97
Suidical ideation/suicidal thoughts, 79, 228
Suicide:
  adolescent, 228
  attempts, 228–229
  attitudes toward, 228–229
  cultural differences in, 72
  defined, 227
  depression and, 188
  future research directions, 229–230
  risk factors, 80, 228
  survivors, 229
  youth prevention in Indian and Alaska Native community, 234–237
Suicide prevention, 80–81, 234–237
Sullivan, Harry Stack, 88
Super Kids, 27
Support, importance of:
  chronic mental illness and, 169–170

pregnancy and, 93
psychosocial adjustment and, 104–105
in stress management, 127–128
Support groups, 32, 38, 127–128
Symptoms, *see specific types of disorders and illnesses*

Taxonomy on Infant Mental Health, 10
Teaching Kids to Cope (TKC), 28–29
Texas Inventory of Grief, 47
Therapeutic alliance, 78. *See also* Nurse-patient relationship
Therapeutic Puppet Theatre, 100
Therapeutic touch, 33, 110, 114
Trail Making Test, 172
Traumatic events, response to:
emotional, 6–7
human, 230–231
posttraumatic stress disorder (PTSD), 231, 234
research examples:
accidental trauma, 232
human-made disasters, deliberate, 232–234
natural disasters, 231–232
Treatment, *see specific types of disorders and illnesses*
Tricyclic antidepressants, 32
Twin studies, 189
Type I/Type II traumatic events, 230–231

Validation therapy, 174
Violence:
adolescent, 131
battered women:
children of, 130–131
dating violence, 130
domestic violence, 130
prevalence of, 129
child abuse, 131
elder abuse, 132
future research directions, 132
intimate partner, 198
during pregnancy, 128–129, 198–199
violence, defined, 128–129
weapons and, 131, 235
in the workplace, *see* Workplace violence

Way of Coping Questionnaire, 38
Well-being, 37, 103, 113, 128
Women:
abused as children, 27–28
alcoholism in, 151–152
depression in, 138–139
eating disorders in, 193–197
grandmother caregivers, 43–45
violence and, *see* Violence
Workplace mistreatment, 133–134
Workplace violence:
employee training programs, 137–138
environmental risk factors, 136–137
fatal assaults, background of, 134–135
health care workers and, 135
mental health and, 135–136
non-fatal assaults, background of, 134–135
prevention programs, 137
risk factors:
environmental, 136–137
patient characteristics in mental health settings
World Health Organization, 112, 188

Yoga, 32, 111

Zen, 111